URINARY TRACT BLEEDING

Diagnosis and Control by Medical, Radiologic, and Surgical Techniques

Edited By

MURRAY M. BERN, M.D.

Section Chief of Hematology
New England Deaconess Hospital
Assistant Professor of Medicine
Harvard Medical School
Boston, Massachusetts

FUTURA PUBLISHING CO., INC.
Mount Kisco, New York
1985

Library of Congress Cataloging-in Publication Data
Main entry under title:

Urinary tract bleeding.

Includes bibliographies and index.
1. Urinary organs—Hemorrhage. I. Bern, Murray M.
[DNLM: 1. Hemorrhage—diagnosis. 2. Hemorrhage—therapy. 3. Urologic Diseases—complications. WJ 100 U763]
RC872.U75 1985 616.6 85-80319
ISBN 0-87993-236-8

Published by:
Futura Publishing Company, Inc.
295 Main Street
Mount Kisco, New York 10549

L.C.#: 85-80319
ISBN#: 0-87993-236-8

To Ruth S. Bern
and
In Memory of Hymie Bern
and
Devra B. Finkelstein

Contributors

Edward S. Amis, Jr., M.D.: Department of Radiology, Naval Hospital; Associate Professor of Surgery and Radiology, Uniformed Services University of the Health Sciences, Bethesda, Maryland

Birger Astedt, M.D.: Department of Obstetrics and Gynecology and Coagulation Laboratory, Professor, University of Lund, Allmanna Sjukhuset, Malmo, Sweden

Christos A. Athanasoulis, M.D.: Head of Section of Vascular Radiology, Massachusetts General Hospital, Professor of Radiology, Harvard Medical School, Boston, Massachusetts

Murray M. Bern, M.D.: Chief of Clinical Hematology, New England Deaconess Hospital, Assistant Professor of Medicine, Harvard Medical School, Boston, Massachusetts

Robert E. Desautels, M.D.: Urological Surgeon, New England Deaconess Hospital and Brigham and Women's Hospital, Assistant Clinical Professor of Surgery, Harvard Medical School, Boston, Massachusetts

Laura Feldman, M.D.: Assistant in Radiology, Massachusetts General Hospital, Instructor In Radiology, Harvard Medical School, Boston, Massachusetts

Mark S. Huberman, M.D.: Attending Physician in Oncology, New England Deaconess Hospital, Instructor in Medicine, Harvard Medical School, Boston, Massachusetts

Antoine Kaldany, M.D.: Attending Physician in Nephrology, Joslin Clinic and New England Deaconess Hospital, Assistant Professor of Medicine, Harvard Medical School, Boston, Massachusetts

John Libertino, M.D.: Chief of Surgery, Department of Urology, Lahey Clinic Medical Center, Burlington, Massachusetts, Clinical Assistant Professor in Surgery, Harvard Medical School, Boston, Massachusetts

Peter N. Madras, M.D.: Co-Director of Vascular Laboratory Department of Surgery, New England Deaconess Hospital, Assistant Professor of Surgery, Harvard Medical School, Boston, Massachusetts

H. David Mitcheson, M.D.: Urologist, Assistant Professor, Tufts University School of Medicine, Urologist, New England Medical Center, Boston, Massachusetts

Anthony P. Monaco, M.D.: Director of Division of Organ Transplantation, Department of Surgery, New England Deaconess Hospital, Professor of Surgery, Harvard Medical School, Boston, Massachusetts

Inga Marie Nilsson, M.D.: Professor, Department of Coagulation Disorders, University of Lund, Allmanna Sjukhuset, Malmo, Sweden

Lester Persky, M.D.: Clinical Professor of Urology, Case Western Reserve University School of Medicine, Cleveland, Ohio

Richard C. Pfister, M.D.: Head, Section of Uroradiology, Department of Radiology, Massachusetts General Hospital, Associate Professor of Radiology, Harvard Medical School, Boston, Massachusetts

Miljenko V. Pilepich, M.D.: Associate Professor of Radiology, Division of Radiation Oncology, Washington University School of Medicine, St. Louis, Missouri

Martin Schiff, Jr., M.D.: Attending Urologist, Yale-New Haven Hospital, Professor of Surgery/Urology, Yale University School of Medicine, New Haven, Connecticut

Elaine M. Sloand, M.D.: Fellow in Hematology, New England Deaconess Hospital, Clinical Fellow in Medicine, Harvard Medical School, Boston, Massachusetts

Sabina R. Wallach, M.D.: Attending Physician in Hematology-Oncology, New England Deaconess Hospital, Clinical Instructor in Medicine, Harvard Medical School, Boston, Massachusetts

David C. Yoburn, M.D.: Attending Physician in Nephrology, Joslin Clinic and New England Deaconess Hospital, Clinical Instructor in Medicine, Harvard Medical School, Boston, Massachusetts

Leonard Zinman, M.D.: Chairman, Department of Urology, Lahey Clinic Medical Center, Burlington, Massachusetts, Clinical Assistant Professor in Surgery, Harvard Medical School, Boston, Massachusetts

Introduction

Urinary tract bleeding can be a major clinical problem, which when severe can cause damage to tissues, can cause organ failure, and if uncontrolled can be life-threatening. The timely diagnosis and control of such bleeding can reduce morbidity, reduce permanent structural and functional damage to the tract and its surrounding tissues, and save lives. Toward this goal it is essential to have the capacity to apply a wide range of diagnostic and therapeutic tools. The appropriate basic and applied sciences are summarized, with emphasis given to practical management principles. The text is designed to serve everyone treating patients with urologic disease wherein hemorrhage is a potential complication.

This text describes the techniques used for the diagnosis and treatment of urologic bleeding drawing upon medical, surgical, as well as diagnostic and therapeutic radiologic disciplines. It is divided into broad general categories beginning with the medical issues. The first two chapters explore the coagulopathies as they present in the presence of renal disease. The next two chapters review the events within the systemic blood or kidneys that may create the appearance of hematuria. Finally in this section there is a discussion of fibrinolysis and the application of antifibrinolytic therapy.

The second section includes an outstanding discussion of the application of diagnostic radiology in the diagnosis and control of urinary tract hemorrhage. The first chapter of this section reviews the noninvasive radiologic manifestations of hemorrhage. The second chapter describes the roles of invasive radiology in the diagnosis and control of these various events. Both chapters are extensively illustrated, offering excellent pictorial examples of the events being described.

The third section discusses the surgical approaches available for the control of renal, ureteral, bladder, and post-prostatectomy hemorrhage. These chapters offer insight into the surgical skills to be applied and the equipment needed to support these skills.

The fourth section covers various subjects not heretofore explored wherein urinary tract hemorrhage can occur. Attention is given to the application of chemotherapy and radiotherapy to urinary tract neoplasms when they are primary or secondary to the urinary tract. There are discussions of systemic as well as instillation therapy for the various diseases. The radiotherapy chapter includes a description of the application to neoplastic diseases as well as a short discussion of the application of radiation therapy to benign diseases. Finally, two chapters discuss unique problems associated with patients having advanced renal failure. One of these latter chapters deals with the hemorrhagic complications associated with renal transplantation including access procedures. The last chapter discusses the management of dialysis in patients at high risk for hemorrhage.

The text, therefore, offers a broad overview of the issues and mechanics involved with supporting these very complicated patients, written by outstanding clinicians involved in the field. The text should serve the practicing physicians and surgeons well as they serve their patients.

Murray M. Bern, M.D.
Boston, Massachusetts

Notes of Appreciation

Each of the contributors are thanked for their energetic and timely work for this book. The author is extremely appreciative for the efficient, careful, and thorough work by Mary Lawless in preparing the final manuscripts and bibliographies. The author is also appreciative for the editorial advice offered by Leonard Zinman, M.D., John Chaffey, M.D., and Melvin Clouse, M.D., regarding the scope and contributors for this book, and for the generous assistance of Karoly Balogh, M.D., and Urmila Khettry, M.D., in selecting and preparing photographs of pathologic specimens. We also thank the Radiology Department of the New England Deaconess Hospital for their permission to reproduce the x-rays from their teaching file collection. We acknowledge the generosity of the Center for Devices and Radiological Health of the Food and Drug Administration for permission to reproduce several x-rays of the Genitourinary Section from their Learning File.

Contents

Chapter 1

Coagulation and Coagulopathies in Patients With Renal Disease

Murray M. Bern, M.D.

Coagulation is a complex coalescence of chemical and physical events that lead to the formation of a secure hemostatic plug. The system involves soluble plasma substances, circulating platelets, and immobilized endothelial cells on the vessel walls. The entire system is buffered by procoagulant and anticoagulant modulators. Once formed, the clots are dissolved by the fibrinolytic system. Alteration of any part of this scheme can cause failure to clot, an inability to prevent clotting, or excessive lysis of clots already formed, causing inappropriate hemorrhage or thrombosis. Figure 1 demonstrates a broad overview of the system. Patients with renal failure have changes in this coagulation system, with defects of the soluble plasma coagulants, the plasma anticoagulants, the fibrinolytic system, platelets, and endothelial cells, each of which can be dissected and managed selectively. Table I lists therapies available for many of these lesions.

I. Coagulation

A. Activation Phase of Coagulation

Coagulation of plasma begins with the Fletcher factor (prekallikrein), the Williams, Flujac, or Fitzgerald factor (high molecular weight kininogen), factor XII (Hageman factor), and factor XI (plasma thromboplastin antecedent, PTA). Coagulation begins with activation on surfaces and from endothelium, with positive feedback loops to accentuate the activities. Figure 2 depicts the activation phase. Lesions of this early activation phase cause dramatic *in vitro* effects but are not associated with clinical bleeding until the level of factor XI where deficiency does cause bleeding potential. As an example, Fletcher factor defi-

From Bern MM (ed.): *Urinary Tract Bleeding: Diagnosis and Control by Medical, Radiologic, and Surgical Techniques*. Mount Kisco, NY, Futura Publishing Co., Inc., 1985.

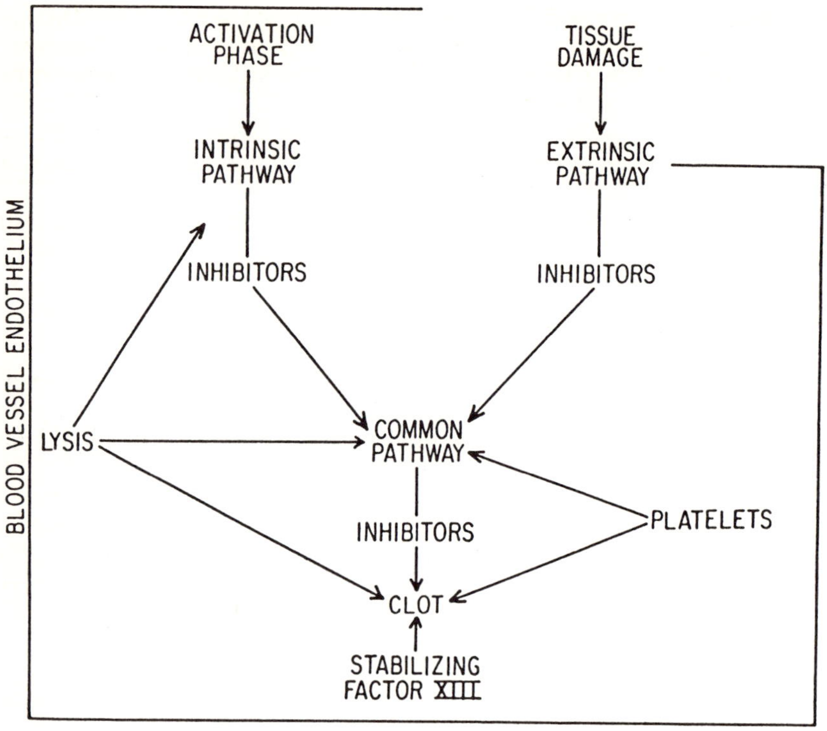

Figure 1: *An overview of the coagulation system, demonstrating the contributions made by blood vessel endothelium, damage to the blood vessels releasing tissue thromboplastin, platelets, fibrinolysis, and the so-called intrinsic and extrinsic clotting materials.*

ciency causes prolonged partial thromboplastin times (PTT), which can be "auto corrected" by incubating the plasma with a phospholipid for a few minutes. Deficiencies of factors XII and XI will not be corrected by this *in vitro* maneuver. Patients with factor XII deficiency do not have clinical bleeding disorders.

Deficiencies of activation phase substances are due to congenital lesions, advanced liver disease, or renal disease. Factor XI deficiency is an autosomal recessive trait that is associated with surgical or trauma-related hemorrhage. Spontaneous bleeding is uncommon. In fact, many of these patients will have no history of bleeding problems. They are detected by finding a prolonged PTT, activated (aPTT), or whole blood clotting time. Management requires fresh frozen plasma (FFP) transfusion preoperatively and postoperatively. Adequacy of replacement therapy can be monitored by measuring factor XI levels or by measuring the aPTT after transfusion.

Activation Phase in Renal Failure

Factor XII deficiency by functional and antigenic assays has been associated with nephrotic syndrome.[1–7] This acquired deficiency can normalize after recovery from the nephrotic syndrome.[1–7] These depletions may be due to urinary losses, consumption, *in vivo* activation, or loss of function of the antigen, i.e. an acquired dysfunction.[4,5] No inhibitors to factor XII have been identified, nor were changes of crossed-immunoelectrophoresis seen,[7] even though the level of XII antigen is greater than the level of XII coagulant.[4,5] Patients with decreased factor XII have had minimal lesion, membranous, membranoproliferative, or amyloid renal disease.[2–5,7,8]

Occasionally the nephrotic patient may also have partial deficiency of factor XI.[3,9] Rarely patients are reported as having decreased prekallikrein or kallikrein inhibitor.[3,5,7]

An excellent summary of coagulation defects found in nephrotic syndrome is available by Vaziri.[10]

B. Intrinsic Pathway of Coagulation

Activation of factors XI and XII lead to the activation of the intrinsic and probably of the extrinsic pathway, which then activates the common pathway (see Fig. 3). Besides factors XI and XII, the intrinsic pathway is made of factor IX (Christmas or Hemophilia B factor) and factor VIII (Hemophilia A and von Willebrand's factors). Tissue thromboplastin and factor VII compose the extrinsic pathway. These cooperate with factors V (labile or proaccelerin factor) and calcium and phospholipids to initiate the common pathway, via the activation of factor X to Xa. Deficiencies of these factors lead to increased hemorrhagic potential, and they require specific diagnosis for safe care of the patients.

Patients with significant factor IX or VIII deficiency have histories of bleeding, the magnitude of which is inverse to the level of the factors. Patients with less than 10% of either substance will have some clinical bleeding, with very obvious problems when the factor concentrations are less than 5% of normal. Both hemophilia A (factor VIII deficiency) and B (factor IX deficiency) are sex-linked recessive genetic defects affecting males predominantly. It is very important to remember that a female may have either disease if her father has one of these diseases and if her mother is a carrier for the same disease. Von Willebrand's disease (factor VIII deficiency with an associated platelet defect) is an autosomal dominant disease and affects males and females.

These diseases demand precise diagnosis since treatments differ. The aPTT will be prolonged. Factor IX deficiency is clinically identical to hemophilia A, though less common. The diagnosis is made by measuring factor IX. Factor VIII deficiency due to hemophilia A is due to deficiency of VIII coagulant activity (VIII:C) and the VIII coagulant antigen (VIII:Cag), but the VIII-related antigen (VIII:Rag) is normal. Von Willebrand's disease is due to deficiency of VIII:C, plus deficiencies of the factor VIII-related antigen (VIII:Rag) and of the ristocetin cofactor (VIII:cof). The ristocetin or von Willebrand factor also mediates adhesion of platelets to endothelial cells, a deficiency of which causes prolonged bleeding times.

1. *Factor IX in Renal Failure*

Factor IX deficiency has been found in some[9,11–14] but not all patients with nephrotic syndrome.[1,14] Those with deficiencies of factor IX have had a variety of histopathologic diagnoses, including sickle cell nephropathy, minimal change disease, focal glomerulosclerosis, and amyloidosis. Urinary losses of factor IX may account for the very short plasma half disappearance rate, especially with large protein losses.[6,11,13] The normal values for plasma half disappearance is

Table I

Partial List of Coagulopathies Encountered in Surgery and their Available Emergency Therapies

Coagulopathy		**Emergency Therapy**	
	1st Choice	**2nd Choice**	**3rd Choice**
HMW Kininogen Deficiency	None needed	—	—
Fletcher Factor Deficiency	None needed	—	—
Factor XII Deficiency	None needed	—	—
Factor XI Deficiency	Plasma	—	—
Factor IX Deficiency	Plasma	II, VII, IX, X Concentrate* **	—
Factor VIII Deficiency { Hemophilia A	Cryoprecipitate or VIII Concentrate*	Plasma	—
Factor VIII Deficiency { von Willebrand	Cryoprecipitate*	Plasma	VIII Concentrate*
Factor VIII Antibody	II, VIII, IX, X Concentrate* **	DDAVP***	Androgens***
Factor VII Deficiency	Plasma	II, VII, IX, X Concentrate* **	—
Factor X Deficiency	Plasma	II, VII, IX, X Concentrate* **	—
Factor V Deficiency	Plasma	—	—
Factor II Deficiency	Plasma	II, VII, IX, X Concentrate* **	—
Factor I Deficiency Dysfibrinogenemia	{Cryoprecipitate*	Plasma	Fibrinogen Concentrate*
Vitamin K Deficiency	Plasma	Vitamin K Replacement	—
Warfarin	Plasma	Vitamin K Replacement	II, VII, IX, X Concentrate* **

Heparin	Protamine Sulfate	Time	—
Liver Disease			
Chronic	Vitamin K Replacement	Plasma	II, VII, IX, X Concentrate* **
Acute PIVKA	Plasma	Plasma Exchange	
Fibrinolysis	Epsilon Amino Caproic Acid	AMCHA	AMCA or Trasylol
Circulating Anticoagulants	Steroids, If appropriate	Plasma Exchange	—
DIC	Remove Precipitating Cause	Heparin/Plasma	ATIII Concentrate
Hemolytic Uremia Syndrome	Plasma	Heparin	ATIII Concentrate
Amyloidosis (Factor X Deficiency)	Plasma	—	—
Nephrotic Syndrome (Factor Deficiencies)	Plasma	—	—
Thrombocytopenia: Acquired			
Drug-induced	Platelet Transfusion	Withdraw Offending Drug	—
Immune	Platelet Transfusion	Steroids***	Azathioprine***
Dilutional	Platelet Transfusion	Delay Procedure	—
Post-transfusion Purpura	Plasma Exchange	PL^{AI} Negative Platelets	—
Aplastic Marrow	Platelet Transfusion	—	—
Malignant Invasion of Marrow	Platelet Transfusion	—	—
Cyclic thrombocytopenia	Delay Procedure	Platelet Transfusion	—
Paroxysmal Nocturnal Hemoglobinuria	Plasma Free Platelet Transfusion	—	—
Merritt-Kasabach	Platelet Transfusion	Control Local Consumption	—
Hypersplenism	Platelet Transfusion	Splenectomy	—
Hypothermia	Platelet Transfusion	Warming/Heparin	—
TTP	Plasma Exchange	Plasma Infusion	(?) Antiplatelet Agents
Platelet Dysfunction of Cellular Origin			
Thrombosthenia	Platelet Transfusion	—	—
Thrombopathia	Platelet Transfusion	—	—
Leukemia	Platelet Transfusion	Treat Leukemia***	—
Myelofibrosis	Platelet Transfusion	Splenectomy Occasionally	—

(continued)

Table I

Partial List of Coagulopathies Encountered in Surgery and their Available Emergency Therapies

Coagulopathy	**Emergency Therapy** 1st Choice	2nd Choice	3rd Choice
Platelet Dysfunction of Metabolic Origin			
Drugs	Platelet Transfusion	Delay Procedure	—
Uremia	Platelet Transfusion	DDAVP; Cryoprecipitate, Dialysis	—
Hyperbilirubinemia	Platelet Transfusion	Correct Bilirubinemia	—
Fibrin Degradation Products	Control Fibrinolysis	—	—
Hyperglobulinemia	Plasmapheresis	Control Cause	—
Vascular Defects			
Ehlers-Danlos	Surgical Hemostasis	—	—
Scurvey	Surgical Hemostasis	Vitamic C	—
Retained Clot	Irrigation	Surgical Evacuation	—

*These products may transmit blood-transmitted diseases such as hepatitis or AIDS since they are pooled plasma products.
**They are also capable of causing intravascular coagulation (see text).
***Slow onset of activity; will be less useful in emergency.

From: Bern M: Management of hemorrhage during surgery. *Surgical Rounds* 3:36–40, 1980. Used with permission of the publisher.

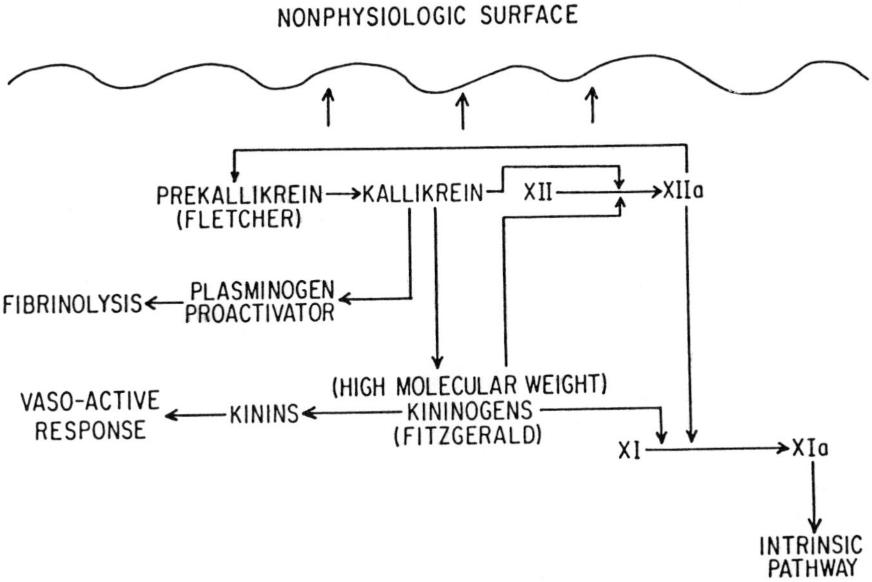

Figure 2: *A schematic figure of the activation phase of coagulation.*

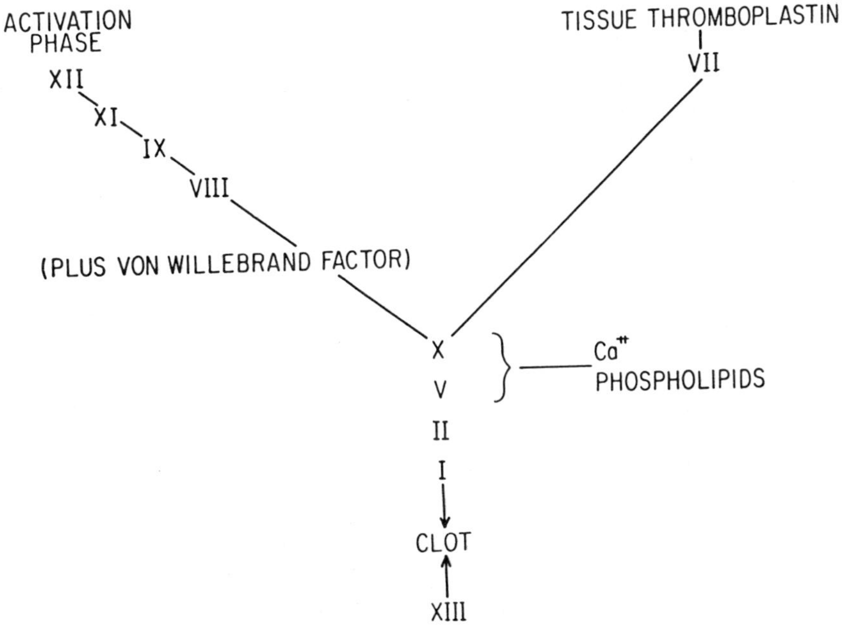

Figure 3: *A simplified diagram of the coagulation system indicating how the intrinsic and extrinsic pathways lead to activation of the common pathway.*

20–30 h. In patients with factor IX losses with nephrotic syndrome, even with protein losses of only 5 gm/d, the factor IX T½ may be less than 2 hours.[13] However, not all patients with excessive proteinuria will have the deficiency.[1] Plasma or factor concentrate replacement therapy may not be adequate to control or prevent hemorrhage.[13] Therapy for the basic disease, for example with steroids, may end the factor IX deficiency.[9] This can be useful even if the neuropathy is due to the sickle cell disease.[11]

2. *Therapy for Factor IX Deficiency*

Therapy for factor IX deficiency is to infuse the factor by giving FFP or concentrates of factor IX (with factors II, VII, and X). The latter products pose significant problems since the available concentrates are products of pooled plasma and can transmit hepatitis. Also, the concentrates often contain some activated factors such as Xa and VIIa, which pose a risk of acute thrombosis.[15–17] Use of FFP can be complicated by fluid overload, especially in renal failure. While replacement therapy is adequate therapy for congenital absences, it may not suffice in those with nephrotic syndrome. Due to rapid clearance in some of these patients, therapeutic levels may be hard to sustain.

3. *Factor VIII in Renal Failure*

There are complex changes of factor VIII in chronic renal failure. The factor VIII complex is actually elevated in patients with chronic renal failure. The VIII-related antigen, the VIII-ristocetin cofactor, and the VIII-coagulant levels can all rise.[18–26] These elevations may be due to release from damaged endothelial cells or due to slow clearance from plasma of the molecules. Kazatchkine et al, proposed and it was later argued that the factor VIII was defective based upon disproportionate differences between the antigen and coagulant levels.[18,20] There is some evidence that lends support to the original suggestion.[27,28] Twenty-two of 38 patients with renal failure had increased electrophoretic mobility of their isolated factor VIII.[28] The larger multimeric forms of factor VIII are distributed normally in renal failure.[29] Paradoxically, the changes of factor VIII may actually contribute to the atherosclerosis seen in patients with chronic uremia (see below).

Factor VIII coagulant activity rises in patients with nephrotic syndrome, even in the absence of uremia.[14,30–32] There is no correlation between factor VIII elevation and levels of serum albumin, or even the causes for the nephrotic syndrome.[30] When the nephrosis is controlled, the factor VIII level falls.[32]

4. *Therapy for Factor VIII Deficiency*

Therapy for factor VIII deficiency is based also upon replacement with FFP or with concentrates of factor VIII (cryoprecipitate or lyophilized factor VIII). The adequacy of replacement is monitored by measuring factor VIII at peak and trough levels, so as to keep the plasma VIII:C greater than 20% of normal. For von Willebrand's disease, the level of VIII:Rag can be transiently boosted by giving the patient either FFP or the cryoprecipitate. The VIII:C will rise concomitantly, and remain elevated for longer periods of time than due to the replaced material alone. Since the bleeding time lesion is not corrected by lyophilized factor VIII, cryoprecipitate or the plasma are the best therapies for von Willebrand's disease. Adequacy of therapy for von Willebrand's disease requires measurements of the factor VIII coagulant and the bleeding time. (Cryoprecipitate also corrects the bleeding time lesions seen in uremia. This is discussed in the section of this chapter dealing with platelets and in Chapter 2.)

5. Factor VIII in Atherosclerosis in Renal Failure

Patients with chronic renal failure have accelerated atherosclerosis. The several possible mechanisms for this are discussed throughout this chapter. One cause may be that the elevated factor VIII complex is seen in renal failure. The factor VIII-ristocetin cofactor facilitates platelet adhesion to damaged endothelial surfaces, and may contribute to pathological arterial thrombosis. Factor VIII may contribute to some glomerular lesions. One report indicates that infusion of prostacyclin during hemodialysis blocks the release of factor VIII during dialysis,[25] in addition to protecting the platelets.[33]

C. Extrinsic Pathway

Tissue thromboplastin plus factor VII comprise the extrinsic pathway. Factor VII deficiency is an autosomal recessive genetic trait capable of causing hemorrhage. Here the PT (prothrombin time) is abnormal while the aPTT is normal. A specific diagnosis is established by measuring the factor VII level. Common causes for factor VIII deficiency are liver disease, oral anticoagulants, fat malabsorption, and malnutrition.

Factor VII in Renal Failure

Patients with nephrotic syndrome rarely have a deficiency of factor VII, and then can have a hemorrhagic diathesis.[34,35] Other patients will have elevated factor VII levels in the nephrotic syndrome.[14,32,34] Factor VII may be lost into the urine[34] even though the rate of disappearance of the factor from plasma is normal.[13] In the rare nephrotic patient with factor VII deficiency, the deficiency improves in parallel with improvement of the nephrotic syndrome.

D. Common Pathway

Congenital deficiencies of factors X, V, II, or I of the common pathway are due to autosomal recessive defects. They are not common problems, but can be very problematic when present. The magnitude of the bleeding diathesis corresponds to the magnitude of the deficiency. Histories of bruising, epistaxis, menorrhagia, hemarthrosis, and surgical or trauma-induced bleeding are usually present. Lesions in the common pathway cause prolonged PT *and* aPTT. Except for factor X deficiency, these are not corrected by addition of Russell's viper venom in the Styphven test. Factor X deficiency will be corrected by addition of aged serum, since X is not consumed during the clotting process. Absorbed plasma made deficient of factor II and X will correct factor V and factor I deficient plasmas. Individual factor assays in the common pathway should be performed when bleeding occurs with prolongation of the PT and the PTT.

Acquired defects due to reduced synthesis of these factors are the most common causes of combined prolongations of the PT and the aPTT. These synthetic defects, including factors I and V deficiency, are most commonly due to advanced hepatic disease. Acquired deficiency of vitamin K due to starvation, vitamin K-depleted diets, or malabsorption, especially for fats, can lead to loss of vitamin K-dependent factors II, VII, IX, and X. This tends to occur when patients are malnourished due to inadequate oral intake, as can occur postoperatively, and is worsened when antibiotics are given concomitantly.[36,37] This can be worsened by concomitant renal failure.[38–40] Coagulopathies such as this can appear in patients after only one week of vitamin K depletion. Spurious ingestion of oral anticoagulants such as warfarin, another cause of these deficiencies, is not a rare event among persons with access to the drugs.

Advanced parenchymal liver disease is commonly associated with renal failure, and thus deserves discussion. Defects associated with liver disease include deficiencies of factors I, II, V, VII, IX, and X, uninhibited fibrinolysis, acquired inhibitors, or consumptive coagulopathy. Beside the inhibition created by the fibrin lysis degradation products (FDPs), inhibitors appear that are incomplete precursor forms of the factors II, VII, IX and X molecules. This inhibitor syndrome is clumped under the eponym PIVKA (Prothrombin in Vitamin K Antagonist/Absence).[34] These incomplete molecules have active binding sites but no coagulant activity, due to the absence of the terminal gamma carboxyglutamic acid residues, which are normally attached with the help of vitamin K. They are released from hepatocytes following acute hepatic damage following infection, trauma, or anoxia. The latter often appears with ATN following hypotension from bleeding, heart failure, etc. The PIVKA syndrome is treated by plasma replacement and by improving the liver function. Patients with renal failure and factor deficiency may not tolerate the volumes of plasma required for replacement. In severe circumstances plasma exchange may be required.

Fibrin(ogen) lysis degradation products (FDP/fdp) tend to accumulate in liver failure due to decreased clearance by the reticulo-endothelial system. High liters of FDP/fdp inhibit fibrin polymerization and interfere with platelet function. There is a greater degree of fibrinolysis in liver failure due to loss of inhibitors to fibrinolysis. Thrombocytopenia is also commonly seen in this setting due to splenic sequestration associated with portal hypertension.

Thus, patients with liver disease may have a combination of defects, of which the dominant one is not discernible until selective studies or selective therapeutic maneuvers have been conducted to which the response is monitored. Emergencies, on the other hand, may require platelet and plasma replacement first, and thereafter, judicious use of other agents, including fibrinogen, epsilon aminocaproic acid (EACA), or even heparin. In very selected cases, it is useful to use concentrates of factors II, VII, IX, and X. However, the risks following use of these products should be cause for concern as discussed above.

Common Pathway in Renal Failure

Factor X is generally normal in patients with renal failure with or without nephrotic syndrome.[2,14,30] despite the more rapid clearance of the molecule.[13]

Factor V levels tend to be normal or elevated in those with nephrotic syndrome.[14,30–32] The levels of factor II, prothrombin, tend to be normal or low in patients with nephrotic syndrome[30,32] despite urinary losses.[13] By immunologic assays, factor II is low in nephrotic patients.

E. Fibrinogen (Factor I) and Fibrin Stabilizing Factor (Factor XIII) in Renal Failure.

Fibrinogen tends to rise above normal in chronic renal failure.[25] Those with nephrotic syndrome also have hyperfibrinogenemia, the levels of which correlate inversely with albumin and directly with cholesterol levels.[6,30,31] Prothrombin is converted to thrombin by factor Xa, and thrombin then lyses the terminal peptides from fibrinogen to create soluble fibrin monomers. These soluble fibrin monomers then polymerize into lengthy chains, which are then cross-linked by the transaminase factor XIII, (the fibrin stabilizing factor). This process appears to be defective in renal failure.[42] This forms (α)-glutamyl-E-lysyl bonds (see Fig. 4). The (α) component of the fibrin chains polymerize poorly in the presence of uremia, while the other chains have a similar but less profound defect. In uremic plasma, the factor XIII functions normally, but its substrates, the fibrin monomers, appear to be defective. In one study, urea acted as a false substrate for the esterase activity of factor XIII.[43] In these experiments, urea penetrated the clot and disturbed the substrate-transaminase relationship, disturbing the isopeptide linkages. In uremia, the level of factor XIII varies from low to normal to high.[44] It tends to fall in patients with acute post-streptococcal glomerulonephritis and with Henock-Schonlein nephritis, but rises in those with nephrotic syndrome.[44–47] Others have found factor XIII levels to be normal.[43]

Drugs may interfere in these late steps of fibrin formation. Penicillins (or their metabolic by-products) given to uremic patients may act synergistically with the uremia to prolong the recalcification time, the thromboplastin time of

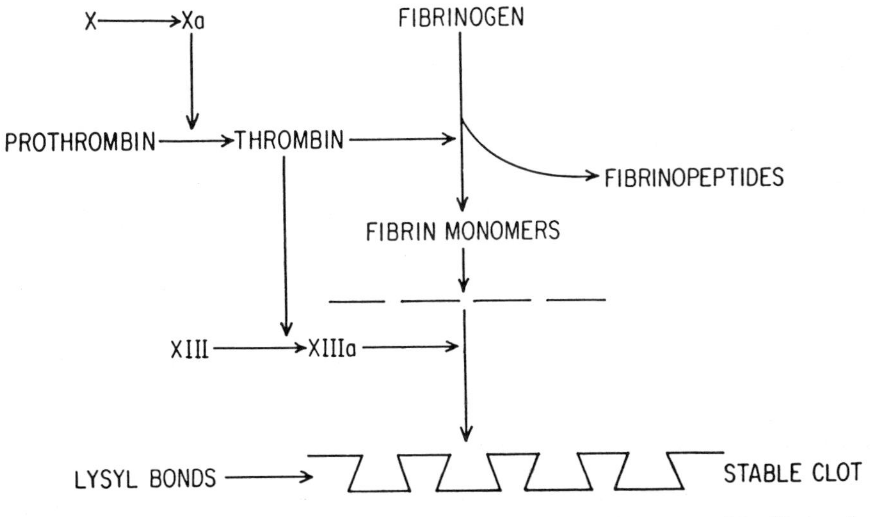

Figure 4: *Diagram of the final steps of coagulation leading to stable fibrin clot.*

Quick, the thrombin time, the reptilace time, and to change the shape of the thromboelastrogram.[48,49] Carbenicillin, penicillin, ampicillin, and methicillin have similar effects to varying degrees. Cephalothin, dicloxacillin, and flucloxicillin did not cause these changes in the experiments reported.[49] Protamine chloride corrected the defects, while penicillinase was useless.[49] High doses of penicillin derivatives, such as carbenicillin, also worsen the bleeding time lesion which is already a problem in uremic patients.

Low molecular weight dextrans can cause acute renal failure with extremely elevated specific gravities.[50–52] In this condition, the offending agent remains in the circulation for prolonged times, causing further renal damage and coagulopathy.[50–53] In addition to the dextrans causing reduction of platelet adhesion, they also cause reduction of fibrin polymerization and the clots' susceptibility to lysis,[54] adding to the uremic coagulopathy acquired during renal failure.[55] Plasma exchange is a useful therapy.[50]

F. Inhibitors of Coagulation in Renal Failure

Changes of the natural or acquired inhibitors of coagulation in patients with renal failure can create either hemorrhagic or thrombotic potential. The primary natural inhibitiors of coagulation in plasma is antithrombin III (AT III), alpha-2-macroglobulin, and alpha-1-antitrypsin, with AT III being dominant.[56] Depletion of AT III is associated with an increased prevalence of venous and arterial thrombi. Patients receiving hemodialysis have normal, slightly increased, or low normal to low levels of AT III by functional and immunologic assays.[30,31,57–65] Low levels of AT III are more likely to be seen in patients with nephrotic syndrome where the frequency of thrombotic complications correlates with the AT III deficiency.[63,64] The drop of AT III parallels falls of alpha-1-antitrypsin and albumin in nephrotic, dialyzed, and transplanted patients.[63–66] AT III is found in the urine of nephrotic patients.[63,64] A compensatory, possibly protective, rise of the alpha-2-macroglobulin occurs.

AT III replacement may be therapeutic. Patients with hemolytic uremic syndrome (HUS) have been treated successfully with AT III replacement.[67,68] Prevention of AT III consumption is also of potential benefit. Agents such as warfarin or sulfinpyrazone appear to give some protection.[60,69]

Other inhibitors may be as common as fibrin(ogen) degradation products, FDP/fdps, which appear following fibrin(ogen) lysis, or as uncommon as antibodies to coagulation factors, as may occur with autoimmunity syndromes. Less potent and nonspecific inhibitors can appear in patients with hyperglobulinemia of IgG or IgM types. While many of these inhibitors do have *in vivo* activity, it is not uncommon for acquired inhibitors to have greater *in vitro* influence than clinical importance.[70] The latter occurs in patients with autoimmune disease, but also in patients receiving drugs capable of causing biologically false-positive ANA. Drugs often used in patients with renal failure, such as pronestyl and methyldopa, can prolong the aPTT due to an inhibitor to the phospholipids used in the *in vitro* assay.[70] When the patient's platelets are substituted as a source of that phospholipid in the coagulation assay, the results are normal. The activated whole blood clotting times using silica to activate, will also be normal since there is no need of exogenous phospholipid in the assay. On the other hand, in using this system, a true biologically important lesion can be missed since a functional deficiency to less than 20% of normal is needed before the WBCT is prolonged. A more precise though still nonspecific assay is to make serial dilutions of the test plasma or the phospholipid by saline in the aPTT assay. The resultant curve distinguishes true from artifactual inhibitors. Another assay could be a platelet-mediated thromboplastin generation time. Assays using anticardiolipin have some specificity for the defect. When present, thrombosis is a greater potential clinical problem than is bleeding.

Protein C is another *in vivo* inhibitor of coagulation.[71] It is modulated by Protein C and thrombin.[72] It acts to dampen the activities of factors VIII:C and V.[71] A deficiency of Protein C may cause an excessive thrombosis syndrome. In a limited series of patients so far studied with chronic renal failure, on and off hemodialysis, the Protein C levels were normal.[22] As greater experience is acquired, patients have been found with depletion of Protein C in the presence of severe renal diseases.[274]

II. Platelets

Platelets create the primary hemostatic plug defects. The process begins by the adherence of the platelets to exposed subendothelial substances. The platelets then release their intracellular contents, including calcium, ADP, 5-hydroxytryptamine (5-HT), phospholipids platelet factor 3 (PF3), the heparin-neutralizing substance platelet factor 4 (PF4), and other materials. The released PF3 becomes soluble cofactor for factors V, VII, VIII, and X in the presence of calcium and can activate factor X to Xa. The platelets become intertwined with fibrin polymers within the clot. The released 5-HT causes local and possibly distal vasospasm, which further reduces the blood flow.

A. Platelet Disorders in General

Qualitative and quantitative deficiencies of platelets can lead to increased bruising, intracutaneous hemorrhage (petechia), or site-specific bleeding such as epistaxis, hemoptysis, melena, hematuria, etc. Petechial bleeding is often seen in areas of increased hydrostatic pressure. For ambulatory patients, this is usually in the legs. For the coughing patients, the petechia may be around the head and face. For patients receiving positive end expiratory pressure ventilation, they appear on the chest and upper abdomen and back. These lesions are usually nonpalpable, beginning as red lesions and fading to purple and to brown in 2–5 days. Palpable petechia traditionally suggest vasculitis, or bacterial or fungal emboli.

Thrombocytopenia and thrombocytopathies present as an immediate hemostatic defect in patients with surgery or trauma. On the other hand, patients with normal platelets, but with defects in other phases of coagulation, often have reasonable early hemostasis, but subsequently fail to secure the clot and have slightly delayed bleeding.

Many diseases cause thrombocytopenia or defects in platelet function and can cause microscopic or gross hematuria. The following paragraphs introduce the problem. Subsequent sections in this and the next chapter deal with the platelets in renal failure.

1. Congenital Platelet Disorders

Several congenital platelet lesions exist, and hematuria can be a manifestation of these diseases. Von Willebrand's disease causes prolonged bleeding times due to failure of the platelets to adhere. This defect usually but not always occurs in the presence of low factor VIII:C and low factor VIII:Rag levels, with the attendant prolongation of aPTT (see above). Glanzman's thrombocytopathy is marked by decreased clot retraction, prolonged bleeding time, poor platelet adhesion to glass, and no platelet aggregation in response to ADP, thrombin, and collagen. The Bernard-Soulier syndrome involves very large platelets with dense granular condensations and decreased levels of PF3. Storage pool defect is marked by poor collagen-induced aggregation, poor PF3 release, and normal response to ADP-induced aggregation. The May-Hegglin syndrome has giant platelets, Dohle bodies in the granulocytes, and possible thrombocytopenia. The Wiskott-Aldrich syndrome includes eczema, frequent infections, dense granules in the polymorphonuclear cells and platelets, and thrombocytopenia. Complete descriptions and bibliographies of these lesions can be found in standard hematology and coagulation textbooks.

2. Acquired Platelet Disorders

Many acquired diseases can cause defects of platelet function or count, and can lead to hematuria. A full listing of these diseases is beyond the scope of this text. Pharmaceutical agents are the most common cause for suppressed platelet function or platelet count. Among the drugs, aspirin and other nonsteroidal anti-inflammatory drugs can become common clinical problems. When used in uremic patients, these drugs have an additive effect upon the dysfunction of uremia. These agents block the membrane-bound cyclo-oxygenase or prostaglandin synthesis in the prostaglandin pathway. Aspirin binding to the cyclo-oxygenase is irreversible, and causes platelet failure for the life of the platelet. Correction of this defect can take up to 7 days, though for most clinical situations, 3 or 4 days is generally adequate. Blockade of the prostaglandin synthetase is reversible, and for these, it is usually adequate to stop the drug for about 24–36 hours. For emergenices, platelets can be transfused after plasma clearance of the offending drug. For elective procedures, it is wisest to delay surgery until the drug-induced lesions clear. These defects can be confirmed by assaying of platelet aggregation in response to arachidonic acid or by measuring the prostaglandin synthesis by-product, malondialdehyde.

Other pharmaceuticals also suppress platelet function. Dipyridamole suppresses platelets by modulating the 3'5'-cycle AMP concentration. Sulfinpyrazone probably exerts its suppressive influence by way of its metabolites.

Numerical deficiencies of platelets occur from marrow failure or marrow displacement. A wide variety of diseases exist in these categories that need not be listed here. Deficiencies of folic acid or vitamin B_{12} occur due to poor intake, malabsorption, or increased losses. Suppression of marrow function may follow response to drugs and environmental exposures such as radiation, benzene, and many therapeutic agents. Predictably, thrombocytopenia follows chemotherapeutics and some immunosuppressants. Azathioprine, a commonly used immune suppressant in renal transplantation, can suppress marrow, as can the more cytotoxic agents such as cyclophosphamide. Cyclosporin has been linked causally to thrombocytopenia in rare cases. Severe uremia alone can cause mild to moderate marrow suppression.

Peripheral overutilization of platelets also causes thrombocytopenia. Consumption may be immune-mediated, or due to anatomical, infectious, or thrombotic diseases. Drug-related or autoimmune thrombocytopenias are relatively common. Thrombotic consumption syndromes include thrombotic thrombocytopenic purpura (TTP), diffuse intravascular coagulopathy (DIC), and Kasabach-Merritt syndrome, among others. TTP and DIC frequently appear with hematuria and renal failure. Hemolytic uremic syndrome is a closely linked relative of TTP. Systemic infections with bacteria, viruses, and parasites create thrombocytopenia; measles vaccinations can also cause thrombocytopenia. Hypersplenism due to many underlying diseases is also a major problem. Heparin occasionally causes thrombocytopenia with a devastating thrombotic potential. Dilutional thrombocytopenia follows large transfusion therapy if platelets are not given simultaneously. Post-transfusion purpura due to Pl^{A1} antibody acquired during transfusion must be considered. Paroxysmal nocturnal hemoglobinemia and cyclic thrombocytopenia are other causes.

Scurvy is associated with prolonged bleeding times due to vascular fragility despite normal platelet counts. There are additional causes for nonthrombocytopenic purpura, such as vasculitis and Henoch-Schönlein syndrome, which effect renal function.

B. Platelet Disorders in Renal Failure

Platelet counts and functions are often abnormal in patients with renal failure. Understanding these abnormalities often allows for correction of the hemorrhage or the hemorrhagic potential.

As already discussed, many drugs cause thrombocytopenia and platelet dysfunction. Since the clearance of these drugs in patients with renal failure varies, additional precautions are necessary. An example is cimetidine. Cimetidine can cause thrombocytopenia due to marrow suppression more frequently in uremic patients by virtue of its slowed clearance.[73] Patients receiving cimetidine clear other drugs more slowly when their normal clearance mechanisms involve the liver.

Patients receiving hemodialysis lose greater amounts of folic acid to the dialysate than they ingest in their diets.[74–76] Losses up to 75 μg per dialysis occur, while the average daily intake among uremic patients is 32 μg per day. The Recommended Daily Allowance is 400 μg per day.[74] Folate losses to peritoneal dialysate is much less, though it does occur at about 9 μg per day. The pharmacologic route of the folate explains the problems. The monoglutamate of folic acid binds to albumin, leaving the free plasma folate available for clearance by dialysis. Thus, the combination of amount ingested, the albumin present, displacement of folate off albumin by other drugs, and dialysis create the need for supplemental folic acid.

Patients with acute and chronic renal failure have defects of platelet function that can be altered further by hemodialysis. A variety of causes for these defects have been described (see Chapter 2).[77–82] The platelet defects cause defective primary hemostasis with abnormal capillary fragility, prolonged bleeding times, poor clot retraction, and poor platelet aggregation.[78] There is also reduction of support for the coagulation process due to less release of PF3.[83]

This in turn causes decreased prothrombin consumption and decreased thromboplastin generation.[78-84]

Probably the most consistently changed platelet function in uremic patients is the bleeding time.[84-87] It occasionally becomes prolonged even in nonuremic patients but with acute glomerulonephritis.[88] The prolongation of the bleeding time is a reasonable but not altogether reliable predictor for excessive bleeding.[84,87,89] While platelet aggregation to ADP and epinephrine can be defective,[80,81] defective aggregation response to collagen did correlate best with prolonged bleeding times and did identify patients with excessive clinical bleeding.[89] The platelet response to arachidonic acid is variable in chronic renal failure, with greater response to low doses, but poorer response to higher doses.[89] Platelet adhesion to glass is depressed and may not improve following dialysis.[61,79,85,87,90-92]

Platelet survival is reduced in chronic renal failure, in some cases possibly due to the primary renal lesion. With shortened survivals, rates of platelet production go up when the marrow can respond. These abnormalities normalize during dialysis.[93]

C. Platelets During Dialysis

Platelet counts can fall during hemodialysis.[94] The platelets are deposited along with fibrin on the membrane, reducing the efficiency of the membrane.[95-97] No increase of circulating platelet aggregates was demonstrated following dialysis, even though there are increased screen filter pressures of venous efferent blood.[98]

Platelet function may actually decay during dialysis.[94] Effluent venous platelets during dialysis may actually become unresponsive even to high doses of ADP.[93] However, upon their return to the systemic circulation, they seem to recover somewhat from this dialysis-associated defect. Adhesion can improve.[87,92]

The magnitude and importance of these changes vary according to dialysis systems being used. The effect upon platelets thus should be measured in each dialysis unit so as to be better equipped to manage complications that may occur in the patients.

Similar but not identical changes are induced by hemofiltration.[99] With hemofiltration there is a loss of platelets, which recover toward but not to normal during the procedure. In addition, fibrinogen is lost and fibrin monomers are increased.

D. Causes of Abnormal Platelet Function in Renal Failure

Platelets are biochemically damaged due to the uremic environment. Uptake and release of 5-hydroxytryptamine (serotonin) is defective.[86,100] ADP and Mg^{++}-ATPace levels are decreased though the ATP levels are normal. The 5-HT and ADP defects are corrected by dialysis and transplantation, though the Mg^{++}-ATPace defect is not. The storage pool of ADP, and probably not the metabolic pool, is defective.[86] Platelet cyclic-AMP and platelet adenyl cyclase is higher than normal.[101]

A wide variety of substances have been incriminated and then have been refuted as being the cause for the platelet disorders in uremia. Major shifts in the platelet and endothelial cell prostaglandin and endothelial prostacyclin metabolism occur and appear key to our understanding of uremia-associated platelet defects. These are discussed in detail in Chapter 2. Included among the incriminated agents have been urea,[86] guanidinosuccinic acid.[78,100,102,103] phenols, and parahydrocyphenylactic acid.[86,104] Recent interest has developed for the "middle molecules," which are about 1000 daltons in weight, accumulate in the plasma of patients receiving hemodialysis, and suppress the first phase of ADP-induced aggregation in a dose-dependent fashion.[77,105–108]

E. How to Correct the Problem—Sometimes

Dialysis can improve platelet function. It generally improves aggregation response to ADP and epinephrine,[80,81,85,106] and may improve overall platelet function.[78,87,109] On the other hand, hemodilaysis can actually cause problems.

While hemodialysis improves the plasma milieu, it is at the expense of exposing the platelets to artificial surfaces and sheer forces, causing clinical results that are not always gratifying. Markers of platelet damage during dialysis are available. Platelet-derived thromboxane A_2 plus β-thromboglobulin (β-TG) rise during hemodialysis.[110] Sulfinpyrazone, PGI_2, or PGE_1 tend to protect the platelets from the effects of these traumas.[61,110–113] As a matter of fact, uremia, which is normally associated with low PGI_2 plasma levels, causes a rise of PGI_2 during hemodialysis.[78]

Caution is needed when using β-TG as a monitor of platelet damage in patients with renal failure. Normally, β-TG is cleared by the kidneys. Thus, elevation of β-TG plasma levels may be due to suppressed clearance and not simply due to platelet damage.[114] This is despite the fact that azotemic platelets release less β-TG than do normal platelets.[114] PF4, on the other hand, is unaffected by renal failure.[115–117] The β-TG is 36,000 daltons with a plasma clearance of about 100 minutes. PF4 is about 8,000 daltons and is cleared in about 30 minutes by nonexcretory mechanisms.[118]

Peritoneal dialysis avoids these problems and improves bleeding time more reliably. This advantage is probably due to the hypoalbuminemia created during peritoneal dialysis.[119] Peritoneal dialysis improves platelet function as indicated by response to epinephrine and ADP, possibly due to an improved plasma microenvironment or due to the lowered albumin.[80] Platelet functions also improve following renal transplantation.[120]

Managing prolonged bleeding times that are resistant to dialysis or when dialysis is not being used can be particularly difficult. For an emergency and for temporary benefit, transfusion of freshly prepared platelets give "microbandaid" effect. Unfortunately, the transfused cells soon acquire the same uremic lesion as the native platelets. Cryoprecipitate causes a delayed and transient improvement of the bleeding time.[25,121] Nadir bleeding times are seen 1 to 12 hours after the infusion of 10 bags of cryoprecipitate infused over 30 minutes. The improvement in bleeding times disappears in 24–36 hours. This response is not being observed consistently in our hands, and thus the efficacy of this approach must be tested before proceeding with invasive procedures. The mechanism of action is unknown. Another approach requires infusion of 1-deamino-8-D-arginine vasopressin (DDAVP), a derivative of vasopressin.[28,122] This agent causes release of factor VIII von Willebrand factor from storage sites into the plasma.

When given at 0.3 or 0.4 μg/kg body weight in saline and infused over 30 minutes, DDAVP corrects the bleeding time within 1 to 2 hours, and the improvement lasts up to 8 hours after the infusion. There was a further increase of factor VIII coagulant and related antigen, with a shift toward the larger factor VIII von Willebrand factor multimers. Some patients will have mild flushing or headache following the treatment,[28] but will have much less smooth muscle activity as compared to the native vasopressin. Water retention will occur. It can be reported in 36–48 hours.

III. Clinical Situations

A. Acute Renal Failure

The coagulopathies associated with acute renal failure differ slightly from those associated with chronic renal failure. Even though these differences are detectable in large groups of patients, they are not so distinctive as to preclude evaluations of individual patients.[123–126] Acute tubular necrosis is the most common cause of acute nephropathy and occurs with a variety of diseases including traumatic, surgical, infectious, cardiac, or obstetrical catastrophes. Diffuse intravascular coagulation (DIC) not infrequently complicates these catastrophes, and thus greatly complicates the coagulopathy. Moreover, the volume expanders, broad spectrum antibiotics, blood replacements, anticoagulants, etc., can add primary coagulopathies of their own.

In acute renal failure, significant bleeding is seen in about half of the patients with acute renal failure.[123] The platelet counts are low and the bleeding times are prolonged. Platelet adhesion is decreased. The whole blood clotting times and thrombin times can be prolonged in both acute and chronic failure. Factors I and VIII rise in both.[123] The plasminogen levels are normal in acute renal failure. The inhibitors of activation are elevated—more in acute than chronic failure—lowering the total fibrinolytic capacity.[123] Elevated FDPs in acute renal failure may reflect intravascular coagulation due to the primary disease.[123]

B. Amyloidosis

Amyloidosis can cause bleeding that can be life-threatening. The amyloid infiltrates blood vessel walls, causes primary coagulopathies, and causes renal failure with its associated coagulopathies. In a series of 100 patients, three patients had hematuria.[127] The most frequently encountered coagulopathy (51% of the cases) was prolongation of the thrombin time, for which there is no clear explanation.[127,128]

Purpura due to vascular fragility is seen often in patients with diffuse amyloidosis.[129] The bleeding time can be prolonged due to amyloid in the vessels of the skin. Thus, an analysis of platelet function is needed before concluding whether the problem is due to platelet defects of uremia, due to the skin defects, or both. Platelet aggregation, platelet-mediated prothrombin consumption, or platelet-mediated thromboplastin generation times may be useful in this analysis.

Amyloidosis is associated with factor X deficiency[130–143] and rarely with factor IX deficiency,[131] factor XII deficiency,[8] or intravascular coagulation.[144] Factor X appears to bind to the amyloid causing the factor deficiency.[145–147] The bleeding does not correlate well with the level of factor X in amyloidosis.[128] Infusion of factor X does not correct or only transiently corrects the lesion, presumably due to rapid binding of the molecule to the amyloid.[130,132,135,147,148] The amount of factor X found probably relates inversely to the bulk of amyloid present.[149]

The amyloid is also a cause of renal failure, with or without nephrotic syndrome. Patients may be maintained by either peritoneal dialysis or hemodialysis.[150] Transplantation has also been used successfully.[151] Alkylating agents, with or without prednisone, have been reported as useful, especially when the amyloid is associated with plasma cell dyscrasias.[152–154] Penicillamine or colchicine may also have roles.[154]

C. Cardiopulmonary Bypass Surgery in Uremic Patients

Patients with acute and chronic renal failure are often candidates for surgery, including coronary artery bypass graft surgery. These procedures require the cooperative efforts of physicians, surgeons, anesthesiologists, and the blood bank. The patients requiring heparin during cardiac bypass circulatory assistance have received various preparative techniques. Preoperative efforts should be made to reduce any fluid overload and correct electrolyte imbalances. Full heparinization has been used but preferably with as much preoperative correction of coagulopathy as possible.[155] No particular effort to correct the platelet lesions has thus far been reported. It is not clear from the literature how many of these patients have had intra- or postoperative complications due to hemorrhage. From our experience, it appears that anticoagulation with heparin is feasible in patients with renal failure without encountering exceptional hemorrhagic problems. During and following heparin therapy, the effects upon coagulation parameters should be monitored. Heparin reversal with protamine sulfate should be planned and monitored carefully.

Of importance, but yet without data available, is how to best protect the continued patency of the coronary artery vein graft or peripheral vessel grafts placed into uremic patients. The combined influences of suppressed platelet function, altered fibrinolysis, chronically elevated factor VIII ristocetin cofactor, changed lipid metabolism, and diabetes mellitus when present need to be taken into account when studying the survival of the bypass grafts. Much work needs to be performed in this area.

D. Intravascular Coagulation Involving Kidneys - DIC, TTP, and HUS

Intravascular coagulopathies and secondary fibrinolysis cause systemic and/or organ specific disease, which manifest clinically as organ failures, or hemorrhage.[82] Hemorrhage occurs following full consumption of the procoagulant materials and/or following fibrinolysis. The kidneys are commonly involved in these processes, and hematuria with or without renal failure is common. Diffuse intravascular coagulopathy (DIC), and thrombotic thrombocytopenia purpura (TTP) are examples of systemic diseases that often involve the kidneys.

Hemolytic uremic syndrome (HUS) is an organ specific disease that closely mimics TTP involving the kidneys selectively. The renal expressions of these diseases are worsened by concomitant vasoative stimuli[156–158] and angiotensin activity wherein ATN can follow the pursuant renal parenchymal anoxia.[159–163] Mesangial cells swell and vacuoles appear, while organelles and free ribosomes increase.[164] Cellular proliferation in the mesangium gives the appearance of mesangial proliferative glomerulonephritis. Glomeruli also hyalinize, [164–166] and local fibrinolysis increases.[165] The review of Kincaid-Smith describes these lesions and their experimental counterparts.[167]

DIC, which involves all phases of coagulation and fibrinolysis, can complicate already established syndromes such as sepsis, hypotension, acidosis, hyperthermia, trauma, neoplasms, progranulocytic leukemia, abruptio placenta, dead fetus syndrome, and many others. TTP, and possibly HUS, involve platelets and endothelium and are presently not explained by a single defect but may involve prostaglandin synthesis or release from the endothelial cells of platelet-agglutinating factor VIII.[168–171]

In DIC and TTP, all tissues may be involved, including skin, brain, and kidneys with hematuria. Thrombocytopenia is present. Circulating platelets are physiologically "exhausted" from having been activated and having released intracellular granules.[172–174] Platelet survival is shortened. With DIC, prothrombin fragments and fibrin monomers are in the plasma. Fibrinolysis leads to dissolution of fibrin and lysis of fibrinogen to create fibrin(ogen) degradation products.

HUS shares many microscopic characteristics with TTP, including thrombocytopenia, microangiopathic hemolytic anemia, and platelets mixed with fibrin in the small vessels of the kidneys, giving the appearance of focal glomerulonephritis.[175] The level of thrombocytopenia does not correlate well with the severity or duration of HUS. Clinically, proteinuria, hematuria, hypertension, and edema are commonly seen in HUS.[176,177] While HUS is predominantly a childhood disease, it is not uncommon among adults, especially pregnant or recently pregnant women.[177–179]

In HUS, platelet counts are low and platelet survival is shortened.[180] Platelet counts tend to return to normal if nephrectomy is performed. Systemic fibrinogen and plasminogen kinetics appear to be normal,[180–184] while glomerular fibrinolysis appears to be inhibited.[185] Many mechanisms of HUS have been suggested, but most have been called ultimately into question. Recently, defects of PGI_2 release have received the most attention.[170,172,186–189] Platelet-derived β-TG appears to suppress PGI_2 release.[190]

Therapies specific for these syndromes remain moderately controversial, while the primary therapies to support the patient's blood pressure, reverse hypotension, correct acidosis, control infection, correct metabolic abnormalities, and remove necrotic tissues are not controversial. Beyond the general supportive measures, therapy should be tailored to the situation. For example, DIC most often can be managed by replacing the missing procoagulants with FFP, cryoprecipitate, or platelets, while the underlying causative problems are controlled. If this is not successful, heparin therapy can be used.

Therapy for TTP and HUS are somewhat more controversial. Therapy for HUS and TTP is based on the presumed pathophysiology. Heparin,[187–192] platelet suppression[197–200] and plasma infusion or exchange[186,201–204] have been advocated. Splenectomy has been credited with occasional successes in TTP. Based on the current understanding of these syndromes, plasma infusion and/or exchange appear to be the most reasonable therapies. This approach either replaces, stabilizes, or provokes production of PGI_2. Antithrombin III (AT III) replacement has also been useful in treating HUS when AT III deficiency is present.[68,69] However, not many patients with HUS have AT III deficiency, especially children with epidemic form.[68]

Current investigations indicate a role for PGI_2 replacement therapy. Agents with similar activities to PGI_2 but which are more stable, such as PGE_1, are now being investigated. Drugs that enhance PGI_2 production or block its catabolism will also be available for study in these diseases.

E. Pregnancy-Associated Renal Diseases Associated with Coagulopathies

Pre-eclampsia, eclampsia, and hemolytic uremic syndrome (discussed above) are among the diseases that can complicate pregnancy and can cause simultaneous alterations of renal function and coagulation. These alterations extend from subclinical observations to lethal clinical events. Hathaway and Bonner have prepared an excellent monograph on these subjects.[205] Gibson et al. have described nicely the contribution of platelets to these events.[206]

A problem in discussing the reports on the cause(s) and treatment(s) of these syndromes is that a significant number of patients thought to have pre-eclampsia or eclampsia are found by biopsy to have other diseases.[207,208] Thus it must be kept in mind that therapeutic studies and their conclusions can be contaminated by sampling errors. However, for practical reasons the diagnosis is usually based on clinical parameters.

Many pathologic and pathophysiologic changes have been described in eclampsia and pre-eclampsia.[209] That cne or more of these changes cause the syndrome, or are a consequence of the syndrome, remains for the most part controversial. The fact that the kidney is often a target organ also is unexplained.[203,209] For the purpose of this text, coagulation is the focus of attention, but not without awareness of the roles played by genetics, immunology, and renin-aldosterone-angiotensin systems.[210]

The renal microcirculation is affected by platelets and fibrin that accumulate in the kidneys.[164,211–215] Systemic platelet counts fall inversely to rise of uric acid.[210,214] Platelet counts less than $100{,}000/mm^3$ are not uncommon.[215,216] Maternal platelet survival is shortened.[218] Antithrombin III falls paralleling the severity of the disease.[219] Some patients have suppressed fibrinolysis with loss of plasminogen.[206,220–222] Microangiopathic hemolysis is seen. The overall pattern is that of an intravascular thrombotic disease.[223] An underlying cause for these changes has been ascribed in some studies to an endothelial defect in which prostacyclin (PGI_2) production, release, or function is depressed.[168,224–230]

Based upon these findings, it is reasonable to consider treatments with anticoagulants if appropriate in the overall context of the patient's care. After supplying appropriate general medical or surgical therapies, anticoagulant can be selected based on the patient's specific coagulation defects. Any single approach will fail in a significant proportion of patients if applied to all patients without discrimination regarding the coagulatin lesion(s) present. Heparin,[231,232] aspirin,[233] PGI_2- or PGI_2-like agents,[234] AT III replacement, fibrinolytic therapy, and oral anticoagulants can be considered with due respect for the inherent risks and the individuality of each patient.[235]

F. Renal Transplant Rejection

Chapter 11 discusses surgical management of hemorrhagic lesions seen in renal transplantation. A review of the mechanism of renal rejection is beyond the intent of this text. Changes that do occur in coagulation, and which are discussed here, exist in a milieu of other immune-mediated events and should not be viewed as occurring in an isolated environment.

Intrarenal thrombosis is often involved in hyperacute and may be involved in acute or delayed-acute rejections.[236–238] Intravascular fibrin and platelet deposits are detectable, and glomeruli contain fibrin.[239–241] PMNs and endothelial necrosis appear. Fibrinogen accumulates in the kidney and can be monitored by radiolabel techniques.[242,243] Platelet survival is shortened, sometimes to the point of causing thrombocytopenia.[239,244,245] Plasma levels of platelet releasates rise[246,247] (see discussion of renal failure and the platelet releasates above). These changes can occur in well cross-matched kidneys and are ascribed to circulating antibodies.[239,240,246–249]

Blood samples taken from afferent arteries (A) and efferent veins (V) of the transplanted kidneys give clearer pictures of coagulation than can be seen after dilution in systemic blood. There are significant A-V gradients for fibrinogen, prothrombin, platelets, and factors V and VIII.[237,250,251] Fibrin-split products appear in urine.[180,252] While these changes may be mediated by the immune-mediated rejection, care must be used to exclude perfusion defects due to defective vascular anastomosis.[253–255]

These events can be treated with anticoagulants with the goal of preserving renal function. Before applying any such therapy, three elements must be correctly established by experts in renal transplantation and coagulation. First, it must be determined that the apparent rejection is not due to a perfusion deficiency. Second, it must be determined that correct immunotherapy has been applied, including appropriate immune suppressant drugs, antilymphocyte globulins, and radiotherapy. Third, it should be determined which elements of coagulation are involved in the rejection process. Selective anticoagulation therapy offers better chances for success, and less risk of complicating hemorrhage. Heparin,[256–260] platelet suppressants,[180,258,261–263] warfarin plus dipyridamole,[263] and defibrinating agents have been used.[264,265] These are areas where additional clinical investigations are needed.

G. Tendency Towards Atherosclerosis During Chronic Renal Failure

Curiously, there is a tendency for patients with chronic renal failure to acquire arterial thrombosis with atherosclerosis, despite their hemorrhagic tendencies.[120,266,267] The processes leading to accelerated atherosclerosis associated with renal failure may include the effects of hypertension, hyperlipidemia, diabetes mellitus, endothelial cell damage by uremic plasma, smooth muscle proliferation, loss of antitrypsin or alpha-2-macroglobulins, hypercalcemia of secondary hyperparathryoidism, in addition to changes of platelets, coagulation, and fibrinolysis. The magnitude of the problem is demonstrated by the fact that 20.5% of 293 deaths among 687 patients studied with chronic renal failure were due to coronary artery disease. Nondiabetics with an established history of coronary heart disease had a mortality rate of 25% per year dialysis, with over 40% of the deaths due to acute myocardial infarction.[267–270]

The factor VIII complex is elevated[268,269] in these patients (see above). Since the factor VIII-ristocetin cofactor facilitates platelet adhesion to damaged endothelial surfaces, this change may contribute to the tendency for pathological thrombosis. The released platelet-derived growth factor (PDGF) or other growth stimuli in uremic plasma can then stimulate smooth muscle proliferation.[270,271] The change in factor VIII also possibly contributes to some of the glomerular lesions.[272] Infusion of prostacyclin during hemodialysis appears to block the release of factor VIII during dialysis, in addition to protecting the platelets.[33,78]

Not all patients with renal failure have defects of platelet function. Discriminate assays in one study pointed to important variability in platelet aggregation.[273]

The AT III is the major native *in vivo* inhibitor of thrombin and patients with depressed levels of antithrombin III are at increased risk for thrombin.[57–59] Both normal and decreased levels of AT III have been described in chronic renal failure. The differences in reported levels may be based on differences in the patient populations studied or on the assays used. Some but not all patients with nephrotic syndrome have depressed AT III due to loss into the urine.[62,65] Lowered AT III in nephrotic patients parallels the fall of serum.[63] In this setting, the other inhibitors of thrombin, including α_1 antitrypsin and α_2 macroglobulin, may play important roles.[65] The AT III levels appear to improve during hemodilaysis despite the heparin, an agent that binds to and facilitates clearance of AT III. Prostacyclin infusion can also affect the AT III level during hemodialysis.[273]

References

1. Honig GR, Lindley A. Deficiency of Hageman factor (factor XII) in patients with the nephrotic syndrome. *J Pediat.* 78:633–637, 1971.
2. Green D, Arruda J, Honig G, Meuhrcke R. Urinary loss of clotting factors due to hereditary membranous glomerulonephropathy. *Am J Clin Pathol.* 65:376–383, 1976.
3. Lange LG, Carvalho A, Bagdasarian A, Lahire B, Colman RW. Activation of Hageman factor in the nephrotic syndrome. *Am J Med.* 56:565–569, 1974.
4. Hruby MA, Honig GR, Shapiro E. Immunoquantitation of Hageman factor in the urine and plasma of children with nephrotic syndrome. *J Lab Clin Med.* 96:501–510, 1980
5. Saito H, Goodnough LT, Makker SP, Kallen RJ. Urinary excretion of Hageman factor (factor XII) and presence of nonfunctional Hageman factor in the nephrotic syndrome. *Am J Med* 70:531–534, 1981.
6. Branson HE, Vaziri ND, Slater LM. Adult nephrotic syndrome and acquired coagulopathies: Hageman factor deficiency. *J Natl Med Assoc.* 74:339–343, 1982.
7. Thompson AR. Factor XII and other hemostatic protein abnormalities in nephrotic syndrome patients. *Thromb Haemost.* 48:27–32, 1982.
8. Sabatier JC, Croze M, Genin C, Gonthier R, Berthoux FC. Acquired factor XII (Hageman) deficiency associated with renal amyloidosis. *Kidney Int.* 17:705, 1980. (Abstr.)
9. Handley DA, Lawrence JR. Factor-IX deficiency in the nephrotic syndrome. *Lancet.* 1:1079–1081, 1967.
10. Vaziri ND. Nephrotic syndrome and coagulation and fibrinolytic abnormalities. *Am J Nephrol.* 3:1–6, 1983.
11. Natelson EA, Lynch EC, Hettig RA, Alfrey CP, Jr. Acquired factor IX deficiency in the nephrotic syndrome. *Ann Intern Med.* 73:373–378, 1970.
12. Koshy MC, Kashgarian M, Boreyko C. Factor IX deficiency in nephrotic syndrome. *Conn Med.* 39:472–474, 1975.

13. Rahman F, Zanger B, Natelson EA. Factor IX deficiency in the nephrotic syndrome: Studies with prothrombin complex concentrate. *J Urol.* 113:853–855, 1975.
14. Vaziri ND, Branson HE, Ness R. Change of coagulation factors IX, VIII, VII, X, and V in nephrotic syndrome. *Am J Med Sci.* 280:167–171, 1980.
15. Abildgaard CF, Penner JA, Watson-Williams ED. Anti-inhibitor coagulant complex (Autoplex) for treatment of factor VIII inhibitors in hemophilia. *Blood.* 56:978–984, 1980.
16. Hultin MB. Studies of factor IX concentrate therapy in hemophilia. *Blood.* 62:677–684, 1983.
17. Seligsohn U, Kasper CK, Osterud B, Rapaport SI. Activated factor VII presence in factor IX concentrate and persistence in circulation after infusion. *Blood.* 53: 828–837, 1979.
18. Warrell RP, Jr, Hultin MB, Coller BS. Increased factor VIII von Willebrand factor antigen and von Willebrand factor activity in renal failure. *Am J Med.* 66:226–228, 1979.
19. Ambruso DR, Durante DP, McIntosh RM, Hathaway WE. Factor VIII and renal disease. *Ann Intern Med.* 87:636–637, 1977.
20. Kazatchkie M, Sultan Y, Caen JP, Bariety J. Bleeding in renal failure: A possible cause. *Br Med J.* 2:612–615, 1976.
21. Ruggeri ZM, Ponticelli C, Mannucci PM. Factor VIII and chronic renal failure (Letter). *Br Med J.* 1:1085, 1977.
22. Bern MM, Klumpar DI, Wheeler WE, Davis GL. Factor VIII complex in chronic renal failure: Influence of protein C, fibrinolysis and diabetes mellitus. *Thromb Res.* 31:177–186, 1983.
23. Wegmuller E, Gruninger U, Furlan M, Beck EA, Hodler J, Reubi FC. Factor VIII activity in chronic renal disease. *Nephron.* 28:157–162, 1981.
24. Janson PA, Jubelirer SJ, Weinstein MS, Deykin D. Treatment of the bleeding tendency in uremia with cryoprecipitate. *N Engl J Med.* 303:1318–1322, 1980.
25. Turney JH, Woods HF, Fewell MR, Weston MJ. Factor VIII complex in uraemia and effect of haemodialysis. *Br Med J.* 282:1653–1656, 1981.
26. Shearn SA, Peake IR, Giddings JC, Humphrys J, Bloom AL. The characterization and synthesis of antigens related to factor VIII in vascular endothelium. *Thromb Res.* 11:43–56, 1977.
27. Howard MA, Whitworth JA, Hendrix LE, Thomas KB, Firkin BG, Abnormal factor VIII in chronic renal failure. *Med J Aust.* 1:148–151, 1979.
28. Winter M, Seghatehian MJ, Chauron JS. An abnromal factor VIII molecule in uraemia? *Lancet.* 1:1112, 1983.
29. Mannucci PM, Remuzzi G, Pusineri F, Lombardi R, Valsecchi C, Mecca G, Zimmerman TS. Diamino-8-D-arginine vasopressin shortens the bleeding time in uremia. *N Engl J Med.* 308:8–12, 1983.
30. Kanfer A, Kleinknecht D, Broyer M, Josso F. Coagulation studies in 45 cases of nephrotic syndrome without uremia. *Thromb Diath Haemorrh* 24:562–571, 1970.
31. Thomson C, Forbes CD, Prentice CR, Kennedy AC. Changes in blood coagulation and fibrinolysis in the nephrotic syndrome. *Q J Med.* (N.S.) 43:399–407, 1974.
32. Kendall AG, Lohmann RC, Dossetor JB. Nephrotic syndrome: A hypercoagulable state. *Arch Intern Med.* 127:1021–1027, 1971.
33. Turney JH, Williams LC, Fewell MR, Parsons V, Weston MJ. Platelet protection and heparin sparing with prostacyclin during regular dialysis therapy. *Lancet* 2:224–226, 1980.
34. Yatzides H. Richet G. Activité de certaines protienes de la coagulation dans le plasma et les urines au cours du syndrome nephrotique. *Revue Fr Etiol Clin Biol.* 2:717–727, 1957.
35. Epstein O, Bevan G, Siddiqui N, Ardeman S. Factor VII deficiency associated with nephrotic syndrome. *Br Med J.* 2:1361, 1976.
36. Schwigon CD, Barckow D. Efficacy and tolerance of cefotoxine, cefoperazone, and lamoxactam in intensive care patients. *Program and Abstracts of the Twenty-*

second Interscience Conference on Anti-microbial Agents and Chemotherapy. Oct. 1982. (Abst. 819).
37. Schentag JJ, Wels PB, Reitberg DP, Walczak P, Hawkins Van Tyle J, Lascola RJ. A randomized clinical trial of moxalactam alone versus tobramycin plus clindamycin in abdominal sepsis. *Ann Surg*. 198:35–41, 1983.
38. Natelson EA, Brown CH III, Bradshaw MW, Alfrey CP, Williams TW, Jr. Influence of cephalosporin antibiotics on blood coagulation and platelet function. *Antimicrob Agents Chemother*. 9:91–93, 1976.
39. Lerner PI, Lubin A. Coagulopathy with cefazolin in uremia (Letter). *N Engl J Med*. 290:1324, 1974.
40. Pineo GF, Gallus AS, Hirsh J. Unexpected vitamin K deficiency in hospitalized patients. *Can Med Assoc J*. 109:880–883, 1973.
41. Vaziri ND, Toohey J, Paule P, Hung E, Darwish R, Barton C, Alikhani S. Urinary excretion and deficiency of prothrombin in nephrotic syndrome. *Am J Med*. 77: 433–438, 1984.
42. Losowsky MS, Walls WD. Abnormal fibrin stabilization in renal failure. *Thromb Diath Haemorrh*. 22:216–222, 1969.
43. Klingemann H-G, Egbring R, Havemann K. Structure of fibrin and fibrin monomer in renal and hepatic failure. *Klin Wochenschr*. 58:533–535, 1980.
44. Panicuci F, Sagripanti A, Pinori E, Vispi M, Lecchini L, Barsotti G, Giovannetti S. Comprehensive study of haemostasis in chronic uremia. *Nephron*. 33:5–8, 1983.
45. Alkjaersig NK, Fletcher AP, Lewis ML, Cole BR, Ingelfinger JR, Robson AM. Pathophysiological response of the blood coagulation sysem in acute glomerulonephritis. *Kidney Int*. 10:319–328, 1976.
46. Henriksson PL, Hedner U, Nilsson IM. Factor XIII (fibrin stabilising factor) in Henock-Schonlein's purpura. *Acta Paediat Scand*. 66:273–277, 1977.
47. Yoshioka K, Miyata H, Uraoka Y, Maki S. Plasma factor XIII levels in children with renal disease. *Nephron*. 27:19–24, 1981.
48. Romo JMT, Corbacho L, Sanchez S, Rodriguez JL, Macias JF, Del Canizo C, De Castro S. Effects of carbenicillin on blood coagulation: a study in patients with chronic renal failure. *Clin Nephrol*. 11:31–34, 1979.
49. Andrassy K, Weischedel E, Ritz E, Andrassy T. Bleeding in uremic patients after carbenicillin. *Thromb Haemost*. 36:115–126, 1976.
50. Van Den Berg CJ, Pineda AA. Plasma exchange in the treatment of acute renal failure due to low molecular-weight dextran. *Mayo Clin Proc*. 55:387–389, 1980.
51. Mailloux L, Swartz CD, Capizzi R, Kim KE, Onesti G, Ramiriz O, Brest AN. Acute renal failure after administration of low-molecular-weight dextran. *N Engl J Med*. 277:1113–1118, 1967.
52. Chinitz JL, Kim DE, Onesti G, Swartz C. Patholphysiology and prevention of dextran-40-induced anuria. *J Lab Clin Med*. 77:76–87, 1971.
53. Feest TG. Low molecular weight dextran: A continuing cause of acute renal failure. *Br Med J*. 2:1300, 1976,
54. Muzaffar TZ, Stalker AL, Bryce WA, Dhall RD. Dextrans and fibrin morphology. *Nature* (London). 238:288–290, 1972.
55. Atik M. Dextran 40 and dextran 70: A review. *Arch Surg*. 94:664–672, 1967.
56. Abildgaard U, Fagerhol MK, Egeberg O. Comparison of progressive antithrombin activity and the concentrations of three thrombin inhibitors in human plasma. *Scand J Clin Lab Invest*. 26:349–354, 1970.
57. von Kaulla E, von Kaulla KN. Antithrombin 3 and diseases. *Am J Clin Pathol*. 48:69–80, 1967.
58. Jorgensen KA, Stoffersen E. Antithrombin III in Uremia. *Scand J Urol Nephrol*. 13:299–303, 1979.
59. Woods HF, Dawson A, Ash G, Weston MJ. Heparin-induced decrease in circulating antithrombin III. *Lancet*. 1:208–209, 1978.
60. Bern MM, Green J. Effect of sulfinpyrazone upon antithrombin III and platelet factor 4 in chronic renal failure. *Thromb Res*. 27:457–466, 1982.

61. Brandt P, Jespersen J, Sorenson LH. Antithrombin-III and platelets in haemodialysis patients. *Nephron.* 28:1–3, 1981.
62. Bern MM, Cavalieri BM, Lukas G. Plasma levels and effects of sulfinpyrazone in patients requiring chronic hemodialysis. *J Clin Pharmacol.* 20:107–116, 1980.
63. Kauffman RH, de Graeff J, de la Rivierie GB, van Es LA. Unilateral renal vein thrombosis and nephrotic syndrome. Report of a case with protein selectivity and antithrombin III clearance studies. *Am J Med.* 60:1048–1054, 1976.
64. Kauffman RH, Veltkamp JJ, van Tilburg NH, van Es LA. Acquired Antithrombin III deficiency and thrombosis in the nephrotic syndrome. *Am J Med.* 65:607–613, 1978.
65. Boneu B, Bouissou F, Abbal M, Sie P, Caranobe C, Barthe P. Low levels of antithrombin III and plasma antithrombin activity in nephrotic syndrome. *Kidney Int.* 22:428, 1982. (abs. 427)
66. Zazgornik J, Balcke P, Schmidt P, Kopsa H, Hysek H, Lenz K. Alpha-1-Antitrypsin und Fibrinogenspiegel bei chronischer Niereninsuffizienz und nacn Nierentransplantation. *Klin Wochenschr.* 59:1261–1265, 1981.
67. Monnens L, deJong M, van Oostrom C, van Munster P. Antithrombin III levels in children with the epidemic form of hemolytic-uremic syndrome. *Nephron.* 32: 261–262, 1982.
68. Brandt P, Jespersen J, Gregersen G. Post-partum haemolytic-uraemic syndrome treated with antithrombin-III. *Nephron.* 27:15–18, 1981.
69. Bern MM, Bothe A, Jr, Bistrian B, Batist G, Haywood E, Blackburn G. Effects of low-dose warfarin on anti-thrombin III levels in patients with morbid obesity. *Surgery* 94:78–83, 1983.
70. Shapiro S, Thiagarajan P, DeMarco L. Mechanism of action of the lupus anticoagulant. *Ann NY Acad Sci.* 370:359–365a, 1981.
71. Marlar RA, Kleiss AJ, Griffin JH. Mechanism of action of human activated protein C, a thrombin-dependent anticoagulant enzyme. *Blood.* 59:1067–1072, 1982.
72. Comp PC, Jacocks RM, Ferrell GL, Esmon CT. Activation of protein C in vivo. *J Clin Invest.* 70:127–134, 1982.
73. Ma KW, Brown DC, Masler DS, Silvis SE. Effects of renal failure on blood levels of cimetidine. *Gastroenterology.* 74:473–477, 1978.
74. MacKenzie JC, Ford JE, Waters AH, Harding N, Cattell WR, Anderson BB. Erythropoiesis in patients undergoing regular dialysis treatment (RDT) without transfusion. In: *European Dialysis and Transplant Assoc. Dialysis and Renal Transplantation:* Proc. of the Fifth Annual Conferences, Dublin, Ireland, June 1968. Kerr DNS, Ed. Excerpta Medica, International Congress Series #179. Proc. 5:172–178, 1968.
75. Hampers CL, Streiff R, Nathan DG, Snyder DS, Merrill JP. Megaloblastic hematopoiesis in uremia and in patients on long-term hemodialysis. *N Engl J Med.* 276:551–554, 1967.
76. Andersen KEH. Folic acid status of patients with chronic renal failure maintained by dialysis. *Clin Nephrol.* 8:510–513, 1977.
77. Ylikorkala O, Huttunen K, Jarvi J, Biinikka L. Prostacyclin and thromboxane in chronic uremia: Effect of hemodialysis. *Clin Nephrol.* 18:83–87, 1982.
78. Rozenberg MC, Stewart JH. The bleeding disorder of uraemia: A qualitative platelet defect. *Lancet.* 2:66–69, 1966.
79. Horowitz HI, Stein IM, Cohen BD, White JG. Further studies on the platelet-inhibitory effect of guanidinosuccinic acid and its role in uremic bleedings. *Am J Med.* 49:336–345, 1970.
80. Nenci GG, Berrettini M, Agnelli G, Parise P, Buoncristiani U, Ballatori E. Effect of peritoneal dialysis, hemodialysis and kidney transplantation on blood platelet function. I. Platelet aggregation by ADP and epinephrine. *Nephron.* 23:287–292, 1979.
81. Bemis J, Rigney J, Sosin A, Deane N. Enhanced platelet aggregation in chronic renal failure patients receiving hemodialysis treatment. *Trans Am Soc Artif Int Org.* 23:48–52, 1977.

82. Lindsay RM, Clark WF. Platelet destruction in renal disease. *Semin Thromb Hemost.* 8:138–155, 1982.
83. Rabiner SF, Hrodek O. Platelet factor 3 in normal subjects and patients with renal failure. *J Clin Invest.* 47:901–912, 1968.
84. Eknoyan G, Wacksman SJ, Glueck HI, Will J. Platelet function in renal failure. *N Engl J Med.* 280:677–681, 1969.
85. Castaldi PA, Rozenberg MC, Stewart JH. The bleeding disorders of uremia: A qualitative platelet defect. *Lancet.* 2:66–69, 1966.
86. Eknoyan G, Brown CH III. Biochemical abnormalities of platelets in renal failure: Evidence for decreased platelet serotonin, adenosine diphosphate and MG-dependent adenosine triphosphatase. *Am J Nephrol.* 1:17–23, 1981.
87. Remuzzi G, Livio M, Marchiaro G, Mecca G, de Gaetano G. Bleeding in renal failure: Altered platelet function in chronic uremia only partially corrected by haemodialysis. *Nephron.* 22:347–353, 1978.
88. Linné T. Prolonged bleeding time in non-uremic acute glomerulonephritis. *Thromb Haemost.* 42:1060–1061, 1979.
89. Steiner RW, Coggins C, Carvalho ACA. Bleeding time in uremia: A useful test to assess clinical bleeding. *Am J Hematol.* 7:107–117, 1979.
90. Remuzzi G, Benigni A, Dodesini P, Schieppati A, Gotti E, Livio M, Mecca G, Donati B, deGaetano G. Platelet function in patients on maintenance hemodialysis: Depressed or enhanced? *Clin Nephrol.* 17:60–63, 1982.
91. Salzman EW, Neri LL, Adhesiveness of blood platelets in uremia. *Thromb Diath Hemorrh.* 15:84–92, 1966.
92. Stewart JH, Castaldi PA. Uremic bleeding: A reversible platelet defect corrected by dialysis. *Q J Med.* 36:409–423, 1967.
93. Lusvarghi E, Curci G, Sacchi S, Baraldi P, Baraldi A, Cappelli G, Landini S, Malmusi G, Orlandini G, Savazzi AM, Vandelli L, Quaglino D. Evaluation of platelet kinetics in chronic renal failure (conservative and regular dialysis treatment). *Haematologica.* 64:747–758, 1979.
94. Levin RD, Kwaan HC, Ivanovich P. Changes in platelet function during hemodialysis. *J Lab Clin Med.* 92:779–786, 1978.
95. Lindsay RM, Prentice CRM, Davidson JF, Burton JA, McNicol GP. Haemostatic changes during dialysis associated with thrombus formation on dialysis membranes. *Br Med J.* 4:454–458, 1972.
96. Stewart JH, Farrell PC, Dixon M. Reduction of platelet/fibrin deposition in hemodialysis by aspirin administration. *Aust NZ J Med.* 5:117–122, 1975.
97. Farrell PC, Eschbach JW, Vizzo JE, Babb AL. Hemodialyzer reuse: Estimation of area loss from clearance data. *Kidney Int.* 5:446–450, 1974.
98. Bischel MD, Orrell FL, Scoles BG, Mohler JG, Barbour BH. Effects of microemboli blood filtration during hemodialysis. *Trans Am Soc Artif Int Org.* 19:492–497, 1973.
99. Knostering H, Girndt J, Matthaei D, Naidu R, Quellhorst E. Alterations of clotting factors and platelets during hemofiltration. *J Dialysis.* 1:607–617, 1977.
100. Kamoun P, Kleinknecht D, Ducrot H, Jerome. Platelet-serotonin in uraemia. *Lancet.* 1:782, 1970.
101. Vlachoyannis J, Schoeppe W. Adenylate cyclase activity and c-AMP content of human platelets in uremia. *Eur J Clin Invest.* 12:379–381, 1982.
102. Saito H, Ratnoff OD, Donaldson VH. Defective activation of clotting, fibrinolytic, and permeability-enhancing systems in human Fletcher trait plasma. *Circ. Res.* 34:641–651, 1974.
103. Stein IM, Cohen BD, Kornhauser RS. Guanidinosuccinic acid in renal failure, Experimental Azotemia, and Inborn Errors of the Urea Cycle. *N Engl J Med.* 280:926–930, 1969.
104. Rabiner SF, Monlinas F. The role of phenol and phenolic acids on the thrombocytopathy and defective platelet aggregation of patients with renal failure. *Am J Med.* 49:346–351, 1970.

105. Horwitz HI, Cohen BD, Martinez D, Papayoanou MF. Defective ADP-induced platelet factor 3 activation in uremia. *Blood.* 30:331–340, 1967.
106. Wathen R, Smith M, Keshaviah P, Covity C, Shapiro F. Depressed *in vitro* aggregation of platelets of chronic hemodialysis patients (CHDP): a role for cyclic AMP. *Trans Am Soc Artif Int Org.* 21:320–328, 1975.
107. Furst P, Bergstrom J. Uremic toxins with special regard to middle molecules and their effect on hematopoiesis and platelet function. In: *Niere Blutgerinnung Haemostase Hamb Symposium 21.* Stuttgart, Germany, Schattauer, 1978.
108. Gallice P, Fournier N, Crevat A, Saingra S, Frayssinete R, Murisaco A, Sicardi F. In vitro inhibition of platelet aggregation by uremic middle molecules. *Biomedicine.* 33:185–188, 1980.
109. Rabiner SF. The effect of dialysis on platelet function of patients with renal failure. *Ann NY Acad Sci.* 201:234–242, 1972.
110. Green D, Santhanam S, Krumlovsky FA, del Greco F. Elevated beta-thromboglobulin in patients with chronic renal failure: effect of hemodialysis. *J Lab Clin Med.* 95:679–685, 1980.
111. Woods HF, Ash G, Parsons V, Weston MJ. Reduction of dialyzer fibrin deposition with sulphinpyrazone. *Clin Nephrol.* 12:122–126, 1979.
112. Woods HF, Ash G, Weston MJ, Bunting S, Moncada S, Vane JR. Prostacyclin can replace heparin in haemodialysis in dogs. *Lancet* 2:1075–1077, 1979.
113. Lindsay RM, Prentice CRM, Ferguson D, Burton JA, McNicol GP. Reduction of thrombus formation on dialyzer membranes by aspirin and RA 233. *Lancet.* 2: 1287–1290, 1972.
114. Guzzo J, Niewwiarowski S, Musial J, Bastl C, Grossman RA, Rao A, Berman I, Paul D. Secreted platelet proteins with antiheparin and mitogenic activities in chronic renal failure. *J Lab Clin Med.* 96:102–113, 1980.
115. Adrassy K, Deppermann D, Ritz E, Koderisch J, Seelig H. Different effects of renal failure on beta-thromboglobulin and high affinity platelet factor 4 (HA-PF4)-concentrations. *Thromb Res.* 18:469–475, 1980.
116. Depperman D, Andrassy K, Seelig H, Ritz E, Post D. Beta-thromboglobulin is elevated in renal failure without thrombosis. *Thromb Res.* 17:63–69, 1980.
117. Kurihara Y, Nakayama H, Nakagawa S. Plasma β-thromboglobulin and platelet factor 4 in renal insufficiency. *Thromb Res.* 18:557–560, 1980.
118. Endo Y, Mamiya S, Satoh M, Takahashi K, Harada T. Plasma β-thromboglobulin and platelet factor 4 in patients with chronic renal failure and effect of hemodialysis. *Tokyo J Exp Med* 135:349–358, 1981.
119. Lindsay RM, Friesen M, Koens F, Linton AL, Oriopoulos D, DeViber G. Platelet function in patients on long-term peritoneal dialysis. *Clin Nephrol.* 6:335–339, 1976.
120. Lindner A, Charra B, Sherrard DJ, Scribner BH. Accelerated atherosclerosis in prolonged maintenance hemodialysis. *N Engl J Med.* 290:697–701, 1974.
121. Janson PA, Jubelirer SJ, Weinstein MJ, Deykin D. Treatment of the bleeding tendency in uremia with cryoprecipitate. *N Engl J Med.* 303:1318–1322, 1981.
122. Watson AJS, Keogh JAB. Effect of 1-diamino-8-argenine vasopressin on the prolonged bleeding time in chronic renal failure. *Nephron.* 32:49–52, 1982.
123. Larsson SO, Hedner U, Nilsson IM. On coagulation and fibrinolysis in acute renal insufficiency. *Acta Med Scand.* 189:443–451, 1971.
124. Donner L, Neuwirtova R. The hemostatic defect of acute and chronic uremia. *Thromb Diath Haemorrh.* 5:319–328, 1961.
125. Kendall AG, Lowenstein L, Morgen RO. The hemorrhagic diathesis in renal disease (with special reference to acute uremia). *Can Med Assoc J.* 85:405–411, 1961.
126. Wardie EN, Taylor G. Fibrin breakdown products and fibrinolysis in renal disease. *J Clin Pathol.* 21:140–146, 1968.
127. Yood RA, Skinner M, Rubinow A, Talarico L, Cohen AS. Bleeding manifestations in 100 patients with amyloidosis. *JAMA.* 249:1322–1324, 1983.

128. Greipp PR, Kyle RA, Bowie EJW. Factor-X deficiency in amyloidosis: A critical review. *Am J Hematol.* 11:443–450, 1981.
129. Kyle RA, Bayrd ED. Amyloidosis: Review of 236 cases. *Medicine* (Baltimore). 54:271–299, 1975.
130. Korsan-Bengtsen K, Hjort PF, Ygge S. Acquired factor X deficiency in a patient with amyloidosis. *Thromb Diath Haemorrh.* 7:558–566, 1962.
131. McPherson RA, Onstad JW, Ugoretz RJ, Wolf PL. Coagulopathy in amyloidosis: Combined deficiency of factors IX and X. *Am J Hematol.* 3:225–235, 1977.
132. Menache D, Boivin P. Deficit acquis en facteu X chez un malade atteint d'amylose primitive: Injection d'une fraction C.S.B. *Nouv Rev Fr Hematol.* 2:868–887, 1962.
133. Cordonnier D, Puglisi JC, Shaerer R, Kolodie L, Debru JL. Syndrome nephrotique et deficit acquis de en facteur Stuart revelateurs de l'association amylose-myelome. *J Urol Nephrol* (Paris). 78:760–764, 1972.
134. Jacobson RJ, Sandler SG, Roth CE. Systemic amyloidosis associated with microangiopathic haemolytic anaemia and factor X (Stuart factor) deficiency. *S Afr Med J.* 46:1634–1637, 1972.
135. Maroy B, Mottier D, Saleun JP, Bergeret G. Deficit acquis en facteur X associe' a une amyloidose: Un cas. *Nouv Presse Med.* 7:3441–3442, 1978.
136. Andre R, Duhamel G, Bergoz D, Rochant H. Syndrome hemorrigique par deficit acquis en facteur Stuart-Prower. Amylose. Maladie de Waldenstrom. *Bull Soc Med Hop Paris.* 117:41–48, 1966.
137. Josso F, Boussen M, Prou-Wartelle O, Piguet H. Sultan Y, Bousser J. Anomalies complexes de la coagulation dans deux cas de maladie de Kahler avec syndrome hemorrhagique. Signification due deficit en facteur Stuart au cours du myelome. *Nour Rev Fr Hematol.* 6:739–744, 1966.
138. Galbraith PA, Sharma N, Parker WL, Kilgour JM. Acquired factor X deficiency: Altered plasma antithrombin activity and association with amyloidosis. *JAMA* 230:1658–1660, 1974.
139. Krause JR. Acquired factor X deficiency and amyloidosis. *Am J Clin Pathol.* 67:170–173, 1977.
140. Wick A, Sulser H, Pflugshaupt R. Erworbener isolierter Faktor-X-defect bei generalisierter Amyloidose. *Schweiz Med Wochenschr.* 102:1799–1803, 1972.
141. Howell M. Acquired factor X deficiency associated with systematized amyloidosis: A report of a case. *Blood.* 21:739–744, 1963.
142. Pechet L, Kastrul JJ. Amyloidosis associated with factor X (Stuart) deficiency case report. *Ann Intern Med.* 61:315–318, 1964.
143. Bernhardt B, Valletta M, Brook J, Lejnieks I. Amyloidosis with factor X deficiency. *Am J Med Sci.* 264:411–414, 1972.
144. Bowie EJW, Maldonado JE, Brown AL, Didisheim P, Owen CA, Jr. Intravascular coagulation in systemic amyloidosis. *Thromb Diath Haemorrh.* (Suppl) 36:305–312, 1969.
145. Fishleder A, Cavalier D, Lucas F, Tubbs R, Bukowski R, Triplett D. Pathogenesis of acquired factor X deficiency in primary amyloidosis. *Clin Res.* 28:728A; 1980. (Abstr.)
146. Fair DS, Plow EF, Edgington TS. Combined functional and immunochemical analysis of normal and abnormal human factor X. *J Clin Invest.* 64:884–894, 1979.
147. Furie B, Greene E, Furie BC. Syndrome of acquired factor X deficiency and systemic amyloidosis. In vivo studies of the metabolic rate of factor X. *N Engl J Med.* 297:81–85, 1977.
148. Spero JA, Lewis JH, Hasiba U, Ellis LD. Treatment of amyloidosis associated factor X deficiency. *Thromb Haemost.* 35:377, 1976.
149. Zeitler KD, Blatt PM. Amyloidosis and factor X deficiency. *South Med J.* 75:306–308, 1982.
150. Stone WJ, Latos DL, Lankford PG, Baker AS. Chronic peritoneal dialysis in a patient with primary amyloidosis, renal failure, and factor X deficiency. *South Med. J.* 71:764–767, 1978.

151. Jacob ET, Bar-Nathan N, Shapira Z, Gafni J. Renal transplantation in the amyloidosis of familial mediterranean fever. *Arch Intern Med.* 139:1135–1138, 1979.
152. Kyle RA, Greipp PR. Primary systemic amyloidosis: Comparison of melphalan and prednisone versus placebo. *Blood.* 52:818–827, 1978.
153. Cohen HJ, Lessin LS, Hallal J, Burkholder P. Resolution of primary amyloidosis during chemotherapy. Studies on a patient with nephrotic syndrome. *Ann Intern Med.* 82:466–473, 1975.
154. Corkery J, Bern MM, Tullis JL. Resolution of amyloidosis and plasma-cell dyscrasia with combination chemotherapy, (Letter). *Lancet.* 2:425–426, 1978.
155. Connors JP, Shaw RC. Considerations in the management of open-heart surgery in uremic patients. *J Thorac Cardiovasc Surg.* 75:400–404, 1978.
156. Whitaker AN, McKay DG, Csavossy I. Studies of catecholamine shock. I. Disseminated intravascular coagulation. *Am J Pathol.* 56:153–176, 1969.
157. Grandchamp A, Ayer G, Truniger B. Pathogenisis of redistribution of intrarenal blood flow in haemorrhagic hypotension. *Eur J Clin Invest.* 1:271–276, 1971.
158. Spink WW, Reddin J, Zak SJ, Peterson M, Starzecki B, Seljeskog E. Correlation of plasma catecholamine levels with hemodynamic changes in canine endotoxin shock. *J Clin Invest.* 45:78–85, 1966.
159. Gavras H, Brown JJ, Lever AF, Macadam RF, Robertson JIS. Acute renal failure, tubular necrosis, and myocardial infarction induced in the rabbit by intravenous angiotensin II. *Lancet.* 2:19–22, 1971.
160. Grandchamp A, Veyrat R, Rosset E, Sherrer JR, Truniger B. Relationship between renin and intrarenal hemodynamics in hemorrhagic hypotension. *J Clin Invest.* 50:970–978, 1971.
161. Brown JJ, Gleadle RI, Lawson DW, Lever AF, Linton AL, Macadam RF, Prentice E, Robertson JIS, Tree M. Renin and acute renal failure: Studies in Man. *Br Med J.* 1:253–258, 1970.
162. Koffler D, Paronetto F. Fibrinogen deposition in acute renal failure. *Am J Pathol.* 49:383–391, 1966.
163. Clardson AR, MacDonald MK, Fuster V, Cash JD, Robson JS. Glomerular coagulation in acute ischaemic renal failure. *Q J Med.* 39:585–599, 1970.
164. Vassalli P, Simon G, Rouiller C. Electron microscopic study of glomerular lesions resulting from intravascular fibrin formation. *Am J Pathol.* 43:579–617, 1963.
165. Humair L, Potter EV, Kwaan HC. The role of fibrinogen in renal disease. I. Production of experimental lesions in mice. *J Lab Clin Med* 74:60–71, 1969.
166. Kincaid-Smith P. The role of coagulation in the obliteration of glomerular capillaries. In: *Glomerulonephritis.* Kincaid-Smith P, Mathew TH, Becker EL, Eds. New York, John Wiley and Sons.
167. Kincaid-Smith P. Coagulation and renal disease. *Kidney Int.* 2:183–190, 1972.
168. Remuzzi G, Marchesi D, Mecca G, Misiani R, Livios M, de Gaetano G. Haemolytic-uremic syndrome: Deficiency of plasma factor(s) regulating prostacyclin activity? *Lancet.* 2:871–872, 1978.
169. Grunfeld JP, Ganeval D, Bournerias F. Acute renal failure in pregnancy. *Kidney Int.* 18:179–191, 1980.
170. Hensby CN, Lewis PJ, Higard P, Mufti GJ, Hows J, Webster J. Prostacyclin deficiency in thrombotic thrombocytopenia purpura (Letter). *Lancet.* 2:748, 1979.
171. Kelton JG, Moore J, Santos A, Sheridan D. Detection of a platelet-agglutinating factor in thrombotic thrombocytopenic purpura. *Ann Intern Med.* 101:589–593, 1984.
172. Fong JS, Kaplan BS. Impairment of platelet aggregation in hemolytic uremic syndrome: Evidence for platelet "exhaustion." *Blood.* 60:564–570, 1982.
173. Parbtani A, Cameron JS. Platelet and plasma serotonin concentrations in glomerulonephritis I. *Thromb Res.* 15:109–125, 1979.
174. Pareti FI, Capitanio A, Mannucci L, Ponticelli C, Mannucci PM. Acquired dysfunction due to the circulation of "exhausted" platelets. *Am J Med.* 69:235–240, 1980.
175. Gianantonio C, Vitacco M. Mendilaharzu F, Rutty A, Mendilaharzu J. The hemolytic-uremic syndrome. *J Pediatr.* 64:478–491, 1964.

176. Montgomery RR, Hathaway WE. The Hemolytic-uremic syndrome. In: *Kidney Disease, Hematologic and Vascular Problems.* McIntosh RE, Guggenheim SJ, Schrier RW, Eds. New York, John Wiley and Sons, 1977, p. 89.
177. de Chadarevian JP, Kaplan BS. The hemolytic uremic syndrome of childhood. In: *Perspectives in Pediatric Pathology*, Vol. 4, Rosenberg HS, Bolande RP, Eds. Chicago, Year Book Medical, 1978, pp. 465–502.
178. Calvert GD. Postpartum haemolytic uraemic syndrome: Case report and brief review. *J Obstet Gynaecol Br Commonw.* 79:244–249, 1972.
179. Gianantonio CA, Vitacco M, Mendilaharzu F, Gallo GE, Sojo ET. The haemolytic-uremic syndrome. *Nephron.* 11:174–192, 1973.
180. George CRP, Slichter SJ, Quadracci LJ, Striker GE, Harker LA. A kinetic evaluation of hemostasis in renal disease. *N Engl J Med.* 291:1111–1115, 1974.
181. Avalos JS, Vitacco M. Molinas F, Penalver J. Gianantonio C. Coagulation studies in the hemolytic-uremic syndrome. *J Pediatr.* 76:538–548, 1970.
182. Katz J, Lurie A, Kaplan BS, Krawitz S, Metz J. Coagulation findings in the hemolytic-uremic syndrome of infancy: Similarity to hyperacute renal allograft rejection. *J Pediatr.* 78:426–434, 1971.
183. Harker LA, Slichter SJ. Platelet and fibrinogen consumption in man. *N Engl J. Med.* 287:999–1005, 1972.
184. Katz J, Krawitz S, Sacks PV, Levin SE, Thompson P, Levin J, Metz J. Platelet, erythrocyte, and fibrinogen kinetics in the hemolytic-uremic syndrome of infancy. *J Pediatr.* 83:739–748, 1973.
185. Bergstein JM, Kuederli U, Bang NU. Plasma inhibitor of glomererular fibrinolysis in the hemolytic-uremic syndrome. *Am J Med.* 73:322–327, 1982.
186. Remuzzi G, Misiani R, Marchesi D, Livio M, Mecca G, de Gaetano G, Donati MB. Treatment of the hemolytic uremic syndrome with plasma. *Clin Nephrol.* 12: 279–284, 1979.
187. Remuzzi G, Marchesi D, Mecca G, Misiani R, Livio M, de Gaetano G, Donati MB. Haemolytic-uraemic syndrome: Deficiency of plasma factor(s) regulating prostacyclin activity? *Lancet.* 2:871–872, 1978.
188. Webster J, Rees AJ, Lewis PJ, Hensby CN. Prostacyclin deficiency in haemolytic-uraemic syndrome (Letter). *Br Med J.* 281:271, 1980.
189. Brain MC, Dacie JV, Hourihane DOB. Microangiopathic haemolytic anaemia: The possible role of vascular lesions in pathogenesis. *Br J Haematol.* 8:358–374, 1962.
190. Hope W, Martin TJ, Chesterman CN, Morgan FJ. Human B-thromboglobulin inhibits PGI_2 production and binds to a specific site in bovine aortic endothelial cells. *Nature.* 282:210–212, 1979.
191. Kaplan BS, Thompson PD. Heparin for the hemolytic uremic syndrome. *N Engl J Med.* 294:846, 1976.
192. Hall GH, Caldwell RA, Shaldon C, Bisson PG. Heparin-treated haemolytic-uraemic syndrome simulating Fabry's disease. *Br Med J.* 2:317–318, 1971.
193. Proesmans W, Eeckels R. Has heparin changed the prognosis of the hemolytic-uremic syndrome. *Clin Nephrol.* 2:169–173, 1974.
194. Tune BM, Leavett TJ, Gribble TJ. The hemolytic uremic syndrome in California: A review of 28 nonheparinized cases with long-term follow-up. *J Pediatr.* 82:304–310, 1973.
195. Vitacco M, Sanchez Avalos J, Gianantonio CA. Heparin therapy in the hemolytic-uremic syndrome. *J Pediatr.* 83:271–275, 1973.
196. Myers TJ, Wakem CJ, Ball ED, Tremont SJ. Thrombotic thrombocytopenic purpura: Combined treatment with plasmapheresis and antiplatelet agents. *Ann Intern Med.* 92:149–155, 1980.
197. Thorsen CA, Rossi EC, Green D, Carone FA. The treatment of the hemolytic-uremic syndrome with inhibitors of platelet function. *Am J Med.* 66:711–716, 1979.
198. Amorosi EL, Karpatkin S. Antiplatelet treatment of thrombotic thrombocytopenia purpura. *Ann Intern Med.* 86:102–106, 1977.

199. Arenson EB, Jr, August CS. Preliminary report: treatment of the hemolytic-uremic syndrome with aspirin and dipyridamole. *J Pediatr.* 86:957–961, 1975.
200. Eckel RH, Crowell EB, Waterhouse BE, Bozdech MJ. Platelet-inhibiting drugs in thrombotic thrombocytopenia purpura. *Arch Intern Med.* 137:735–737, 1977.
201. Harden LB, Gluck RS, Salcedo JR. Simultaneous haemodialysis and exchange transfusion in hemolytic uremic syndrome. *Clin Pediatr.* 19:640–642, 1977.
202. Pisciotta AV, Garthwaite T, Darin J, Aster RH. Treatment of thrombotic thrombocytopenia purpura by exchange transfusion. *Am J Hematol.* 3:73–82, 1977.
203. Byrnes JJ, Khurana M. Treatment of thrombotic thrombocytopenic purpura with plasma. *N Engl J Med.* 297:1386–1389, 1977.
204. Gordon BR, Saal SD. Post-partum hemolytic uremic syndrome: Treatment with plasma exchange. *Clin Exper Dialysis Apheresis.* 7:169–176, 1983.
205. Hathaway WM, Bonner J, In: *Perinatal Coagulation.* Monographs in Neonatology. New York, Grune and Stratton, 1978.
206. Gibson B, Hunter D, Neame PB, Kelton JG. Thrombocytopenia in preeclampsia and eclampsia. *Semin Thromb Hemost.* 3:234–247, 1982.
207. Lindheimer MD, Fisher KA, Spargo BH, Katz AI. Hypertension in pregnancy: A biopsy study with long-term follow-up. *Contrib. Nephrol.* 25:71–77, 1981.
208. Lindheimer MD, Katz AI. Pathophysiology of preeclampsia. *Ann Rev Med.* 32: 273–289, 1981.
209. Burden RP, Boyd WN, Ober GM. Structural and functional changes in renal circulation after complicated pregnancy. *Nephron.* 24:183–192, 1979.
210. Bonnar J, Redman CW, Denson KW. The role of coagulation and fibrinolysis in preeclampsia. *Perspect Nephrol Hypertension.* 5:85–93, 1976.
211. Kincaid-Smith P. The similarity of lesions and underlying mechanism in preeclamptic toxaemia and post-partum renal failure. Studies in the acute stage and during follow-up. In: *Glomerulonephritis.* Proc. Int. Symp. part 2. Kincaid-Smith P, Mathew TH, Becker EL, Eds. New York, John Wiley and Sons, 1973, pp. 1013–1026.
212. Al-Khader AA, Stewart C, Aber GM. Pregnancy-associated disease of the renal microcirculation. *Clin Sci.* 56:189–192, 1979.
213. McKillop CA, Howie PW, Forbes CD, Prentice CRM. Sequential studies in preeclampsia using plasma fibrinogen chromatography. *Br J Obstet Gynecol.* 84:909–918, 1977.
214. Redman CW, Bonnar J, Beilin L. Early platelet consumption in pre-eclampsia. *Br Med J.* 1:467–469, 1978.
215. Vassalli P, Morris RH, McCluskey RT. The pathogenic role of fibrin deposition in the glomerular lesions of toxemia of pregnancy. *J Exp Med.* 118:467–478, 1963.
216. Giles C. Inglis TCM. Thrombocytopenia and macrothrombocytosis in gestational hypertension. *Br J Obstet Gynecol.* 88:1115–1119, 1981.
217. Kleckner HB, Giles HR, Corrigan JS. The association of maternal and neonatal thrombocytopenia in high-risk pregnancies. *Am J Obstet Gynecol.* 128:235–238, 1977.
218. Rakoczi I, Tallian F, Bagdany S, Gati I. Platelet life-span in normal pregnancy and preeclampsia as determined by a nonradioisotope technique. *Thromb Res.* 15: 553–556, 1979.
219. Weiner CP, Brandt J. Plasma antithrombin III activity: An aid in the diagnosis of preeclampsia-eclampsia. *Am J Obstet Gynecol.* 142:275–281, 1982.
220. Astedt B. On Fibrinolysis. A. In pregnancy, labour, puerperium and during treatment with sex hormones. B. In human ontogenesis and in human organ culture. *Acta Obstet Gynecol Scand* 51(Suppl). 18:1–45, 1972.
221. Bonnar J, McNicol GP, Douglas AS. Fibrinolytic enzyme system and pregnancy. *Br Med J.* 3:387–389, 1969.
222. Wardle EN, Menon ES. Fibrinolysis and pre-eclamptic toxaemia of pregnancy. *Br Med J.* 2:625–627, 1969.
223. Kleiner GJ, Greston WM. Current concepts of defibrination in the pregnant woman. *J Reprod Med.* 17:309–317, 1976.

224. Brussolino F, Benedetto C. Massobrio M, Camussi G. Maternal vascular prostacyclin activity in pre-eclampsia (Letter). *Lancet.* 2:702, 1980.
225. Demers LM, Gabbe SG. Placental prostaglandin levels in pre-eclampsia. *Am J Obstet Gynecol.* 126:137–139, 1976.
226. Lewis PJ, Boylan P, Friedman LA, Hensby CN, Downing I. Prostacyclin in pregnancy. *Br Med J.* 280:1581–1582, 1980.
227. Lewis PJ, Shepherd GL, Ritter J, Chan SM, Bolton PJ, Jogee M, Myatt L, Elder MG. Prostacyclin and pre-eclampsia (Letter). *Lancet.* 1:559, 1981.
228. Remuzzi G, Marchesi D, Zoja C, Muratore D, Mecca G, Misiani R, Rossi E, Barbatao M, Capetta P, Donati MB, de Gaetano G. Reduced umbilical and placental vascular prostacyclin in severe pre-eclampsia. *Prostaglandins.* 20:105–110, 1980.
229. Downing I, Shepherd GL, Lewis PJ. Reduced prostacyclin production in preeclampsia (Letter). *Lancet.* 2:1374, 1980.
230. Carreras LO, Defreyn G, van Houte E, Vermylen J, van Assche A. Prostacyclin and pre-eclampsia (Letter). *Lancet.* 1:442, 1981.
231. Brain MC, Kauph K-B, Dixon HG. Heparin treatment of haemolysis and thrombocytopenia in pre-eclampsia. *J Obstet Gynaecol Br Commonw.* 74:702–711, 1967.
232. Fairley KF, Adey FD, Ross IC, Kincaid-Smith P. Heparin treatment in severe preeclampsia and glomerulonephritis in pregnancy. *Perspect Nephrol Hypertension* 5:103–112, 1976.
233. Goodlin RC, Haesslein HO, Flemming J. Aspirin for the treatment of recurrent toxemia (Letter). *Lancet.* 2:51, 1978.
234. Fidler J, Bennett MJ, deSwiet M, Ellis C, Lewis PJ. Treatment of pregnancy hypertension with prostacyclin (Letter). *Lancet.* 2:31–32, 1980.
235. Pauli RM, Hall JG, Wilson KM. Risks of anticoagulation during pregnancy. *Am Heart J.* 100:761–762, 1980.
236. Rosenberg JC, Broersma RJ, Bullemur G, Mammen EF, Linagham R, Rosenberg BF. Relationship of platelets, blood coagulation, and fibrinolysis to hyperacute rejection of renal xenografts. *Transplantation.* 8:152–161, 1969.
237. von Kaulla KN. *Coagulation Problems in Transplanted Organs.* Charles C. Thomas, Springfield, 1972.
238. Starzl TE, Boehmig HJ, Amemiya H, Wilson CB, Dixon FT, Giles GR, Simpson KM, Holgrimson CG. Clotting changes, including disseminated intravascular coagulation, during rapid renal-hemograft rejection. *N Engl J Med.* 283:383-390, 1970.
239. Busch GJ, Braun WE, Carpenter CB, Carson JM, Galvaneck ER, Reynolds ES, Merrill JB, Dammin GJ. Intrarenal vascular coagulation (IVC) in human renal allograft rejection. *Trans Proc.* 1:267–270, 1969.
240. Kincaid-Smith P. The pathogenesis of the vascular and glomerular lesions for rejection in renal allografts and their modification by antithrombotic and anticoagulant drugs. *Aust Ann Med.* 19:201–214, 1970.
241. Mowbray JF, Pariyananda A. Platelet thrombi in rejection of renal allografts. *Thromb. Diath Haemorrh.* (Suppl) 45:183–190, 1971.
242. Salaman JR. A technique for detecting rejection episodes in human transplant recipients using radioactive fibrinogen. *Br J Surg.* 59:138–142, 1972.
243. Straub PW. Labelled fibrinogen in renal transplantation (Letter). *Br Med J.* 4: 746–747, 1970.
244. Landis F, von Felten A, Berchtold H. Thrombocytopenic episodes in patients with well-functioning renal allografts. *Acta Haematol.* 61:2–9, 1979.
245. Mobray JF. Methods of suppression of immune responses: Integration in internal medicine. In: *Proc. 9th International Congress of Medicine.* Dunning AJ, Ed. Amsterdam, Excerpta Medica, 137:106–110, 1967.
246. Kissmeyer-Nielson F, Olsen S, Peterson VP, Fjeldborg O. Hyperacute rejection of kidney allografts, associated with pre-existing antibodies against donor cells. *Lancet.* 2:662–665, 1966.
247. Kanfer A, Delarue F, Languille T. Transient platelet factor 3 activation during human renal allograft rejection. *Transplantation.* 18:78–81, 1974.

248. Colberg JE, McGrath P, Cress H, Lempert N, Eckert C. The crossmatch profile and other extended crossmatch methods in clinical transplantation. *Arch Surg*. 104: 237–241, 1972.
249. Patel R, Terasaki PI. Significance of the positive crossmatch test in kidney transplantation. *N Engl J Med*. 280:735–739, 1969.
250. Pultavituma A, Azcarate J, Mammen EF, Rosenberg B, Rosenberg JC. Coagulation and platelet changes in rejected renal allografts. *Arch Surg*. 105:255—259, 1972.
251. Claes G. Studies on platelets and fibrin during rejection of canine renal allografts. *Scand J Urol Nephrol*. (Suppl) 10:1–24, 1972.
252. Clarkson AR, MacDonald MK, Petrie JJB, Cash JD, Robson JS. Serum and urinary fibrin/fbrinogen degradation products in glomerulonephritis. *Br Med J*. 3:447–451, 1971.
253. Curtis JJ, Bhathena D, Lucas BA, et al. Hyperacute rejection due to perfusion injury. *Clin Nephrol*. 7:120–124, 1977.
254. Hill GS, Light JA, Perloff LJ. Perfusion-related injury in renal transplantation. *Surgery*. 79:440–447, 1976.
255. Spector D, Limas C, Frost JL, Zachary JB, Sterioff S, Williams GM, Rolley RT, Sandler JH. Perfusion nephropathy in human transplants. *N Engl J Med*. 295:1217–1221, 1976.
256. Amery AH, Pegrum GD, Risdon RA, Williams G. Nature of hyperacute (accelerated second set) rejection in dog renal allografts and effects of heparin on rejection process. *Br Med J*. 1:455–458, 1973.
257. Williams GM. Clinical course following renal transplantation. In: *Kidney Transplantation Principles and Practice*. PJ Morris, Ed, London, Academic Press, 1979, p. 203.
258. MacDonald A, Busch GJ, Alexander JL, Pheteplace EA, Nemzoian J, Murray JE. Heparin and aspirin in the treatment of hyperacute rejection of renal allografts in presensitized dogs. *Transplantation*. 9:1–7, 1970.
259. Clyne DH, Kincaid-Smith P, Ribush NT, Morris PJ, Marshall VC. Improvement in renal blood flow of rejecting renal allografts during heparin infusion. *Med J Aust*. 1:522–524, 1970.
260. Griffin PJA, Salaman JR. A controlled trial of heparin in renal transplant rejection. *Transplantation*. 32:306–307, 1981.
261. Kincaid-Smith P, Saker BM, Fairley KF. Anticoagulants in irreversible acute renal failure. *Lancet*. 2:1360–1362, 1968.
262. Mathew TH, Hogan GP, Lewers DT, Bauer H, Maher JF, Schreiner GE. Controlled, double-blind trial of antiplatelet aggregating agents in vascular renal allografts. *Rejection Transplant Proc*. 3:901–903, 1971.
263. Mathew TH, Clyne DH, Nanra RS, Kincaid-Smith P, Saker BM, Morris PJ, Marshall VC. A controlled trail of oral anticoagulants and dipyridamole in cadaveric renal allografts. *Lancet*. 1:1307–1310, 1974.
264. Dosekun AK, First MR, Chandran KG, Kant KS, Glas-Greenwalt P, Weiss MA, Alexander JW, Pollak VE. Successful treatment by defibrination with Ancrod in a patient with hyperacute renal allograft failure and a deficiency of plasma prostacyclin stimulating factor. *Clin Nephrol*. 18:101–105, 1982.
265. Glas-Greenwalt P, Goldman MH. Role of fibrinolytic system in renal transplantation. *Thromb Haemost*. 46:63, 1981. (Abstr. #0184).
266. Erikson RV, Williman M, Pendras JP. A true hypercoagulability state in patients on chronic hemodialysis. *Trans Am Soc Artif Int Org*. 12:205–209, 1966.
267. Wing AJ, Curtis JR, DeWardener HE. Reduction of clotting in Scribner shunts by long-term anticoagulation. *Br Med J*. 3:143–145, 1967.
268. Francis GS, Sharma BIM, Collins, AJ, Helseth HK, Comty CM. Coronary-artery surgery in patients with end-stage renal disease. *Ann Int Med*. 92:499–503, 1980.
269. Comty CM, Shapiro FL. Cardiac complications of regular daily treatment. In: *Replacement of Renal Function by Dialysis*. Drukker W, Parson FM, Maher JP, Eds. The Hague, Martinus Neihoff, 1978, pp. 519–520.

270. Bagdade JD. Chronic renal failure and atherosclerosis serum factors stimulate the proliferation of human arterial smooth muscle cells. *Atherosclerosis.* 34:243–248, 1979.
271. Mc Manus JFA, Hughson MD, Hennigar GR, Fitts CT, Rajagopalan PR, Williams AV. Dialysis enhances renal epithelial proliferations. *Arch Pathol Lab Med.* 104:192–195, 1980.
272. Tomura S, IDA T, Kuriyama R, Chida Y, Takeuchi J, Motomiya T, Yamazaki H. Activation of platelets in patients with chronic proliferative glomerulonephritis and the nephrotic syndrome. *Clin Nephrol.* 17:24–30, 1982.
273. Turney JH, Fewell M, Williams LC, Dodd N, Weston MJ. Parodoxical behaviour of antithrombin III during hemodialysis and its prevention with prostacyclin. *Clin Nephrol.* 17:31–35, 1982.
274. Sorensen PJ, Knudsen F, Nielsen AH, Dyerberg J. Protein C activity in renal disease. *Thromb Res.* 38:243–249, 1985.

Chapter 2

Prostaglandins in Uremic Bleeding

Elaine M. Sloand, M.D.

I. Introduction

Platelet plug formation at the site of vascular injury is a critical component of clotting. It first requires platelet adhesion to the damaged vessel, followed by platelet aggregation. Fibrin bridging from coagulation finally secures the plug. Prostaglandins in the vessel wall and in the platelets exert a large influence over the platelet plug formation. Alternation of prostaglandin metabolism by drugs, uremia, or other diseases can contribute to excesses of bleeding or thrombosis.

The prostaglandins are unsaturated fatty acids containing 20 atoms arranged as a cyclopentane ring (Fig. 1).[1] Prostaglandin synthesis begins when arachidonic acid is liberated by phospholipase from cell membranes of platelets or endothelial cells. Cyclo-oxygenase oxidizes arachidonic acid to PGG_2 and PGH_2 which are subsequently reduced to PGE_2 and $PGF_{2\alpha}$. These endoperoxides are then converted in the platelet by thromboxane synthetase to the active molecule thromboxane $A_2(TxA_2)$, which actually sets off aggregation of platelets and the constriction of blood vessels (Fig. 2). [2] Deficiency of thromboxane A_2 due to deficiency of thromboxane synthetase causes a bleeding diathesis.[3]

Platelet aggregation in response to thrombin, epinephrine, and collagen is due in most part to the stimulation of TxA_2 production. The second phase of platelet aggregation can be interrupted by blocking production of TxA_2 production as seen following aspirin ingestion, which blocks cyclo-oxygenase activity. Another platelet aggregation system is independent of TxA_2, which is not abolished by aspirin and is mediated by high doses of thrombin and epinephrine.[4]

Arachidonic acid metabolism in the endothelial cells oppose those of the platelet.[3] Arachidonate is metabolized to prostacyclin (PGI_2) which inhibits platelet aggregation and is a potent vasodilator. This hypotensive effect may be very important whenever the PGI_2 is used, especially for those on hemodialysis. At higher concentrations, PGI_2 also inhibits adhesion of platelets to vessel walls.

From Bern MM (ed.): *Urinary Tract Bleeding: Diagnosis and Control by Medical, Radiologic, and Surgical Techniques.* Mount Kisco, NY, Futura Publishing Co., Inc., 1985.

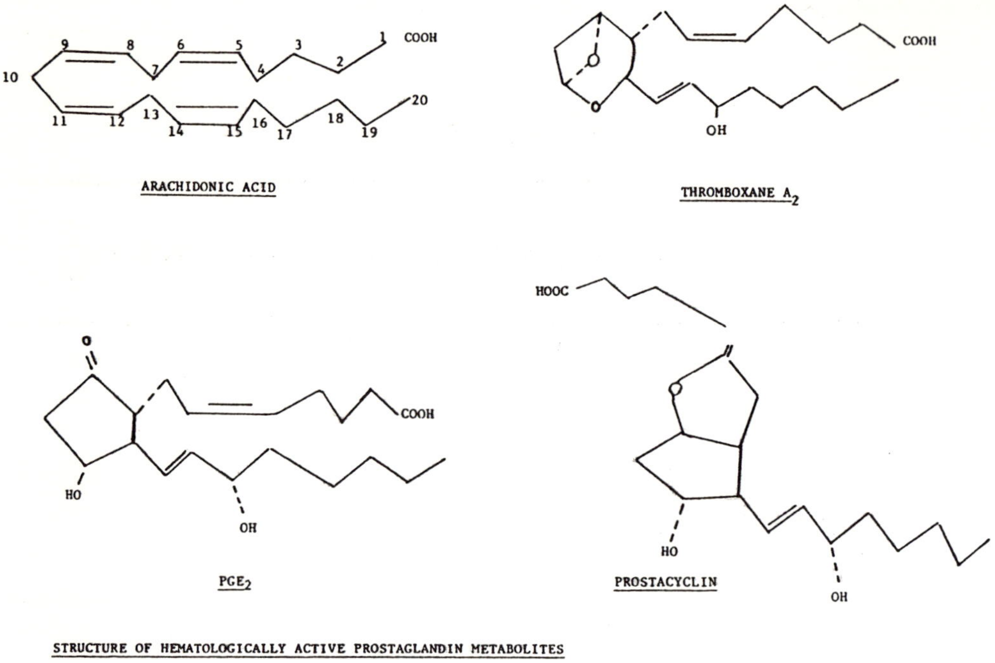

Figure 1: *Molecular structure of arachidonic acid, thromboxane A_2, prostaglandin E_2, and prostacyclin.*

Thromboxane A_2 and prostacyclin exert their control over platelet behavior by modulating the generation of adenyl cyclase (Fig. 3).[5,6] Platelet aggregation is normally inhibited by increasing levels of intracellular 3′,5′ - cyclic AMP. Best et al.[7] demonstrated that incubation of platelet-rich plasma with fresh arterial tissue (a source of PGI_2) leads to an increase in cyclic AMP which then paralleled the inhibition of aggregation. This effect was abolished by treating the vascular tissue with inhibitors of PGI_2. On the other hand, thromboxane A_2 was shown to inhibit cyclic AMP production within the platelets and thus facilitates aggregation.[8]

The hemostatic balance between prostacyclin and thromboxane is still being elucidated, as are the factors that influence their levels. For example, two common proteins, haptoglobin and albumen, inhibit the activities of the prostaglandins.[9,10] Together they account for 96% of the plasma's inhibitory activity toward prostaglandins in platelets.[11] Hypoalbuminemia may actually play a role in production of the hypercoagulable states associated with the nephrotic syndrome. The clinical role of haptoglobin and changes in its concentration have not yet been clarified. In an opposing fashion, a heat labile, nondialyzed plasma fraction stimulates prostacyclin production.[12] Another example is that free radicals generated during PGI_2 synthesis can actually inhibit cyclo-oxygenase, creating a negative feedback loop.[13,14] Interestingly, from the point of view of understanding bleeding in uremia, free radical scavengers such as phenols which appear during uremia can increase PGI_2 synthesis and thus contribute to the coagulopathy of uremia. Thus, there is a complicated balance of prostacyclin metabolism in uremia that is not yet fully elucidated.

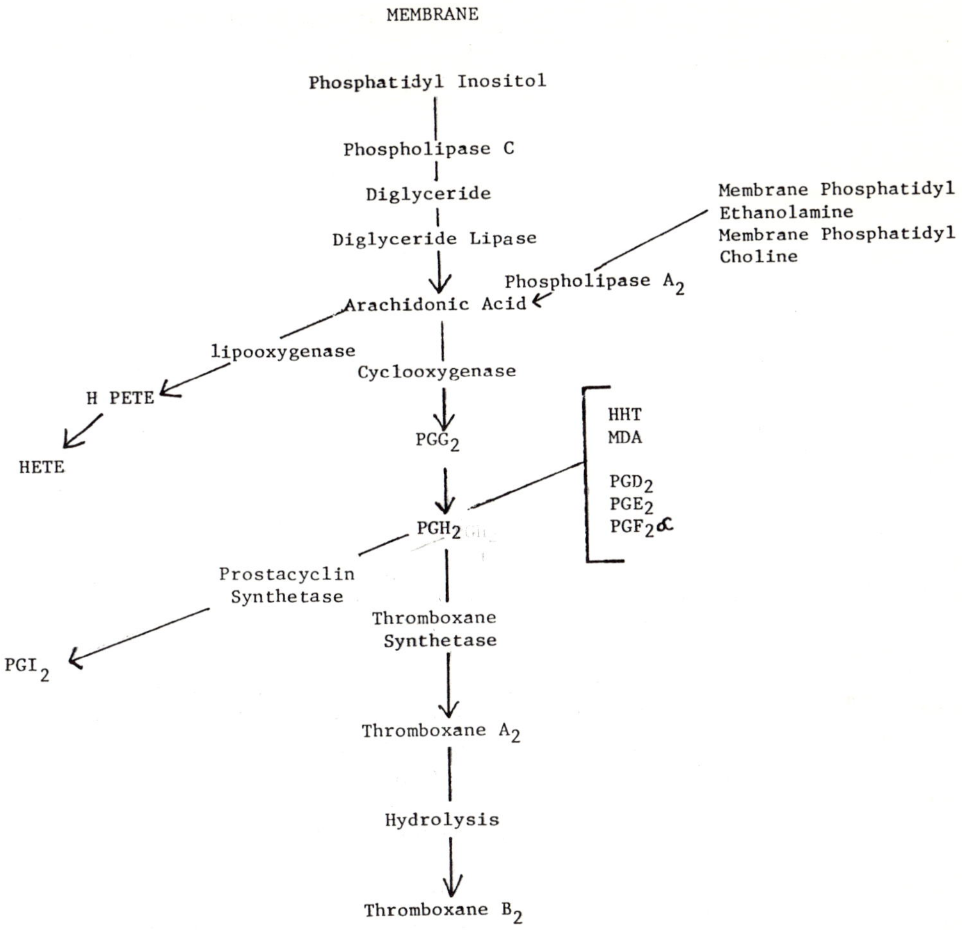

Platelet arachidonic acid metabolism resulting in thromboxane A_2 production.

Figure 2: *The metabolic pathway leading from arachidonic acid to the active moiety thromboxane* A_2. *Some intermediate steps are also demonstrated.*

II. Drugs and Prostacyclins and Prostaglandin

Many drugs taken by patients induce changes in this delicate prostacyclin/thromboxane balance. This is particularly true for the nonsteroidal anti-inflammatory drugs. Aspirin exerts the effect through irreversible acetylation of cyclo-oxygenase. As the platelet is incapable of synthesizing new cyclo-oxygenase, the defect induced by aspirin persists for the lifetime of that platelet. In an adult, inactivation of cyclo-oxygenase occurs with a daily dose of 325 mg or less.[15,16] The endothelial cells are capable of synthesizing new cylco-oxygenase, making

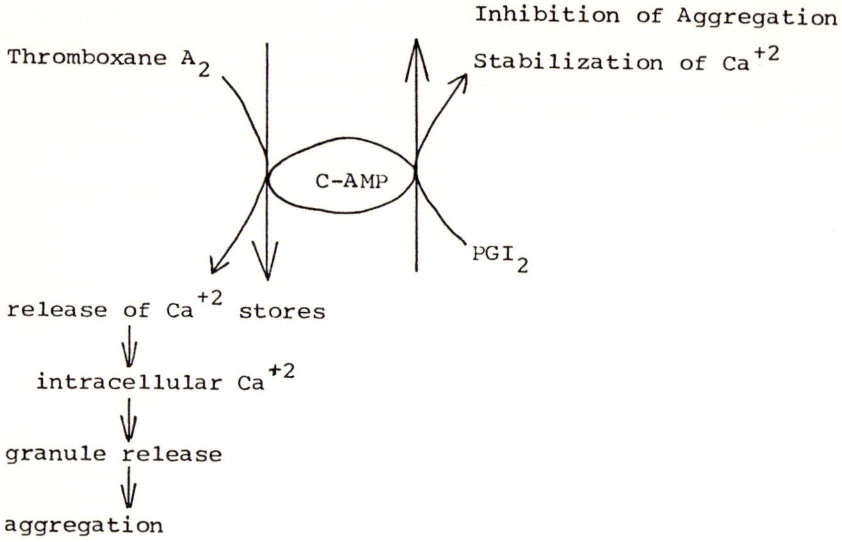

Figure 3: *Platelet cyclic AMP pathway. PGI_2, produced in the vessel wall, elevates platelet C-AMP, which in turn inhibits aggregation. Thromboxane A_2 decreases platelet C-AMP, causing platelet aggregation.*

them more resistant to the effects of aspirin. Thus, low doses of aspirin have been used to suppress TxA_2 synthesis while allowing continued production of prostacyclin in uremic patients undergoing hemodialysis.[16]

There are clinical applications for these findings. When carefully managed, aspirin may be an adequate anticoagulant during hemodialysis.[17] When used with heparin, aspirin reduces thrombus formation on dialyzer membranes. Low dose aspirin (160 mg/day) reduces AV shunt thrombosis in 72% of placebo-treated patients down to 32% of patients treated with aspirin ($p < 0.01$).[18]

Indomethacin and probably all nonsteroidal anti-inflammatory agents have a similar effect on prostaglandin synthesis in the endothelial cells and in the platelets, but the mechanisms differ from that of aspirin. Indomethacin does not bind covalently to cyclo-oxygenase but rather inhibits enzyme acetylation by a competitive and reversible interaction.[19] The degree of prostaglandin inhibition varies with plasma drug levels. Thus, the dose needed for maximal inhibition of platelet prostaglandin is variable, even when dose adjustments are made for patient weight.[20] Upon discontinuing the indomethacin, the platelet function returns to normal linearly. Hence, in contrast to the irreversible effects of aspirin on prostaglandin, indomethacin's effects on platelets is nearly dissipated within 24 hours of the last dose.

Many other classes of drugs with other activities may affect this system as well. Flurbiprofen inhibits platelet granule release by inhibiting platelet phosphodiesterase, an enzyme normally needed to degrade cyclic AMP.[21] Flurbiprofen is excreted through the kidneys and thus requires dose adjustment in renal failure. Sulfinpyrazone inhibits platelet adhesion and release as well as aggregation in response to ADP, epinehprine, and collagen. Sulfinpyrazone[22] or one of its metabolites appears to act as a competitive inhibitor of cyclo-oxygenase. Alone, sulfinpyrazone will not prolong the bleeding time. Of some importance, unlike some other steroidal anti-inflammatory agents, sulfinpyrazone will not alter glomerular filtration rate, and thus it is suitable for use in the uremic patient. Sulfinpyrazone at 600 mg daily has also been useful in diminishing the frequency of shunt thrombosis in patients on chronic hemodialysis.[23] In addition, sulfinpyrazone has been used effectively during hemodialysis to prevent the drop of platelet counts that normally accompany hemodialysis, as well as preventing consumption of antithrombin III.[24]

Glucocorticoids have long been recognized for their hemostatic effect in thromobcytopenic patients. They cause a shortening of the bleeding times before there is an elevation in platelet counts. It has been shown that glucocorticoids inhibit the vessel wall prostacylcin formation by inhibiting phospholipase in the vessel walls.[25]

III. Bleeding and Prostaglandins in Uremia

The role of the prostaglandins in uremic bleeding has been investigated.[9, 23–33] Remuzzi et al. determined that production of a PGI_2-like material was markedly increased in the vein walls of patients with chronic or acute renal failure, with a positive correlation between the length of the bleeding times and peak PGI_2 concentration,[34] though not all uremics studied had elevated PGI_2 levels. No correlation could be found between PGI_2 values and sex, age, or renal diagnosis. Uremic plasma caused an increased release of PGI_2 from bovine aortic endothelial cells grown *in vitro*.[35] Platelet prostaglandin synthesis on the other hand was diminished in uremic patients as compared to control subjects. Platelet aggregation and thromboxane $B_2(TxB_2)$ production in response to ADP were impaired in uremic patients indicating a decrease of platelet production of prostaglandins and of thromboxane A_2.[30] This has been attributed to a decrease

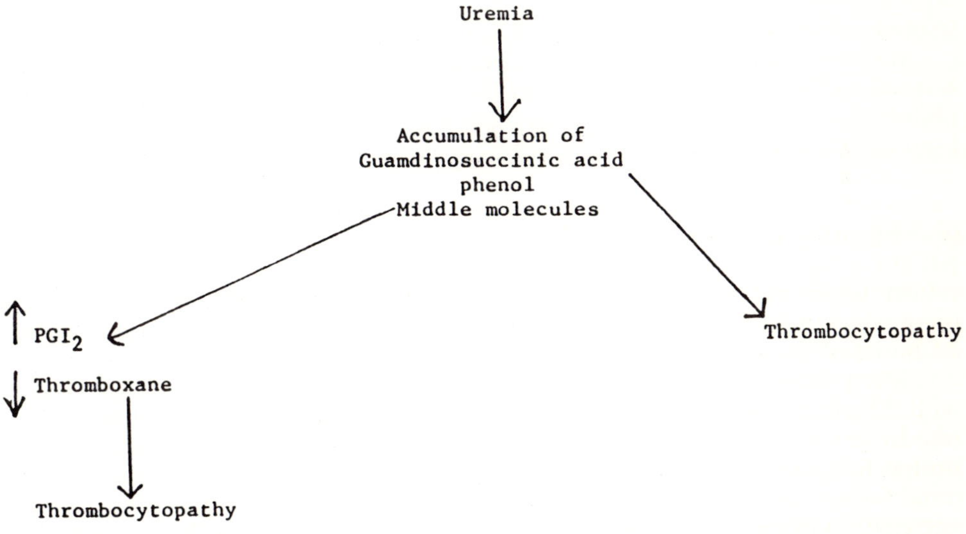

Figure 4: *The effect of uremia upon platelet function. Uremia leads to the accumulation of toxic wastes, some of which produce a thrombocytopathy of themselves. Others may lead to the altered prostaglandin metabolism, which in turn produces a thrombocytopathy.*

of the function of cyclo-oxygenase.[31] This combination increases the potential for bleeding (Fig. 4). It was also demonstrated that normal plasma could partially correct the defect found in uremic platelets, while uremic plasma stimulated PGI_2 production in aortic rings 16 times greater than did normal plasma.

IV. Prostaglandins During Dialysis

Hemodialysis can affect prostaglandin and prostacyclin metabolism. Smith et al. found the levels of TxA_2 measured as the stable metabolic by-product TxB_2 equalled that of control subjects when the patients were adequately dialyzed.[30] There were, however, marked differences of prostaglandin and PGI_2 metabolism when patients were either inadequately dialyzed or treated conservatively as compared to those who were either adequately dialyzed or who were normal.[30] Improvement of prostaglandin metabolism with adequate dialysis parallels other studies that showed improvement of platelet aggregation after intensive dialysis. The etiology of depressed prostaglandin synthesis in uremics is not clear but may relate to the previously mentioned accumulation of free radical scavengers, such as phenols, which inhibit prostacyclin synthetase.

V. Control of Bleeding in Uremia

A. Prostaglandin Metabolism

Therapy for urinary tract bleeding may include manipulation of prostacyclin/thromboxane axes. Blocking agents specific for PGI_2 or stimulants for prostaglandin production will be available soon. In theory, very low doses of aspirin could inhibit the excessive production of PGI_2 of endothelial cells without worsening the already sluggish platelet production of TxA_2. Unfortunately, in studies so far available, inhibition of PGI_2 production occurred but at the expense of exacerbating the bleeding time.[26] Hence, while the idea was an interesting one, rather than being corrected by aspirin, the uremic coagulopathy was made worse with the low doses of aspirin studied.

B. Platelet Transfusion

Platelets may be transfused in an attempt to gain control of bleeding in the uremic patients. It should be remembered that the effect of platelet transfusions is short-lived, as the transfused platelets will soon acquire the same defect as present in native platelets. The duration of any beneficial effect of platelet transfusion, however, has been found to be more effective when given after dialysis.[36] As platelet efficacy is variable from patient to patient, efficacy should be tested by performing a bleeding time after transfusion.

C. Cryoprecipitate

Cryoprecipitate can correct bleeding time in some patients. Janson et al. found that prolonged bleeding times improved in a group of uremic patients

1–12 hours after infusion of 10 bags of cryoprecipitate.[37] Bleeding times remained improved for 24–36 hours. The reason for correction of the bleeding time by cryoprecipitate is not yet known. Why some patients fail to respond is also unknown. The failures may be related to patient selection, concentration and preservation of the factors in the cryoprecipitate, coincidental drug ingestion, or other factors. When using this approach in our institution, we found improvement in about half of the patients. In some, the bleeding times improved but not completely to normal. Thus, an *in vivo* assay, i.e. the bleeding time, should be performed to prove efficacy, before performing invasive procedures. It should also be remembered that correction of bleeding times occurs between 1 and 12 hours after infusion, making cryoprecipitate therapy nonideal for immediate hemostatic control.

D. Dialysis

Intensive hemodialysis or peritoneal dialysis may be used in an effort to correct the uremic bleeding disorder. Dialysis by either means has been shown to improve platelet aggregation. Hemodialysis can cause improvement in platelet TxA_2 production.[32] Peritoneal dialysis has not yet been examined with respect to its role in altering prostaglandin metabolism.

E. Hypoalbuminemia

Rather than being associated with a coagulopathy, the nephrotic syndrome is also associated with a hypercoagulable state, as represented by renal vein thrombosis. Many factors are responsible for this state. In this setting, the prostaglandins have a somewhat paradoxical importance. Understanding the paradox may help in understanding why peritoneal dialysis can help control uremic bleeding. Less arachidonic acid is needed to aggregate platelet-rich plasma from nephrotic patients.[11] These platelets produce more TxA_2. There is also association between low plasma albumin levels and the platelet hypersensitivity to other aggregating agents. This hypersensitivity reverses when albumin is added to plasma *in vitro* (personal observation). By elevating the patients' plasma albumin, by albumin replacement therapy, or by preventing losses, the platelets are made less sensitive. It is believed that the albumin binds to arachidonic acid, thus preventing it from being incorporated into platelet phospholipids, and reducing intracellular TxA_2 synthesis.[38] AT III is also wasted into the urine of nephrotic patients (see Chapter 1).

Another clinical state where hypoalbuminemia may have clinical importance is in those patients undergoing peritoneal dialysis. Peritoneal dialysis can correct the uremia-associated platelet defects.[39] Albumin is lost in large quantities into the peritoneal dialysate, and it is interesting to speculate that low albumin may protect against the defective prostacyclin production normally present in uremia, and these additive effects produce normal platelet aggregation. In the peritoneal dialysis patients we tested, *in vitro* normalization of plasma albumin levels caused significant decrease in the percent aggregation in response to ADP in almost all patients tested.

F. Therapy for Microangiopathic Thrombosis

Hemolytic uremic syndrome and thrombotic thromocytopenic purpura are two disease states in which renal failure occurs and prostaglandin metabolism may play a role. Thrombotic thrombocytopenic purpura is characterized by thrombocytopenia, hemolytic anemia, fluctuating signs of organ failure (especially neurological signs), and renal dysfunction. Histologically, there is widespread microthrombi and reactive endothelial proliferation. Thrombi consist of masses of platelets with little entrapment of erythrocytes and fibrin. The hemolytic anemia is due to the mechanical trauma sustained by the red cells as they pass through the diseased blood vessels. Hemolytic uremic syndrome (HUS) resembles TTP clinically and pathologically, but is characterized by a less fulminant course, more notable renal impairment, and a predominance of children and pregnant women when pregnancy is complicated by pre-eclampsia or eclampsia. The etiology of these disease states is at present unclear. Recent articles have stressed the role of the factor VIII:von Willebrand factor plus an agglutinating factor.[40–42] However, the roles of prostaglandins and prostacyclin are apparently also significant.

Remuzzi and colleagues as well as others have examined the prostacyclin generation in venous tisuses of patients with HUS and TTP and found it decreased.[43,44] Diminished PGI_2 production may be due to its absence or an inhibition of components in plasma which normally stimulate synthesis or release of PGI_2. Plasma from patients stimulated little or no PGI_2 production when exposed to rat aorta. In contrast, normal plasma stimulated production of significant levels of PGI_2.

Release of platelet β-thromboglobulin has been found to inhibit PGI_2 production in blood vessels.[45] Deficiency of prostacyclin stabilizing factor has been found by some,[46] while others have documented presence of factors that inhibit PGI_2 activity within the plasma of patients with microangiopathy.[47] Patients with TTP and HUS recover their ability to synthesize PGI_2 when the disease enters remission.

As with all explanations for these diseases, there are concerns regarding these explanations. Low PGI_2 stimulatory activity persisted into remission of some patients. Also, diminished PGI_2 stimulatory activity can be found even in asymptomatic relatives of a patient with HUS.[48] HUS may occur in members of the same family, suggesting some genetic defect. Thus, since altered prostacyclin production alone may not account totally for the disease, increased platelet production of TxA_2, if present, along with diminished PGI_2 production might provide the missing link in this hypothesis. Platelets from two patients with HUS have been shown to produce significantly greater levels of thromboxane than normal platelets.[49] Damage of endothelial cells may cause the release of factor VIII:von Willebrand factor and loss of PGI_2.

The lack of clear understanding of the pathogenesis of microangiopathic states is reflected in the many treatments that have been advocated. Splenectomy has been associated with remission in a number of cases but no clear rationale has been established for its use. Antiplatelet agents including dextrose, aspirin, dipyridamole, and sulfinpyrazone have been used in their treatment, with benefit to some patients. However, concurrent administration of other potentially effective therapies such as plasma transfusion has often obscured these relationships. It is generally felt that platelet agents used as the only therapy may have questionable benefit. The use of exchange transfusion, plasmophoresis, or plasma exchange was developed after it was observed that repeated whole blood transfusions caused a remission in one patient. Since then many reports have documented the improvement of many but not all patients following plasmaphoresis. Plasma alone can be an effective treatment.[50] It is felt that plasma transfusions provide a component missing in patient's plasma, even when outdated plasma or plasma from which cryoprecipitate is removed is used. *In vitro* experiments have reconfirmed the findings.[51] Plasma exchange therapy has become in recent years our own most frequently applied technique with rather consistent success.

Infusions of prostacyclin have had varied results.[52,53] These irregular results may relate to inadequate PGI_2 infusion, or variations in the causes of the syndrome. As an example, no effect of prostacyclin infusion was seen until the eighth day of infusion in once successful trial. In this successful case, prostacyclin was infused at 4 ng/kg/min for the first 24 hours and at hourly cycles after that at 8 ng/kg/min for 18 days. This prostacyclin infusion markedly reduced the excretion of TxB_2 and the platelet count rose as this urinary metabolite of thromboxane fell. Although PGI_2 infusion may correct the coagulopathy in these cases, it may not alter renal function since the thrombotic damage may be irreversible.

Platelet transfusions have been used in the management of TTP, but their use is controversial. Thrombotic events have been linked to platelet transfusion in some cases. Other ways of altering the PGI_2/TxA_2 axis have not been attempted. As free radicals are capable of inhibiting both PGI_2 synthetase and cyclo-oxygenase, the observation of reduced plasma levels of vitamin E and increased lipid peroxidation in patients with TTP is of interest.[54] Trials with antioxidants have not yet been conducted.

In summary, prostaglandin metabolism of the vessel wall and the platelet have important implications in platelet function as well as in the pathogenesis of thrombosis and bleeding. Diseases associated with altered hemostasis such as TTP, HUS, and uremia may very well have as their common link a derangement in production or degradation of prostaglandin metabolites. Any therapeutic approach to these patients should be based on an understanding of the effect of drugs and other modalities of PGI_2/thromboxane balance.

REFERENCES

1. Moncada S, Flower RJ, Vane JR. Prostaglandins, prostacyclin, and thromboxane A_2. In: *The Pharmacologic Basis of Therapeutics*. Goodman AG, Goodman S, Gilman A, Eds. New York, MacMillan Publishing Co., 1980, pp. 668–681.
2. Marcus, AJ. The role of lipids in platelet function: With particular reference to the arachidonic pathway. *J Lipid Res*. 19:793–826, 1978.
3. Weiss HJ, Lages BA. Possible congenital defect in platelet thromboxane synthetase (Letter). *Lancet*. 1:760–761, 1977.
4. Packham, MA, Kinlough-Rathbone RL, Reimers HJ, Scott S, Mustard JF. Mechanisms of platelet aggregation independent of adenosine diphosphate. In: *Prostaglandins in Hematology*. Silver MJ, et al., Eds. New York, Spectrum, 1977, pp. 247–276.
5. Holmsen H, Karpatkin S. In: *Metabolism of Platelets in Hematology*. William WJ, Beutler F, Erslev AJ, Lichtman MA, Eds. New York, McGraw-Hill, 1983, pp. 1149–1176.
6. Moncada S, Vane JR. Unstable metabolites of arachidonic acid and their role in hemostases and thrombosis. *Br Med Bull*. 43:129–135, 1978.

7. Best LC, Martin TJ, Russell RGG, Preston FE. Prostacyclin increases the cyclic AMP levels and adenylate cyclase activity in platelets. *Nature*. 267:850–851, 1977.
8. Miller OV, Johnson RA, Gorman RR. Inhibition of PGE_1-stimulated cyclic AMP accumulation by thromboxane A_2. *Prostaglandins*. 13:599–609, 1977.
9. Collier HOJ, Denning-Kendall PA, MacDonald-Gibson WJ, Saeed SA. Plasma proteins that inhibit prostaglandin synthesis. In: *Hemostasis, Prostaglandins, and Renal Disease*. Remuzzi G, Mecca G, de Gaetano G, Eds. New York, Raven Press, 1980, pp. 257–267.
10. Saeed SA, McDonald-Gibson WJ, Cuthbert J, Copas JL, Schneider C, Gardiner PJ, Butt NM, Collier HOJ. Endogenous inhibitor of prostaglandin synthetase. *Nature*. 270: 32–36, 1977.
11. Remuzzi G, Mecca G, Marchesi D, Livio G, de Gaetano G, Donati MB, Silver MJ. Platelet hyperaggregability and the nephrotic syndrome. *Thromb Res*. 16:345–354, 1979.
12. MacIntyre DE, Pearson JD, Gordon JL. Localization and stimulation of prostacyclin production in vascular cells. *Nature*. 271:549–551, 1978.
13. Egan R, Paxton J, Kuehl F. Mechanism for irreversible self-deactivation of prostaglandin synthetase. *J Biol Chem*. 251:7329–7335, 1976.
14. Moncada S, Vane JR. Prostacyclin, platelet aggregation and thrombosis. In: *Platelets: A Multidisciplinary Approach*. de Gaetano G, Garattini S, Eds. New York, Raven Press, 1978, pp. 239–259.
15. Pederson AK, Fitzgerald FA. Dose-related kinetics of aspirin. Presystemic actelyzation of platelet cyclooxygenase. *N Engl J Med*. 311:1206–1211, 1984.
16. Weksler BB, Pett SB, Alonso D. Differential inhibition by aspirin of vascular and platelet prostaglandin synthesis in atherosclerotic patients. *N Engl J Med*. 308:800–805, 1983.
17. Lindsay RM, Ferguson D, Prentice CR, Burton JA, McNicol GP. Reduction of thrombosis formation on dialysis membranes by aspirin and RA233. *Lancet*. 2:1287–1290, 1972.
18. Harter HR, Burch JW, Majerus PW, Stanford N, Delmez JA, Anderson CB, Weerts CA. Prevention of thrombosis in patients on hemodialysis by low-dose aspirin. *N Engl J Med*. 301:577–579, 1979.
19. Stanford N, Roth G, Shen T, Majerus PW. Lack of covalent modification of prostaglandin synthetase (cyclo-oxygenase) by indomethacin. *Prostaglandins*. 13:669–675, 1977.
20. Rane A, Oelz O, Frolich JC, Seyberth HW, Sweetman BJ, Watson JT, Wilkinson GR, Oates JA. Relation between plasma concentration of indomethacin and its effect on prostaglandin synthesis and platelet aggregation in man. *Clin Pharmacol Ther*. 23:658–668, 1978.
21. Cockbill SR, Heptinstall S, Taylor PM. A comparison of the abilities of acetylsalicylic acid, flurbiprofen, and indomethacin to inhibit the release reaction and prostaglandin synthesis in human blood platelets. *Br J Pharmacol*. 67:73–78, 1979.
22. Ali M, McDonald JW. Effects of sulfinpyrazone on platelet prostaglandin synthesis and platelet release serotonin. *J Lab Clin Med*. 89:868–875, 1977.
23. Kaegi A, Pineo GF, Shimizu A, Trivedi H, Hirsch J, Gent M. Arteriovenous-shunt thrombosis: Prevention by sulfinpyrazone. *N Engl J Med*. 290:304–306, 1974.
24. Bern M, Cavaliere B, Lukas G. Plasma levels and effects of sulfinpyrazone on patients requiring chronic hemodialysis. *J Clin Pharmacol*. 20:107–116, 1980.
25. Blajchman MA, Senyi AF, Hirsh J, Surya Y, Buchanan M, Mustard JF. Shortening of the bleeding time on rabbits by hydrocortisone caused by inhibition of prostacyclin generation by the vessel wall. *Clin Invest*. 63:1026–1035, 1979.
26. Remuzzi G, Marchesi D, Livio M, Cavenaghi AE, Mecca G, Donati MB, de Gaetano G. Altered platelet and vascular prostaglandin-generation in patients with renal failure and prolonged bleeding times. *Thromb Res*. 13:1007–1015, 1978.
27. Remuzzi G, Livio M, Cavanaghi AE, Marchesi D, Mecca G, Donati MB, de Gaetano G.

Unbalanced prostaglandin synthesis and plasma factors in uraemic bleeding. A hypothesis. *Thromb Res.* 13:531–536, 1978.
28. Remuzzi G, Mecca G, Cavenaghi AE, Donati M, de Gaetano G. Prostacyclin-like activity and bleeding in renal failure. *Lancet.* 2:1195–1197, 1977.
29. Remuzzi G, Marchesi D, Cavenaghi AE, Livio M, Donati MB, de Gaetano G, Mecca G. Bleeding in renal failure: A possible role of vascular prostacyclin (PGI_2). *Clin Nephrol.* 12:127–131, 1979.
30. Smith MC, Dunn MJ. Impaired platelet thromboxane production in renal failure. *Nephron.* 29:133–137, 1981.
31. Remuzzi G, Benigni A, Dodesini P, Schieppati A, Livio M, de Gaetano G, Day JS, Smith WL, Pinca E, Patrignani P, Patrono G. Reduced platelet thromboxane formation in uremia: Evidence for a functional cyclooxygenase defect. *J Clin Invest.* 71: 762–768, 1983.
32. Ylikorkala O, Huttunes K, Jarvi J, Viinikka L. Prostacyclin and thromboxane in chronic uremia: Effect of hemodialysis. *Clin Nephrol.* 18:83–87, 1982.
33. Remuzzi G, Cavenaghi AE, Mecca G, Donati MB, de Gaetano G. Prostacyclin-like activity and bleeding in renal failure. *Lancet.* 2:1195–1197, 1977.
34. Remuzzi G, Benigni A, Dodesini P, Schieppati A, Gotti E, Livio M, Mecca G, Donati MB, de Gaetano G. Platelet function in patients on maintenance hemodialysis: Depressed or enhanced. *Clin Nephrol.* 17:60–63, 1982.
35. DeFreyn G, Dauden V, Machin SJ, Vermylen J. A plasma factor in uremia which stimulates prostacyclin release from cultured endothelial cells. *Thromb Res.* 19: 695–699, 1980.
36. Nakamoto S, Kolff N. Hemorrhagic diathesis in uremia and the avoidance of bleeding problems during dialysis. *Ann NY Acad Sci.* 115:348–356, 1974.
37. Janson PA, Jubelirer SJ, Weinstein MA, Deykin D. Treatment of the bleeding tendency in uremia with cryoprecipitate. *N Engl J Med.* 303:1318–1322, 1981.
38. Smith J, Silver M. Prostaglandin synthesis by platelets and its biological significance. In: *Cell Tissue Physiology* (vol. 1). *Platelets in Biology Pathology.* Gordon JL, Ed. Research monograph, Cardeza Found., Philadelphia. New York, Amsterdam/North Holland Pub. Co., 1976, pp. 331–352.
39. Nenci GG, Berretlin M, Agnell G, Parise P, Buoncristiani U, Ballatori E. Effects of peritoneal dialysis, haemodialysis, and kidney transplantation on blood platelet function, platelet aggregation by ADP and epinephrine. *Nephron.* 23:287–292, 1979.
40. Lian EC-Y, Harkness DR, Byrnes JJ, Wallach H, Nunez R. Presence of a platelet aggregating factor in the plasma of patients with thrombotic thrombocytopenic purpura (TTP) and its inhibition by normal plasma. *Blood.* 53:333–338, 1979.
41. Moake JL, Rudy CK, Troll JH, Weinstein MJ, Colannino NM, Azocar J, Seder RH, Hong SL, Deykin D. Unusually large plasma factor VIII:von Willebrand factor multimers in chronic relapsing thrombotic thrombocytopenic purpura. *N Engl J Med.* 307:1432–1435, 1982.
42. Kelton JG, Moore J, Santos A, Sheridan D. Detection of a platelet-agglutinating factor in thrombotic thrombocytopenic purpura. *Ann Intern Med.* 101:589–593, 1984.
43. Remuzzi G, Misiani R, Marchesi D, Livio M, Mecca G, de Gaetano G, Donati M. Haemolytic-uraemic syndrome: Deficiency of plasma factor(s) regulating prostacyclin activity? *Lancet.* 2:871–872, 1978.
44. Remuzzi G, Misiani R, Mecca G, de Gaetano G, Donati M. Thrombotic thrombocytopenic purpura: A deficiency of plasma factors regulating platelet-vessel-wall interaction? (Letter) *N Engl J Med.* 299:311, 1978.
45. Hope N, Martin TJ, Chesterman CN, Morgan FJ. Human B-thromboglobulin inhibits PGI_2 production and binds to a specific site in bovine aortic endothelial cells. *Nature.* 282:210–212, 1979.
46. Machin SJ, McVerry BA, Parry H, Marrow WJW. A plasma factor inhibition prostacyclin-like activity in thrombotic thrombocytopenic purpura. *Acta Haematol.* 67:8–12, 1982.

47. Wu KK, Hall ER, Papp A. Prostacyclin stabilising factor deficiency in thrombotic thrombocytopenic purpura (Letter). *Lancet.* 2:460–461, 1982.
48. Remuzzi G, Mecca G, Livio M, de Gaetano G, Donati MB, Pearson JD, Gordon JL. Prostacyclin generation by cultured endothelial cells in haemolytic uraemic syndrome (Letter). *Lancet.* 1:656–657, 1980.
49. Remuzzi G, Levio M, Mecca G, de Gaetano G, Donati M. Prostacyclin and kidney disease: Focus on uremia and thrombotic microangiopathy. In: *Clinical Pharmacology of Prostacyclin.* Lewis PJ, O'Grady J, Eds. New York, Raven Press, 1981, pp. 63–68.
50. Bateman SM, Hilgard P, Gordon-Smith EC. Thrombotic thrombocytopenic purpura: A possible plasma factor deficiency. *Br J Haematol.* 43:498, 1979.
51. Lian EC, Harkness DR, Byrnes JJ, Wallach H, Nunez R. Presence of a platelet aggregating factor in the plasma of patients with thrombotic thrombocytopenia purpura (TTP) and its inhibition by normal plasma. *Blood.* 53:333–338, 1979.
52. Budd GT, Bukowski RM, Lucas FV, Cato AE, Cocchetto DM. Prostacyclin therapy of thrombotic thrombocytopenic purpura (Letter). *Lancet.* 2:915, 1980.
53. Fitzgerald GA, Maas RL, Stein R, Oates JA, Roberts LJ. Intravenous prostacyclin in thrombotic thrombocytopenic purpura. *Ann Intern Med.* 95:319–322, 1981.
54. Byrnes J. Thrombotic thrombocytopenic purpura. *Adv Intern Med.* 26:131–157, 1980.

Chapter 3

Systemic Diseases That Manifest as Hematuria, Hemoglobinuria, Pigmenturia, With or Without Renal Failure

Sabina R. Wallach, M.D.

This chapter discusses the systemic diseases that can present as pigmenturia including hemoglobinuria with or without renal failure. Pigmenturia may be confused with hematuria and hemoglobinuria because of similar red or red-orange discoloration of urine. Causes of pigmenturia may be nephrologically inconsequential, such as with beet ingestion or pyridium administration. In contrast, the causes of hemoglobinuria and myoglobinuria require diligent pursuit since these signs often herald significant pathological conditions. Benign pigmenturia may be easily recognized by detailed historical examination. The relationship of these changes with systemic illnesses must be considered when managing the patient.

I. Renal Manifestations of the Hemoglobopathies

The hemoglobinopathies can be linked to several clinically important renal diseases (Table I). These linkages must be contemplated when examining patients for either the red cell disorders or when examining the patients for renal disease.

From Bern MM (ed.): *Urinary Tract Bleeding: Diagnosis and Control by Medical, Radiologic, and Surgical Techniques*. Mount Kisco, NY, Futura Publishing Co., Inc., 1985.

Table I
Renal Manifestations of Hemoglobinopathies

- Hyposthenuria
- Gross hematuria related to submucosal vascular dilatation and extravasation in renal pelvis
- Papillary necrosis
- ↑ Bacteriuria
- Pyelonephritis
- Perirenal hematoma (not in sickle trait)
- Hyperuricaemia (↓ Excretion of uric acid) with urate nephropathy
- Glomerulonephritis and nephrotic syndrome with glomerular microinfarction by plugs of sickled erythrocytes (uncommon)
- Renal infarction
- Renal vein thrombosis (not in sickle trait)
- Chronic renal failure

A. Hemoglobin S Disorders

The sickle cell disorders are commonly associated with hematuria.[1] Hematuria occurs more frequently in the sickle trait (AS) than in sickle cell (SS) disease. The observed difference may reflect the more common sickle trait, which affects two million blacks in the United States (8% of black population).[2] The incidence of hematuria in individuals with sickle trait is uncertain, but ranges from less than 1% in a Jamaican population observed during a 12-year period[3] to 18% in another group observed over a much shorter interval.[4]

Sickle cell trait is not associated with increased mortality in contrast with sickle cell disease. The only well-proven complications of the trait are related to the urinary tract (Table II). These include an increased incidence of asymptomatic bacteriuria in pregnant and nonpregnant women,[5] with an increased incidence of pyelonephritis during pregnancy.[6–9] Massive hematuria, hyposthenuria, and papillary necrosis occur with an increased incidence, presumably

Table II
Genitourinary Abnormalities Associated with Sickle Cell Trait

- Association with sickle trait very likely
    - Bacteriuria
    - Bacteriuria and pyelonephritis in pregnancy
    - Hyposthenuria
    - Hematuria
- Association with sickle trait possible, but more studies needed
    - Renal papillary necrosis
    - Reduced urinary filtration fraction
- Association with sickle trait unlikely or unproven
    - ↓ Renal clearance of creatinine and inulin decreased urinary acidification
    - Renal failure
    - Renal cortical infarction
    - Renal vein thrombosis
    - Perirenal hematoma
    - Priapism

Adapted from Sears DA: *Am J Med.* 64:1021–1036, 1978.[5]

related to similar etiological factors, including sluggish blood flow in the renal medulla with resultant low oxygen tension, acidosis, and hypertonicity. These further contribute to the development of sickling, with obstruction of flow and loss of vascular integrity.[10,11] (Figs. 1 and 2).

Patients with sickle cell disease present with a slightly different incidence and distribution of nephrologic and urologic complications (Table III).[6]

1. *Clinical Presentation*

The hematuria is characteristically microscopic, painless, and total throughout micturition,[12] and is often massive and prolonged.[11,12] Recurrent episodes are common,[12,13] as is a male predominance.[13]

A review by Atkinson[12] of 115 cases of hematuria in 74 patients with a positive sickling test illustrates many of the clinical characteristics:

- The majority of patients had sickle cell trait (AS).
- The bleeding was painless, profuse, and total.
- Clots were uncommon.
- Bleeding was often prolonged: one-third of the patients bled for 2 weeks; one-third of the patients bled up to six months, with occasional episodes lasting longer than 1 year.
- No cause of bleeding other than a positive sickle test could be found in two-thirds of the cases.
- In one-third of cases, causes other than the sickle trait could be identified, e.g. trauma, tumor.
- Bleeding occurred more frequently on the left side.
- Severe anemia was uncommon despite prolonged hemorrhage.

Less common causes of hematuria in the sickle syndromes include papillary necrosis and pyelonephritis.[14] These often appear to be related to well-documented bacteriuria in women with the sickle cell trait.[6–9] The nephrotic syndrome is uncommon, but may develop in association with glomerular micro-infarction due to sludging of sickled erythrocytes. Not surprisingly, it is unresponsive to steroid administration.[14] Major renal infarction may also occur because of sickling in the renal arteries.[14] Occasionally, urate nephropathy occurs in the sickling disorders and may present as microscopic hematuria.[15,16] Renal vein thrombosis probably does not occur with increased frequency in individuals with the sickle trait when compared to the normal population.[5]

Chronic renal failure in patients with sickle cell disease has been managed successfully by maintenance hemodialysis, without an increased incidence of thrombosis of vascular fistulae and without induction of sickling during passage of blood through dialysis tubing.[17]

It is unwise to assume that only one cause exists for hematuria in patients with sickle cell trait or disease. Examination of fresh urinary sediment may reveal the presence of a coexistent glomerulonephritis unrelated to the hemoglobinopathy.[18] Tumors may be identified by intravenous pyelography, which can be performed without risk and with adequate visualization, despite the presence of hyposthenuria.[12] Similarly, papillary necrosis may be found. A concurrent coagulopathy such as von Willebrand's syndrome, a common and treatable disorder, should be considered since it may present with hematuria in the absence of an anatomically defined cause of hemorrhage. In five described

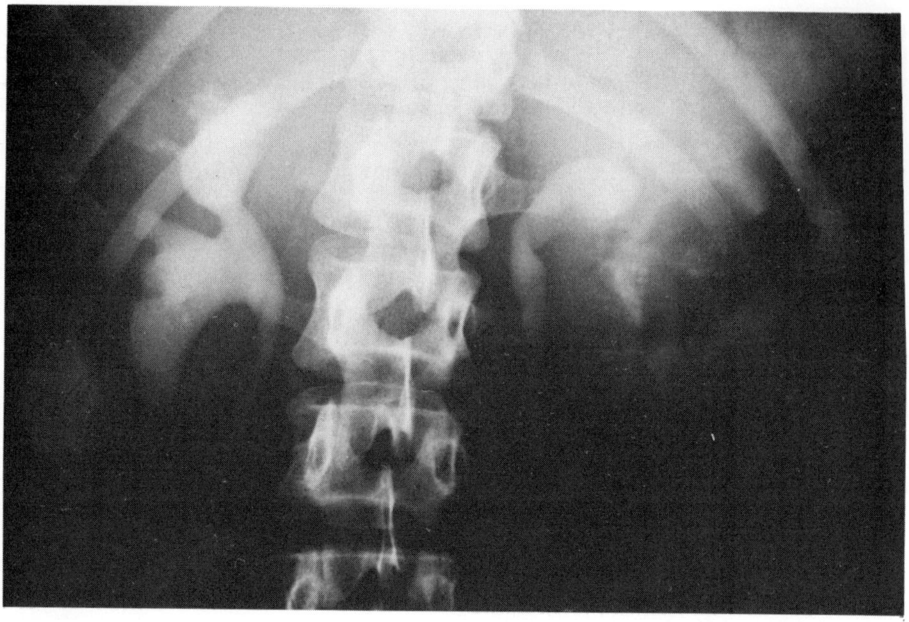

Figure 1: *Intravenous pyelogram demonstrating blunted calyces of papillary necrosis due to sickle cell disease. (From the Learning File of the Center for Devices and Radiological Health, FDA, case GU506.)*

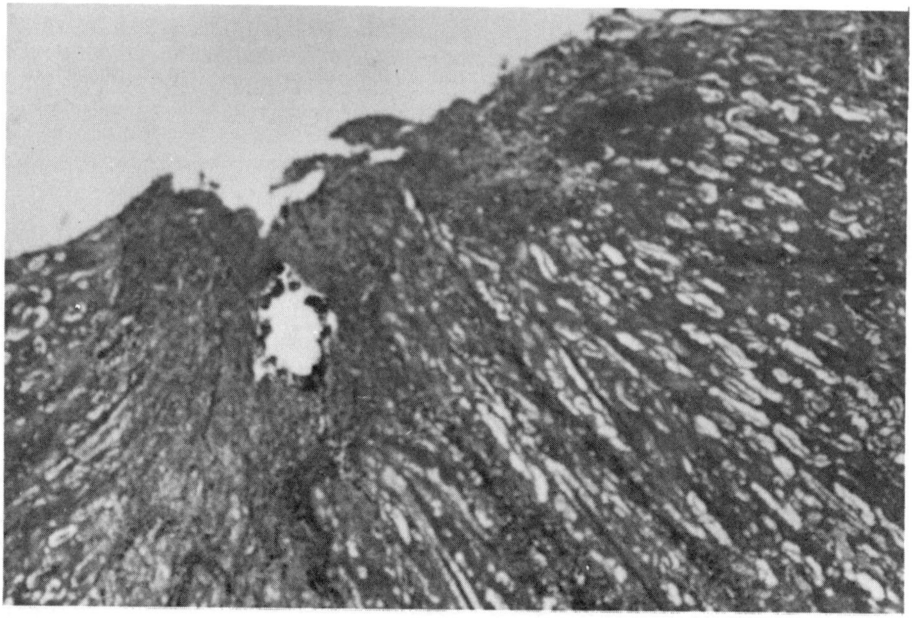

Figure 2: *Photomicrograph of papillary necrosis demonstrating the loss of normal papilla of kidney (40×).*

Table III
Clinical Features of Renal and Genitourinary Abnormalities in 100 Patients with Sickle Cell Disease (SS)

	# Adequate Records	Affected Pts.		Comments
		(#)	(%)	
Pyelonephritis	97	17	18	25 episodes
Nephrotic Syndrome	97	1	1	Bilateral renal vein thrombosis
Priapism	51	5	10	
Hematuria	95	7	7	
IVP	7			
No abnormality		1		
Hydronephrosis		1		
Chronic pyelonephritis		5		

Adapted from Karayalcon G, et al.: *Am J Med Sci.* 269:51–68, 1978.[7]

cases, family histories of bleeding disorders were absent, and hemorrhage was confined to the genitourinary tract.[19]

2. *Pathological Changes*

In addition to hemorrhage, the kidneys undergo many pathological changes in sickle cell nephropathy. They become diffusely enlarged with associated increased blood flow. The glomerular surface area is increased, and glomeruli may become mildly to moderately hypercellular. The glomerular capillaries become dilated and engorged with erythrocytes that appear sickled, especially near the juxtaglomerular apparatus.[20,21] Electron microscopic studies confirm the presence of electron-dense deposits compatible with iron in the glomeruli and tubules.[22]

Similar changes are found in the renal medulla, especially at the cortico-medullary junction. Microradioangiographic studies of this region confirm the presence of dilated capillaries, with ruptured walls and extravasated contrast material.[23] These changes probably reflect the *in vivo* mechanism of peritubular bleeding in the medulla of kidneys removed from patients with sickle cell disorders because of prolonged unilateral hematuria.[21] Similar hemorrhage has been found in the submucosal blood vessels of the renal pelvis and ureters.[20]

3. *Management of Hematuria*

Management of episodes of gross hematuria due to sickle cell disorders should be conservative, with complete bed rest, hydration, and blood transfusion as indicated. Infection should be treated. An anatomical lesion should be considered with an IVP examination. The presence of a coagulopathy should be evaluated. Urinary cytology should be performed. If no other cause of bleeding is found, management should continue to be supportive.

Many therapeutic interventions have been hailed, but most, if not all, are of unconfirmed value. These include:

- oral urea[24]
- urinary alkalinization with distilled water infusion[25] and diuresis[11]
- hyperbaric oxygen[26]
- exchange transfusions.[27]

Agents that primarily affect coagulation are also available. Epsilon amino caproic acid (Amicar®) has been used successfully to control hematuria in this setting.[28] It is a potent inhibitor of activation of the fibrinolytic system.[29] As such, it may induce massive clot formation within the urinary tract, causing obstruction as a complication of therapy (see Chapters 5 and 6). Because of this, only the smallest dose of epsilon aminocaproic acid (EACA) able to control the bleeding should be used. After cessation of bleeding, an intravenous pyelogram should be performed to evaluate the presence of clot.

Recently triglycyl vasopressin (glypressin) has been used successfully to control persistent hematuria in the sickle syndromes.[30] This drug is a synthetic hormonogen of lysine vasopressin, which causes more prolonged vasoconstriction than does vasopressin. It has also been used to control bleeding esophageal varices. Although lysine vasopressin is a potent inducer of plasma plasminogen activation, triglycyl vasopressin is not.[31] Potential side effects of therapy include hypertension, increased intestinal peristalsis, fluid retention, and muscle cramps.[30] Further studies of this drug need to be performed in a larger group of patients to assess its true efficacy.

The development of specific antisickling agents directed towards correction of the intracellular molecular defect remains at an early stage, requiring further study before clinical application.[32,33]

Nephrectomy has been performed in cases of prolonged hematuria.[21,35] Clearly, however, problems may arise if hematuria subsequently occurs in the remaining kidney[13,34,35] so that nephrectomy should be avoided whenever possible.

B. Renal Complication of Other Hemoglobinopathies

Sickle-like syndromes may occur whenever a gene for sickle trait is inherited together with a gene for another variant hemoglobin or for thalassemia. Although mild chronic hemolysis occurs with homozygous hemoglobinopathies such as hemoglobin C disease, renal manifestations are not a feature. However, if hemoglobin S trait is inherited with a second variant hemoglobin such as hemoglobin C, the clinical features of sickle cell disease may be mimicked. Symptoms of hemoglobin S disease (SS) are the most severe, all other combinations being less so. The relative severity of these combined disorders may be predicted by *in vitro* studies of the gelling characteristics of mixtures of hemoglobin S and other variants. Of the combination syndromes, SC disease (SC-Harlem, or SC- α-thalassemia) are the most affected.[33] SO-Arab disease may be clinically indistinguishable from SS disease since hemoglobin O-Arab reacts strongly with hemoglobin S *in vitro*. In addition, this variant hemoglobin migrates with S in acid buffer and has the electrophoretic mobility of C at alkaline pH. However, it is easily distinguishable from SC disease because of the prominence of symptoms, the severity of anemia, and presence of many irreversibly sickled cells on blood smear. SD-Punjab (SD-Los Angeles) has symptoms of mild sickle cell anemia; asymptomatic hematuria may occur.

Hemoglobin S/β thalassemia is clinically similar to sickle cell disease, but is less severe, and has much clinical variation. As expected, β^+ thalassemia heterozygotes have milder disease than those with β^0 thalassemia trait. Hemoglobin S-Lepore (S-Pylos) disease is another sickling disorder of moderate severity.[36]

No sickling occurs in those individuals doubly heterozygote for hemoglobin S and hereditary persistence of fetal hemoglobin (HPFH) since the protective benefit of hemoglobin F is distributed equally among all cells. As the gene for HPFH occurs in 0.1% of blacks,[2] this double heterozygote is not rare and provides another example of "balanced polymorphism." Similarly, no increased morbidity has been identified in those with sickle trait and G6PD deficiency.[37]

II. Metabolic Disorders

A. Renal Manifestations of Paroxysmal Nocturnal Hemoglobinuria

Paroxysmal nocturnal hemoglobinuria (PNH) is a rare acquired chronic disorder of the hemopoietic stem cell characterized by recurrent episodes of intravascular hemolysis and hemoglobinuria. Venous thrombosis is a frequent complication and is a major cause of death. Aplastic anemia, myelofibrosis, and acute nonlymphoblastic leukemia are less common late complications. The underlying red cell abnormality of PNH is a defect of the erythrocyte membrane that causes an increased sensitivity to fixed complement and subsequent cell lysis by either the classic or alternate pathway.[38–40]

The pathognomonic sign of hemoglobinuria occurs only in about 25% of patients. Nocturnal exacerbation is classical but not always present.[41] Episodes that occur at night have been attributed to CO_2 retention and subsequent plasma acidosis. It is probable that acidosis is greater in organs with sluggish blood flow, such as the kidney, particularly in the renal medulla, thereby producing a suitable environment for hemolysis of susceptible cells.[42] A similar mechanism has been proposed to explain exacerbations of hemolysis after strenuous exercise.[43] However, avoidance of CO_2 retention has not prevented episodes of sleep-associated hemolysis.[44]

Since the characteristic episodes of gross hemoglobinuria do not often occur, patients may present only with chronic anemia or hemolysis.[45] Episodes of hemolysis may be asymptomatic but, when severe, abdominal and lumbar back pain may occur. Microscopic hematuria is commonly found. The plasma may be golden brown in color with increased levels of unconjugated bilirubin, free hemoglobin, and methemalbumin if serum haptoglobin has been depleted.[41] Serum LDH may be markedly elevated. The urine contains urobilinogen, albumin, and free hemoglobin during episodes of lysis.

The presence of hemoglobin in the urine can be confirmed by spectroscopic examination. Because of massive hemosiderin deposition in the proximal renal tubular cells, iron is easily identified in the urinary sediment with Prussian blue staining. Dacie has calculated the mean daily urinary iron loss in PNH to be 15.9 mg, even in the absence of hemoglobinuria,[44] compared to less than 0.1 mg per day in normal subjects.

1. *Renal Changes of PNH*

Many chronic changes develop in the kidneys of PNH patients (Table IV) although the renal changes are infrequently of clinical importance. In 21 patients followed by Clark and colleagues[45] over many years, intermittent albuminuria was noted in most patients. Microscopic hematuria was usually present in all patients, even in the absence of hemoglobinuria. Only three patients initially presented with gross hematuria. Urinary concentrating defects were found within 5 years of onset of PNH in all patients and many developed decreased glomerular filtration rates (GFR). Most had enlarged kidneys as shown by intravenous pyelography or isotope scanning with delayed appearance of vascular blush, suggesting a concentrating defect in the absence of outflow obstruction.

2. *Treatment*

Because angiographic dye can activate complement in PNH,[46] radiographic studies should be performed with caution and only for specific indications. Similarly, dehydration should be avoided because it may induce thrombosis in this disorder. Since plasma infusion may precipitate intravascular hemolysis due to complement repletion, this should be avoided whenever possible. Because of this, red cells should be washed before transfusion. Heparin may reduce hemoglobinuria since it appears to block hemolysis of PNH cells *in vitro*. Anticoagulation with heparin or coumadin has a role in the prevention and management of venous thrombosis in PNH.[47]

B. Porphyrias

The porphyrias result from enzyme defects in heme synthesis.[48] Several of these clinical syndromes are associated with pigmented urine.

Table IV
Renal Abnormalities in Paroxysmal Nocturnal Hemoglobinuria

- Hemoglobinuria related to episodes of intravascular hemolysis
- Hemosiderin deposition in proximal tubules and renal tubular acidosis
- Chronic microscopic hematuria
- Proteinuria
- Hyposthenuria
- Cortical infarction due to microvascular obstruction
- Papillary necrosis
- Urate nephropathy
- Chronic progressive impairment of creatinine clearance
- Radiological features:
    - Enlarged kidneys
    - Cortical infarction
    - Cortical thinning
    - Papillary necrosis

Adapted from Clark DA, et al.: *Blood*. 57:83, 1981.[45]

Congenital erythropoietic porphyria (Gunther's disease) is an autosomal recessive condition that presents in early childhood. It causes red urine, hirsutism, and severe bullous cutaneous lesions. Splenomegaly and hemolysis are usually present.[49] The red urine is due to increased formation of uroporphyrin because of lowered levels of uroporphyrinogen III cosynthetase.

Acute intermittent porphyria (AIP), an autosomal dominant disease, is associated with development of dark brown-red urine during characteristic episodes of abdominal pain. However, urine of normal color does not exclude the diagnosis. The urinary chromogen, porphobilinogen (PBG), is colorless and is excreted in increased amounts in AIP. If the urine is acid or is left standing, it will gradually oxidize darker, forming uroporphyrin and porphobilin. Ehrlich's reagent causes porphobilinogen and urobilinogen to turn pink or red. Urobilinogen is colorless but becomes red-brown when oxidized, the basis of the Watson-Schwartz test.

Porphyria cutanea tarda may also be associated with red urine because of increased urophyrin and caproporphyrin excretion.

III. Hemolytic Syndromes That Cause Hemoglobinuria Without Hematuria

Hemoglobinuria, that is, free hemoglobin in the urine, must be distinguished from hematuria, that is, free red cells in the urine. Hemolytic syndromes cause the former, but not the latter. Hemoglobinuria is present when hemoglobin is identified in the cell-free supernatant of centrifuged urine. (Note, however, that red cell lysis in hypo-osmotic stagnant urine may also release hemoglobin.) The presumed source of the red cells can be distinguished by examining the urinary sediment with Wright's stain (see Chapter 4).[50] Laboratory studies can document the presence and magnitude of the hemolysis, which is usually intravascular whenever hemoglobinuria is present. Such studies include Coombs' test, free plasma hemoglobin, LDH, indirect bilirubin, haptoglobin, methemalbumin and, occasionally, hemopexin levels. The peripheral blood smear should always be examined for altered red cell morphology. The reticulocyte count reflects the bone marrow response to increased red cell destruction. Prussian blue stain of the urinary sediment may reveal hemosiderin-laden cells consistent with hemoglobinuria. Further evaluation of the cause of hemolysis should be dictated by the clinical setting after the review of the urinary sediment, Coombs' test, and erythrocyte morphology.

Hemolysis may accompany many diseases (please refer to general texts of hematology for complete discussions). These include congenital diseases, such as G6PD deficiency; acquired diseases, such as infections associated with malaria, *Clostridium welchii*, burns, or microangiopathic anemias; and iatrogenic events, such as drug reactions, transfusion mismatches, water intoxication, or cardiac valve surgery.[51–53]

IV. Myoglobinuria

Muscle damage associated with extensive trauma or crush injury is a well-known cause of pigment-induced renal impairment, although the mechanism of the renal injury remains obscure. Nontraumatic rhabdomyolysis may also cause renal damage and may be due to:

- increased muscle oxygen consumption, e.g. heat stroke, severe exercise or seizures
- decreased muscle energy production, e.g. hypokalemia, hypophosphatemia, genetic enzyme deficiencies (McArdle's disease), or carnitine palmityl transferase deficiency
- muscle ischemia, e.g. arterial insufficiency, anterior pretibial compartment syndrome, sickle cell disease
- infections, e.g. viral influenza, tetanus, gas gangrene
- direct muscle toxins, e.g. alcohol, "Haff" disease.

A rare form of familial myoglobinuria, Meyer-Betz paroxysmal myoglobinuria, may occur following infection or strenuous exertion. In this syndrome, muscle weakness, stiffness, tenderness, or swelling may be variable, and the degree of renal damage determines the outcome, as in other cases of myoglobinuria.

Myoglobinuria may also occur after prolonged EACA administration, used to prevent hemorrhage in hereditary angioneurotic edema,[54] or rebleeding in subarachnoid hemorrhage.[55,56] This is a rare complication, associated with a high total dose of EACA, such as greater than 24 g/day for over 4 weeks.[57] The mechanism by which EACA causes muscle damage is not known.

Table V
Evaluation of Pigmented Urine

- Demonstration that the urinary pigment is a protein
  - Add 3 ml 30 g/liter sulfosalicylic acid to 1 ml supernatant of centrifuged fresh urine. Mix and filter. If pigment is a protein, it will be precipitated.
- Microscopic examination of fresh urine sample
  - Intact erythrocytes: Hematuria.
- Dipstick testing for presence of occult blood
  - "Occultest" or "Hemostix" (Ames), benzidine or orthotoluidine reactions.
  - Hemoglobin and myoglobin produce a positive reaction.
- Inspection of plasma color
  - Normal straw color: myoglobinuria.
  - Pink-red: hemoglobinuria (when plasma hemoglobin > 50 mg/dl).
- Identification of myoglobin in urine
  - Add 2.8 g $(NH_4)_2SO_4$ to 5 ml urine (final solution 80% saturated).
  - Myoglobin remains in solution (filtrate normally colored).
  - Hemoglobin precipitates (filtrate normal color, precipitate pigmented).
- Electrophoresis of urine
  - Paper, starch, acrylamide gels
  - CO increases separation of (carboxy) Hb and (carboxy) Mb bands
- Spectrophotometry of plasma*
  - CO improves separation of (carboxy) Hb and (carboxy) Mb
  - The presence of MetHb is pathomnemonic of intravascular hemolysis.
  - MetHb has maximal absorption at 630 nm.
- Screen for urinary porphyrins

*Differentiation between myoglobin and hemoglobin is difficult in urine, since very small differences are seen by spectrometry and both pigments are rapidly degraded to other compounds of different absorption spectra, e.g. hematin.

Myoglobin, an iron-containing molecule with a molecular weight of 17,000, is released into the circulation whenever striated muscle is damaged. Because of its relatively small size, it is rapidly cleared by the renal glomeruli without altering plasma color. Myoglobin is probably not directly nephrotoxic, although tubular obstruction may occur due to myoglobin precipitation and cast formation.[58] Other muscle breakdown products may be nephrotoxic. Decreased renal perfusion due to concurrent depletion of intravascular volume may contribute further to the acute tubular necrosis of rhabdomyolysis.

Myoglobinuria is often confused with hemoglobinuria, the distinction being of great clinical importance (Table V). Intravascular hemolysis releases hemoglobin into plasma. Hemoglobin is rapidly bound to circulating haptoglobin and the resulting complex is cleared within hours by the reticuloendothelial system. Any excess free hemoglobin will color plasma, in contrast to circulating myoglobin. Whenever the haptoglobin-binding capacity is exceeded, hemoglobinuria will occur, resulting in the formation of colored urine. The color ranges from light pink to red to black and is dependent on the concentration of hemoglobin, its state of oxidation, and the extent of heme dissociation.[59] As with myoglobin, pure hemoglobin is probably not directly nephrotoxic, but obstruction by red cell stroma and renal hypoperfusion may contribute to the development of acute renal failure. Myoglobin and hemoglobin have similar absorption spectra, making identification of each protein by spectrometry difficult in a clinical setting. Therefore, other tests are performed to distinguish between them whenever intravascular hemolysis or rhabdomyolysis is suspected. Confirmation that the urinary pigment is due to protein can be made by adding sulfosalicylic acid to a urine sample: If the pigment is a protein, it will be precipitated[60] (Table V).

V. Pigmenturia

Many ingested agents will cause benign pigmenturia. These agents include foods, drugs, and in some cases, toxins. In the differential management of such cases, it is critical to obtain an accurate history of recent ingestion and to examine urine color. Table VI lists the potential causes for various urine colors.

VI. Renal Manifestations of Hematologic Malignancies

A. Lymphoproliferative Disorders

Renal dysfunction is rarely a presenting problem in myeloma or Waldenstrom's macroglobinemia, but may develop during the course of these disorders, more frequently in the former.[61,62] Hypercalcemia, amyloidosis, Bence-Jones proteinuria, glomerulosclerosis or Fanconi's syndrome due to tubular infiltration or protein deposition, or renal tubular acidosis may be responsible. Hematuria is rare in these conditions. Extensive renal infiltrates of lymphocytes and plasma cells have been reported in one-third of autopsied patients with myeloma, amyloid being found only rarely.[62]

The nephrotic syndrome is an unusual paraneoplastic syndrome. However, Hodgkin's disease, non-Hodgkin's lymphoma, and leukemia have been described in association with it.[63] Lipoid nephrosis is the predominant renal lesion

Table VI
Causes of Urinary Pigments that Can Mimic Hematuria or Hemoglobinuria

Red:	food pigments (beets)
	phenolphthalein
	pyramidon
	sulfonal
	picric acid
	phenazopyridine
Orange:	santonin
	cryptophanic acid
	associated urobilinogen
Red-Brown (if acidic) or Bright Red (if alkaline):	rhubarb
	senna
	chelidonium
	cascara
	aloes
Yellow-Brown to Brown or Black:	acidified hematin
	cutaneous porphyria
	melanin
	phenol
	alkaptonuria (Homogentisic acid)
	ochronosis

Adapted from Urinalysis and Renal Function Tests, *Physician's Hand Book*. Krupp MA, Sweet NJ, Jawitz E, et al. Eds. Los Altos, California, Lang Medical Publications, 1968, p. 108.

in this group of disorders and may be due to impairment of T-lymphocyte functions.[64] Less commonly, immunological mechanisms causing the nephrotic syndrome have been described in Waldenstrom's macroglobinemia[65] and chronic lymphocytic leukemia,[66] with glomerular deposition of complement and immunoglobulin G and M. These may be due to circulating immune complexes, perhaps induced by oncogenic viruses or cellular debris from the malignant cells.[63]

Autopsy studies have revealed frequent microscopic involvement of the kidneys and lymphoma,[67] although this has usually been clinically silent.[68,69] Lymphomatous infiltration of the bladder is far less common, but occurs with extensive visceral involvement or by invasion from adjacent massive pelvic infiltrates. Major bladder involvement is frequently associated with infiltrates of the gonads, uterus, adrenal glands, and kidney at autopsy.[67] Primary lymphoma of the bladder is rare.[68]

Uremia is infrequently associated with lymphomatous involvement of the kidneys but has been described as the presenting problem in lymphocytic lymphoma[70] and Hodgkin's disease.[71] We have recently observed the development of uremia due to occult renal involvement in a patient with chronic lymphocytic leukemia[72] (Fig. 3). More commonly, renal impairment is related to bilateral ureteric obstruction because of massive retroperitoneal adenopathy, nephrocalcinosis with hypercalcemia, or urate nephropathy (Fig. 4). Acute renal failure can follow tumor lysis, presenting with hyperphosphatemia and hyperphosphaturia or with hyperuricemia.[73–76] This may be exaggerated when renal dysfunction is already present.

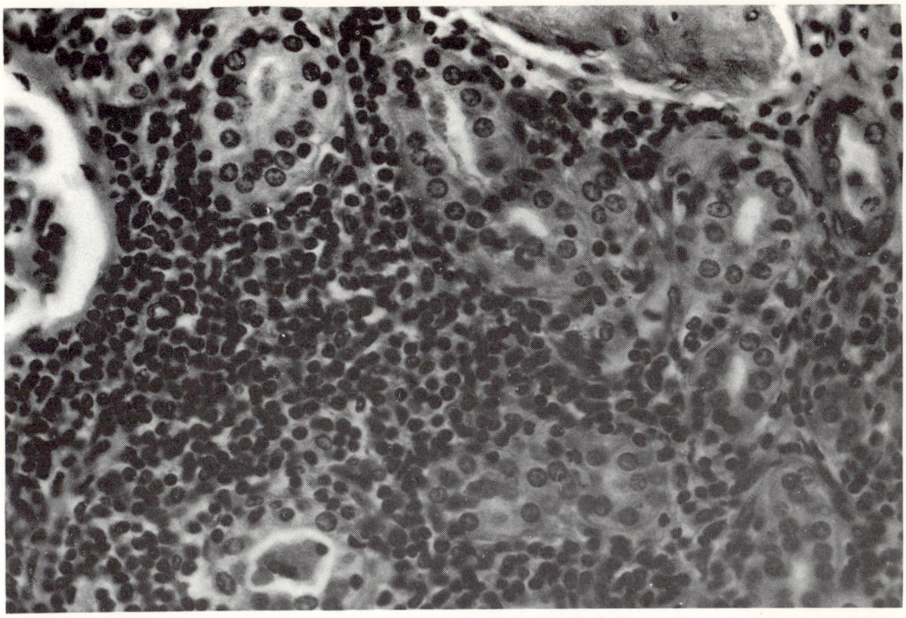

Figure 3: *Photomicrograph demonstrating cellular infiltrates into the kidney by chronic lymphocytic leukemia (100×).*

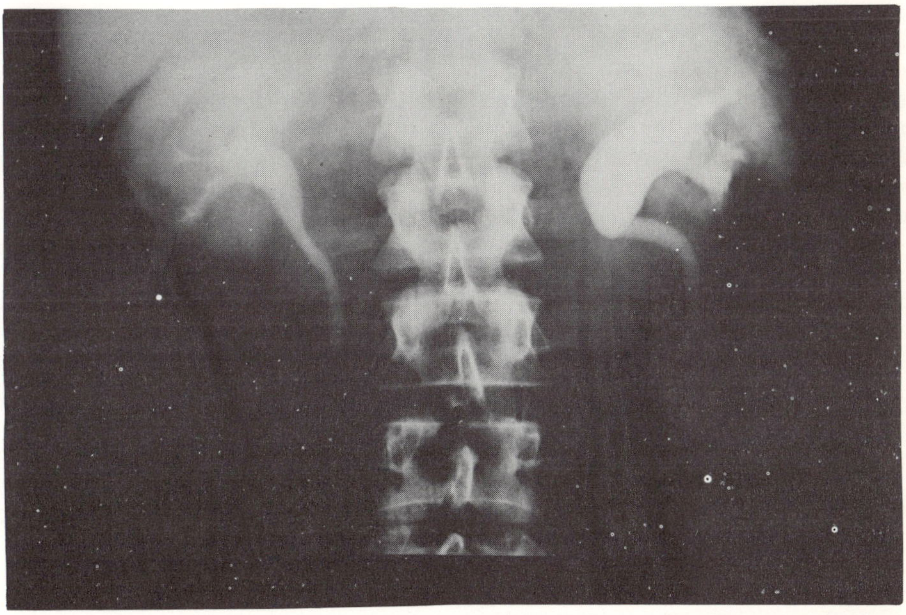

Figure 4: *Excretory phase of intravenous pyelogram demonstrating deplacement of ureters by retroperitoneal lymph nodes enlarged by lymphoma. (From the Learning File of the Center for Devices and Radiological Health, FDA, case GU701.)*

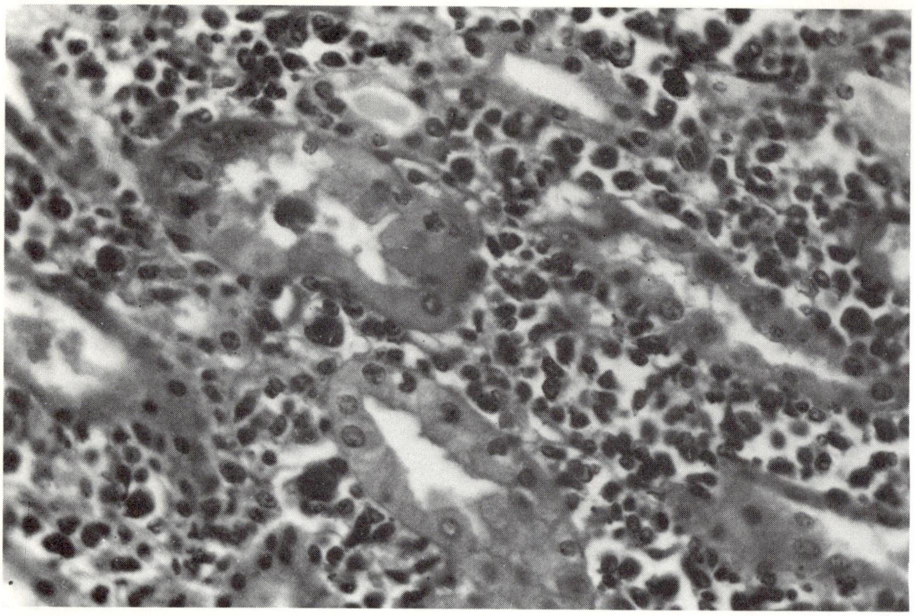

Figure 5: *Photomicrograph demonstrating cellular infiltrate into the kidney by acute nonlymphoblastic leukemia (250×).*

B. Myeloproliferative Disorders

Many renal lesions occur in acute nonlymphoblastic leukemia. These include microscopic or macroscopic hematuria due to thrombycytopenia, disseminated intravascular coagulation, infection, or urate nephropathy. Microscopic leukemic infiltration of the kidneys and the bladder is a common autopsy finding,[67] but it is only of clinical significance if hemorrhage or renal tubular defects occur[77] (Fig. 5). Most infiltrates are not associated with renal impairment. Leukemic infiltration of the kidneys and, to a lesser extent, the bladder, is usually associated with widespread involvement of other extramedullary sites.[67] Such involvement has also been reported in chronic granulocytic leukemia.[67]

REFERENCES

1. Wintrobe MM, Lee GR, Boggs DR, Bithell TC, Foerster J (Eds). Hemoglobinopathies S, C, D, E, and O and associated diseases. In: *Clinical Hematology* (8th Ed). Philadelphia, Lea & Febiger, 1981, pp. 835–868.
2. Motulsky AG: Frequency of sickling disorders in U.S. Blacks. *N. Engl J Med.*288:31–33, 1973.
3. Ashcroft MT, Desai PJ: Mortality and morbidity in Jamaican adults with sickle cell trait and with normal haemoglobin followed up for twelve years. *Lancet.* 2:784–786, 1976.
4. Lewis EL, Ross JR, Cohn JH: Hematuria and sickle cell disorders. *South Med J.* 70:432–433, 1977.

5. Sears DA. The morbidity of sickle cell trait: A review of the literature. *Am J Med.* 64:1021–1036, 1978.
6. Whalley PJ, Martin FG, Pritchard JA: Sickle cell trait and urinary tract infection during pregnancy. *JAMA.* 189:903–906, 1964.
7. Karayalcon G, Rosner F, Kim KY, Chanera P, Aballi AJ. Sickle cell anemia: Clinical manifestations in 100 patients and review of the literature. *Am J Med Sci.* 269:51–68, 1978.
8. McCrudy PR: Abnormal hemoglobins and pregnancy. *Am J Obstet Gynecol.* 90:891–896, 1964.
9. Whalley PJ, Pritchard JA, Richards JR Jr: Sickle cell trait and pregnancy. *JAMA.* 186:1132–1135, 1963.
10. Perille PE, Epstein FH: Sickling phenomenon produced by hypertonic solutions: A possible explanation for the hyposthenuria of sicklemia. *J Clin Invest.* 42:570–580, 1963.
11. Knochel JP: Hematuria in sickle cell trait: The effect of intravenous administration of distilled water, urinary alkalization, and diuresis. *Arch Intern Med.* 123:160–165, 1969.
12. Atkinson DW: Sickling and hematuria. *Blood.* 34:736–737, 1969. (Abstr.).
13. Lucas WM, Bullock WH: Hematuria in sickle cell disease. *J Urol.* 83:733–741, 1960.
14. Berman LB: Sickle cell nephropathy. *JAMA.* 228:1279, 1974.
15. Gold MS, Williams JC, Spivak M, Grann V: Sickle cell anemia and hyperuricemia. *JAMA* 206:1572–1573, 1968.
16. Walker BR, Alexander F: Uric acid excretion in sickle cell anemia. *JAMA.* 215:255–258, 1971.
17. Friedman EA, Rao TKS, Sprung CL, Smith A, Manis T, Bellevue R, Butt KMA: Uremia in sickle-cell anemia treated by maintenance hemodialysis. *N Engl J Med.* 291:431–435, 1974.
18. Susmano S, Lewy JE: Sickle cell disease and acute glomerulonephritis. *Am J Dis Child.* 118:615–618, 1969.
19. Brody JI, Levison SP, Jung CJ: Sickle cell trait and hematuria associated with von Willebrand syndromes. *Ann Intern Med.* 86:529–533, 1977.
20. Buckalew VM Jr, Someren A: Renal manifestations of sickle cell disease. *Arch Intern Med.* 133:660–669, 1974.
21. Mostofi FK, Vorder Bruegge CF, Diggs LW: Lesions in kidneys removed for unilateral hematuria in sickle cell disease. *Arch Pathol.* 63:336–351, 1957.
22. Pitcock JA, Muirhead E, Hatch FE, Johnson JG, Kelly BJ: Early renal changes in sickle cell anemia. *Arch. Pathol.* 90:403–410, 1970.
23. Statius van Eps LW, Pinedo-Veels C, de Vries GH Jr, de Koning J: Nature of concentrating defect in sickle-cell nephropathy. Microradiographic studies. *Lancet.* 1:450–452, 1970.
24. Pariser S: Oral urea treatment of hematuria in sickle-cell trait. *NY State J Med.* 74:2238–2240, 1974.
25. Marynick SP, Ramsey EJ, Knochel JP: The effect of bicarbonate and distilled water on sickle cell trait hematuria and in vitro studies on the interaction of osmolality and pH on erythrocyte sickling in sickle cell trait. *J Urol.* 118:793–796, 1977.
26. Laszlo J, Obenour W Jr, Saltzman HA: Effects of hyperbaric oxygenation on sickle syndromes. *Southern Med J.* 62:453–456, 1969.
27. Harrison FG, Harrison FG Jr: Hematuria with sickle cell disease. *J Urol.* 68:943–949, 1952.
28. Black WD, Hatch FE, Acchiardo S: Aminocaproic acid in prolonged hematuria of patients with sicklemia. *Arch Intern Med.* 136:678–681, 1976.
29. McNicol GP, Fletcher AP, Alkjaersig N, Sherry S: The use of epsilon aminocaproic acid, a potent inhibitor of fibrinolytic activity, in the management of postoperative hematuria. *J Urol.* 86:829–837, 1961.
30. John EG, Schade SG, Spigos DG, Cort JH, Rosenthal IM. Effectiveness of triglycyl vasopressin in persistent hematuria associated with sickle cell hemoglobin. *Arch Intern Med.* 140:1589–1593, 1980.

31. Cash JD, Gader AM, Mulder JL, Cort JH. Structure-activity relations of the fibrinolytic response to vasopressins in man. *Clin Sci Mol Med*. 54:403–409, 1978.
32. Chang H, Ewert SM, Bookshin RM, Nagel RL. Comparative evaluation of fifteen anti-sickling agents. *Blood*. 61:693–704, 1983.
33. Dean J, and Schechter AN: Sickle-cell anemia: Molecular and cellular bases of therapeutic approaches. *N Engl J Med*. 299:863–870, 1978.
34. Lund HG, Cordonnier JJ, Forbes KA: Gross hematuria in sickle cell disease. *J Urol*. 71:151–158, 1954.
35. Bennett MA, Heslop RW, Meynell MJ: Massive haematuria associated with sickle cell trait. *Br Med J*. 1:677–679, 1967.
36. Stamatoyannopoulos G, Fessas P: Observations on hemoglobin "Pylos": The hemoglobin Pylos-hemoglobin S combination. *J Lab Clin Med*. 62:193–200, 1963.
37. Heller P, Best WR, Nelson RB, Becktel J: Clinical implications of sickle cell trait and glucose-6-phosphate dehydrogenase deficiency in hospitalized black male patients. *N Engl J Med*. 300:1001–1005, 1979.
38. Packman CH, Rosenfeld SI, Jenskins DE Jr, Thiem PA, Leddy JP: Complement lysis of human erythrocytes. *J Clin Invest*. 64:428–433, 1979.
39. Ross WF: Paroxysmal nocturnal hemoglobinuria: Present status and future prospects. *West J Med*. 132:219–228, 1980.
40. Wintrobe MM, Lee GR, Boggs DR, Bithell TC, Foerster J (Eds). Paroxysmal nocturnal hemoglobinuria (PNH), In: *Clinical Hematology* (8th Ed). Philadelphia, Lea & Febiger, 1981, pp. 978–990.
41. Harris JH, Kellermeyer RW: *The Red Cell* (Revised Ed). Cambridge, Harvard University Press, 1970.
42. Crosby WH: Paroxysmal nocturnal hemoglobinuria: Plasma factors of the hemolytic system. *Blood*. 8:444–458, 1953.
43. Blum SF, Sullivan JM, Gardner FH: The exacerbation of hemolysis in paroxysmal nocturnal hemoglobinuria by strenuous exercise. *Blood*. 30:513–517, 1967.
44. Dacie JV: *The Haemolytic Anaemias, Congenital and Acquired*. Part IV. New York, Grune and Stratton, 1967.
45. Clark DA, Butler SA, Braren V, Hartmann RC, Jenkins DE Jr. The kidneys in paroxysmal nocturnal hemoglobinuria. *Blood*. 57, 83–89, 1981.
46. Kolb WP, Lang JH, Lasser EC. Nonimmunologic complement activation in normal human serum induced by radiographic contrast media. *J Immunol*. 121:1232–1238, 1978.
47. Hartmann RC, Kolhouse JF: Viewpoints on the management of PNH. *Series Haematol*. 5(3): 42–60, 1972.
48. Tschudy DP. The Porphyrias. In: *Hematology*. Williams WJ, Beutler E, Erslev AJ, et al., Eds. New York, McGraw-Hill, pp. 691–703, 1983.
49. Ippen H, Fuchs T. Congenital porphyria. *Clin Haematol*. 9:323–344, 1980.
50. Chang BS. Red cell morphology as a diagnostic aid in hematuria. *JAMA*. 252:1747–1749, 1984.
51. Beutler E. Hemolytic anemia due to infections with microorganisms. In: *Hematology*. Williams WJ, Beutler E, Erslev AJ, et al., Eds. New York, McGraw-Hill, 1983, pp. 628–631.
52. Landsteiner EK, Finch CA. Hemoglobinemia accompanying transurethral resection of the prostrate. *N Engl J Med*. 237:310–312, 1947.
53. Schen SC, Ham TH, Fleming EM. Studies on the destruction of red blood cells III mechanisms and complications of hemoglobinuria in patients with thermal burns: Spherocytosis and increased osmotic fragility of red blood cells. *N Engl J Med*. 229:701–713, 1943.
54. Frank MM, Sergent JS, Kane MA, Alling DW. Epsilon aminocaproic acid therapy of hereditary angioneurotic edema: A double-blind study. *N Engl J Med*. 286:808–812, 1972.
55. Chowdhary UM, Carey PC, Hussein MM: Prevention of early recurrence of spontaneous subarachnoid hemorrhage by epsilon aminocaproic acid. *Lancet*. 1:741–743, 1979.

56. Nibbelink DW, Torner JC, Henderson WG: Intracranial aneurysms and subarachnoid hemorrhage: A cooperative study. Antifibrinolytic therapy in recent onset subarachnoid hemorrhage. *Stroke*. 6:622–629, 1975.
57. Brodkin HM: Myoglobinuria following epsilon aminocaproic acid (EACA) therapy. *J Neurosurg*. 53:690–692, 1980.
58. Anderson RJ, Schrier RW: Acute renal failure. In: *Harrison's Principles of Internal Medicine* (9th Ed.) Isselbacher KJ, Adams RD, Braunwald E, et al., Eds. New York, McGraw-Hill, 1980.
59. Wintrobe MM, Lee GR, Boggs DR, Bithell TC, Foerster J (Eds). The hemolytic disorders: General considerations. In: *Clinical Hematology* (8th Ed). Philadelphia, Lea & Febiger, 1981, pp. 734–754.
60. Blodheim SH, Margoliash E, Shafrir E: A simple test for myohemoglobinuria (myoglobinuria). JAMA. 167:453–454, 1958.
61. Fudenberg HH, Virella G: Multiple myeloma and Waldenstrom macroglobulinemia: Unusual presentations. *Semin Hematol*. 17:63–79, 1980.
62. MacKenzie MR, Fudenberg HH: Macroglobulinemia: An analysis for 40 patients. *Blood*. 39:874–889, 1972.
63. Gagliano RG, Costanzi JJ, Beathard GA, Arles HE, Bell JD: The nephrotic syndrome associated with neoplasia: An unusual paraneoplastic syndrome. Report of a case and review of the literature. *Am J Med*. 60:1026–1031, 1976.
64. Shalhoub RJ: Pathogenesis of lipoid nephrosis: A disorder of T-cell function. *Lancet*. 2:556–560, 1974.
65. Martelo OJ, Shultz DR, Pardo V, Perez-Stable E: Immunologically-mediated renal disease in Waldenstrom's macroglobulinemia. *Am J Med*. 58:567–575, 1975.
66. Dathan JRE, Heyworth MF, Maciver AG: Nephrotic syndrome in chronic lymphocytic leukemia. *Br Med J*. 3:655–657, 1974.
67. Givler RL: Involvement of the bladder in leukemia and lymphoma. *J Urol*. 105:667–670, 1971.
68. Rosenberg SA, Diamond HD, Jaslowitz B, Craver LF: Lymphosarcoma: A review of 1269 cases. *Medicine*. 40:31–84, 1961.
69. Richmond J, Sherman RS, Diamond HD, Craver LF: Renal lesions associated with malignant lymphomas. *Am J Med*. 32:184–207, 1962.
70. Ellman L, Davis J, Lichtenstein NS: Uremia due to occult lymphomatous infiltration of the kidneys. *Cancer*. 33:203–205, 1974.
71. Champion AE, Coup AJ, Hancock BW: Hodgkin's disease and chronic renal failure. *Cancer*. 38:1867–1868, 1976.
72. Wallach SR, Kaldany A: Personal observation.
73. Monballyu J, Zachee P, Verberckmoes R, Boogaerts MA. Transient acute renal failure due to tumor-lysis-induced severe phosphate loss in a patient with Burkett's lymphoma. *Clin Nephrol*. 22:47–50, 1984.
74. Cohen LF, Balow JE, Margarth IT, Poplack DG, Ziegler JL. Acute tumor lysis syndrome: A review of 37 patients with Burkitt's lymphoma. *Am J Med*. 68:486–491, 1980.
75. Lynch RE, Kjellstrand CM, Coccia PF. Renal and metabolic complications of childhood non-Hodgkins lymphoma. *Semin Oncol*. 4:325–334, 1977.
76. Tsokos GC, Balow JE, Spiegel RJ, Magrath, IT. Renal and metabolic complications of undifferentiated and lymphoblastic lymphomas. *Medicine* (Baltimore). 60:218–229, 1981.
77. O'Regan S, Carson S, Chesney RW, Drummond KN: Electrolyte and acid-base disturbances in the management of leukemia. *Blood*. 49:345–353, 1977.

Chapter 4

Nephritic Causes of Hematuria

Antoine Kaldany, M.D.

The syndrome of "nephritis" refers to inflammatory responses within the nephron where there is injury, possibly progressive destruction, followed by repair and/or scarring of renal capillaries. In acute nephritis, one expects hematuria plus one or more of the following: oliguria, decreased glomerular filtration rate, proteinuria, peripheral edema, and hypertension.

Hematuria, whether gross or microscopic, symptomatic or asymptomatic, must always be considered to be the manifestation of a potentially serious underlying disease until proven otherwise and should never be ignored. The degree of hematuria bears no relationship to the possible cause. We shall review the disease processes involving different segments of the nephron, and analyze the resulting syndromes of hematuria. Table I offers a summary of the diseases to be discussed and their pertinent laboratory findings.

I. Diagnostic Approach to Nephritic Causes of Hematuria

A. Identification and Characterization

The diagnostic approach to the problem of hematuria should be comprehensive. The patient's past and familial history are crucial. Consideration should be given to benign causes of hematuria such as jogging or exercise. The medication history deserves close scrutiny for anticoagulants, bladder irritants (cyclophosphamide, cadmium, etc.) and nephrotoxic chemicals, especially chronic analgesic abuse. One should also rule out any systemic diseases. (Table II).

The famous "three glass test" for the timing of gross hematuria can provide useful clues: (1) Bleeding at onset of urination suggests the presence of lesions

From Bern MM (ed.): *Urinary Tract Bleeding: Diagnosis and Control by Medical, Radiologic, and Surgical Techniques.* Mount Kisco, NY, Futura Publishing Co., Inc., 1985.

Table I
Summary of Nephritic Diseases Causing Hematuria

Renal Disease	Hematuria	Complement	Nephrotic Syndrome	Blood Pressure	Other	Treatment	Outcome
1. Minimal Change Disease	Microscopic	N or low N	Severe	N	Low IgG	Steroids Usually Effective	Usually Favorable
2. Mesangial-Proliferative Glomerulonephritis	Microscopic	N or low N	Severe	N	Low IgG	Steroids Usually Ineffective	Usually Unfavorable
3. IgA Nephropathy	Macro- and Microscopic	N	Rare	N or Elevated	N or High IgA	None	Variable
4. Focal Sclerosis Glomerulonephritis	Microscopic	N or low N	Frequent	N or Elevated	Look for Reflux Nephropathy	None	Progressive Azotemia
5. Membranous Glomerulonephritis	Microscopic	Low or N	Frequent, Severe	N or Elevated		Steroids	Variable
6. Membranoproliferative Glomerulonephritis Type I	Micro- or Macroscopic	Low C_3, C_4 C_{1q} N	Frequent	Elevated	C_3 Nephritic Factor	None Proven Effective	Unfavorable
7. Membranoproliferative Glomerulonephritis Type II	Micro- or Macroscopic	Low C_3, C_4 C_{1q} N	Frequent	Elevated	C_3 Nephritic Factor	None Proven Effective	Unfavorable Recurs in Transplants
8. Rapidly Progressive Glomerulonephritis	Micro- or Macroscopic	Variable	May exist	Elevated		High Doses of Steroids	Variable
9. Systemic Lupus Erythematosis	Micro- or Macroscopic	Low	Frequent	Elevated	Anti-DNA Antibodies	Cytoxic Drugs and Steroids	Variable

N = normal; C = complement

Table II
Factors to Consider in Diagnosis of Hematuria

- Symptoms with bleeding? (pain, colic, voiding problems, etc.)
- Trauma and/or physical exercise
- Familial history of hematuria
- Medications (anticoagulants. . .)
- Systemic illness: fever, skin rashes, purpura, etc.
- Cardiovascular system: hypertension, heart rate
- Hepatic disease? coagulopathy?
- Other: sickle cell disease, hyperuricemia, etc.

below the bladder. (2) Bleeding throughout urination suggests either a renal or a vesical (bladder) etiology. (3) Terminal hematuria suggests trouble at bladder neck or prostrate.

As a rule, patients with glomerular disease have hematuria associated with proteinuria. Some patients with glomerular bleeding do not have proteinuria. If the urinalysis shows red blood cell or hemoglobin casts, especially in the presence of significant proteinuria or azotemia, a glomerular etiology is most likely. Yet even in the absence of red blood cell casts and proteinuria, glomerular bleeding can be distinguished from other causes of hematuria by careful microscopic examination of the urine sediment.[1,2] As far back as 1948, Addis[3] observed "dysmorphic" red blood cells in urine samples from patients with glomerular disease. A recent report by Fairley and Birch[4] expands Addis' observations and showed a very high correlation between glomerular disease and dysmorphic red blood cells in urine sediment ($p < 0.001$). Under phase contrast microscopy, red blood cells found in the urine sediment have alterations and ruptures of their plasma membranes, with alterations in red cell density.[4] These changes are found with all forms of glomerulonephritis, from minimal change disease to membranous to proliferative lesions. Red cells derived from lesions other than glomerular have an appearance similar to that of peripheral blood.[1]

B. Primary Glomerular Disease

1. Minimal Change Disease: (Lipoid Nephrosis)

a. Clinical and Laboratory Features: Although it is seen most often in children between the ages of 2 and 8, minimal change disease can affect all age groups. It is typically associated with heavy proteinuria, including the nephrotic syndrome.[5] Microhematuria is seen in 20–25% of the patients in the early phase of the illness.[6] Renal function may be normal, but mild azotemia is also observed.[7] The serum complement components C_3 and C_4 are usually unchanged, although the total hemolytic complement, CH_{50}, may be slightly depressed in those with severe, persistent hematuria.[8] Serum IgG may be decreased.[8]

b. Pathogenesis: The pathogenesis is still unclear. Idiopathic minimal change disease has recently been associated with HLA-B12 antigen in patients suffering from atopic skin disease.[9] Similar glomerular "lesions" can be found in patients with lymphomas, including Hodgkin's disease.[10]

c. Pathology: On light microscopy, few mesangial proliferative changes, if any, can be identified by even the trained observer.[6] The immunofluorescence studies are usually negative, with an occasional finding of trace IgM staining in the mesangium.[6] The most dramatic changes are observed with the electron microscope: diffuse foot process fusion and presence of scattered small mesangial deposits.[5,11,12]

d. Course and Management: Many patients experience spontaneous remissions.[13] Yet approximately 95% of the patients with minimal change disease ultimately require and usually respond to prednisone therapy.[5,14] Nonresponders often respond to combinations of prednisone with cyclophosphamide or with chlorambucil.[15] Those who fail on these combination therapies will be shown to have focal sclerosis glomerulonephritis. Very few patients with minimal change glomerulonephritis develop chronic renal failure.[16]

2. *Mesangial Proliferative Glomerulonephritis (Mes-Prolif GN)*

a. Clinical and Laboratory Features: This syndrome is seen mostly in young adults and children. Mes-prolif GN may have an acute onset with severe proteinuria, nephrotic syndrome, with micro- and often macroscopic hematuria. Asymptomatic spontaneous hematuria occurs early in the course of the illness. It usually recurs with relapse. Hypertension is quite frequently present, and renal function is often impaired.[17,18]

b. Pathology: The only change observed on light microscopy is a mild increase in mesangial cellularity. Immunofluorescence reveals IgM deposits in the mesangium. Electron microscopy reveals mesangial deposits in most patients.[17]

3. *IgA Nephropathy (Berger's Disease)*

a. Clinical and Laboratory Features: Berger's disease, which is usually observed in young adult males, is characterized by a recurrent macroscopic hematuria often associated with mild proteinuria. Rarely, a full blown nephrotic syndrome may be seen.[19,20] Hematuria may appear at any time, unrelated to the phase or the rate of progression of the disease.

The clinical picture includes lower back pain, diffuse myalgias, and normal or slightly elevated blood pressure.[20,21] Renal function is often normal.[19] In some patients, serum IgA levels may be elevated.[22] Rarely, however, IgA levels may be depressed. Skin biopsy specimens reveal IgA deposits in dermal capillaries in 90% of the patients.[21,23]

b. Pathology: Mesangial proliferation is most often seen. Immunofluorescence reveals IgA, C_3, and properdin deposits.[21,23]

c. Natural History: This disease may slowly progress to azotemia and renal failure. Unfortunately, there is no known effective treatment to date. It may recur in the kidney allograft.[24]

4. *Focal Sclerosis Glomerulonephritis (FSGN)*

a. **Clinical Syndrome:** This includes proteinuria, hypertension, and possibly microscopic hematuria with progressive azotemia.[18,25] In some patients reflux nephropathy may coexist.

b. **Pathology:** Focal and segmental sclerosis and hyalinosis of some glomeruli with deposition of IgM and C_3 seen sometimes by immunofluorescence.[17]

c. **Clinical History and Management:** The proteinuria is often unresponsive to prednisone.[5] Unfortunately, the renal failure is usually progressive and may recur in the renal allografts.

5. *Membranous Glomerulonephritis*

a. **Clinical Syndrome:** Membranous glomerulonephritis often presents with heavy proteinuria and nephrotic syndrome. Microscopic hematuria may be observed at the onset or with relapse of the disease. Hypertension is infrequent. Renal function may remain normal for many years.[26,27] Complement levels are usually normal at the outset.[27]

Idiopathic membranous glomerulonephritis may show an association with HLA-DRW-3. Similar histological changes may be observed in systemic lupus erythematosis and in association with neoplastic diseases, hepatitis B, and certain drugs (penicillamine, gold, etc.).

b. **Pathology:** The immunofluorescence shows granular fluorescence for IgG, C_3, and C_{1q}. Electron microscopy shows diffuse subepithelial deposits and a few mesangial deposits. There is poor correlation between the histological lesion and proteinuria or the degree of azotemia.[11,28]

c. **Natural History and Management:** Approximately 20–25% of patients with idiopathic membranous glomerulonephritis have spontaneous remissions.[26,27] Persistent hematuria may be an unfavorable sign of persistent disease activity. Otherwise, the disease is slowly progressive and leads to end-stage renal disease. Short-term, high-dose steroid therapy may alter the course and either prevent or delay the progression of the disease.[29] Persistence of the nephrotic range proteinuria despite therapy is a bad omen for the prognosis. Up to 30% of the patients are uremic within 10 years from onset.[26,27]

6. *Membranoproliferative (or Mesangio Capillary) Glomerulonephritis*

a. **Clinical Features:** This disease, seen mostly in adolescents and young adults, may present as acute glomerulonephritis with proteinuria, hematuria, and hypertension. In patients with nephrotic syndrome, recurrent microscopic hematuria with red cell casts is usually present. Gross hematuria is not rare.[30,31] Azotemia and progressive renal failure is the rule, with 50% of the patients becoming uremic within 10 years of onset.[32]

The laboratory profile is distinctive due to the presence of the C_3 convertase of the alternative pathway. C_3 levels are invariably low, while C_4 and C_{1q} levels may be low or normal.[33,34] These lesions can recur in the renal allografts.

b. Classification and Histopathology: Mesangial proliferation and interposition of mesangium within the peripheral capillaries give an overall lobular appearance to the glomeruli on light microscopy. Epithelial cell proliferation and crescent formation may be observed. Electron microscopy and immunofluorescence patterns allow a histological classification of this heterogenous disease.[33,34]

Type I: Subendothelial electron-dense deposits are seen by electron microscopy. Diffuse granular deposits along the glomerular basement membrane and in the mesangium are seen by immunofluorescence. IgM of IgG may also be present.

Type II: This is the dense deposit disease. As shown by electron microscopy, there are broad, dense intramembranous deposits in glomerular and tubular basement membranes, coupled with granular deposits in the mesangium. By immunofluorescence, there are broad "sausage-like" (railroad tracks) deposits of C_3 along the glomerular and tubular basement membranes and Bowman's capsule. Rarely, IgM deposits are found with similar distribution. Type II is more likely to recur in the kidney transplants than type I.

7. Crescentic or Rapidly Progressive Glomerulonephritis

a. Clinical Syndrome: This disease is usually associated with systemic diseases such as systemic lupus erythematosis, system vasculitis, Goodpasture's syndrome, or with severe infections such as post-streptococcal or infective endocarditis, and sepsis. Although the onset may be insidious, the renal function declines rapidly, with steadily rising blood pressure, hematuria, red cell casts, and persistent, heavy proteinuria[35–38] (Fig. 1).

b. Pathology: Extensive extracapillary proliferation with crescent formation.[35,36]

c. Course and Management: Without therapy, the prognosis is uniformly poor. In absence of a clear-cut Goodpasture's syndrome, with circulating antiglomerular basement membrane antibodies, the treatment is uncertain.[38] The so-called "pulse therapy," using daily intravenous high doses of methylprednisolone, is probably beneficial, as is plasmapheresis. The combinations of steroids, cytotoxic drugs, anticoagulants, and antiplatelet agents have been abandoned.[39,40]

C. Glomerulonephritis in Systemic Diseases

A variety of infections and multisystem, metabolic, or hereditary diseases can result in significant glomerular involvement. The following is a review of only those diseases that may cause or may be associated with hematuria.

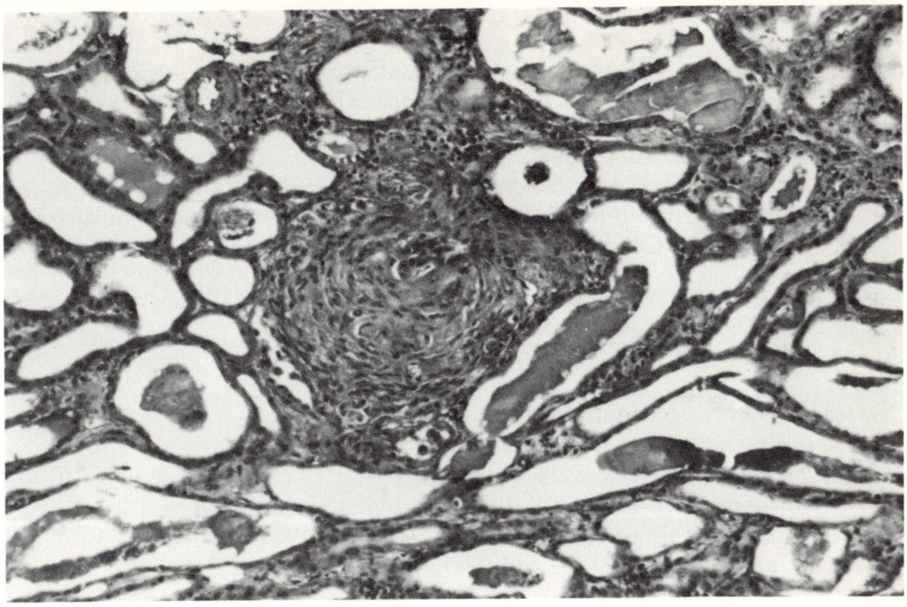

Figure 1: *A photomicrograph demonstrating a glomerulus extensively involved by Goodpasture's syndrome (40×).*

1. Systemic Lupus Erythematosis (SLE)

a. Clinical and Laboratory Features: Although detectable renal involvement has been variably reported in 35–90% of SLE cases,[41] 100% of the patients show histological abnormalities on the biopsy specimens.[42] Virtually any clinical syndrome of glomerular disease can be present in SLE. In some cases, the renal manifestation may uncover the systemic illness while the extrarenal manifestations of SLE have been mild or absent. However, the nephrotic syndrome associated with some degree of renal insufficiency is present in two out of three patients with renal involvement. Renal involvement correlates best with the presence of anti-DNA antibodies of high avidity, circulating immune complexes, low complement levels (particularly C_4), and presence of granular deposits of IgG and C_3 in dermal-epidermal junction capillaries.[43–45]

b. Pathology: Histologically, SLE nephritis presents in four main categories: (1) minimal changes or mild mesangial proliferation,[46] (2) focal proliferative glomerular lesions,[46,47] (3) membranous glomerulopathy,[46] or (4) diffuse endo- and extracapillary proliferative glomerular lesions.[46,47] Active SLE nephritis is underlined by focal necrosis, cellular proliferation, fibrinoid changes, wire loops, hematoxylin bodies, nuclear dusting, hyaline thrombi, and arteriolitis.[43–47]

c. Course: The overall prognosis depends on the histologic type with the diffuse, proliferative glomerulonephritis having the worst prognosis. Yet the overall outcome of SLE has been steadily improving. Now 5-year survival for SLE nephritis is better than 85%.[48–51]

2. *Henoch-Schonlein Purpura*

a. Clinical and Laboratory Features: This clinical syndrome includes hematuria, proteinuria, and azotemia. Rapidly progressive renal failure is uncommon while the nephrotic syndrome with hematuria is found in up to half of the patients.[52,53]

b. Pathology: Histologically, an array of lesions may be observed; the most common being focal and segmental proliferation of the mesangium, or focal and segmental capillary necrosis in glomeruli. The latter offers a poor prognosis. Widespread necrotizing arteritis is rare. Immunofluorescence shows diffuse granular IgA deposits in the mesangium[54]

3. *Systemic Vasculitis Syndrome*

This heading covers a heterogenous group of diseases with several different causative factors and pathogenetic mechanisms. They are characterized by differing clinical symptoms, each resulting from the inflammatory reactions involving vessels of nearly every organ. Hematuria is observed in more than 70% of the patients.

All attempted classifications of the human vasculitides that involve the kidney are hindered by a lack of knowledge of the specific clinicopathological correlations, the immunopathology of the initial lesions, and the pathogenetic mechanisms. In 1953, Zeek[55] proposed a classification of systemic "nonsuppurative" vasculitis based on the histologic features, the size of the vessels involved, and the distribution of the lesions among various tissues (Table III). Since then, additional immune-mediated forms of vasculitides have been identified. In 1976, Conn et al. proposed a classification based on the pathogenetic mechanism that is most evidenced during the illness[56] (Table IV) (Fig. 2).

Table III
Proposed Classification of Systemic Nonsuppurative Vasculitis Based on Histologic Features

1. Polyarteritis Nodosa
2. Hypersensitivity Angitis (microscopic variety of periarteritis)
3. Allergic granulomatous angitis
4. Wegener's granulomatosis

Table IV
Classification of Systemic Vasculitis Based on Pathogenetic Mechanisms

A. *Systemic immune complex vasculitis without respiratory tract involvement:*
   Polyarteritis Nodosa
   Cryoglobulinemia
B. *Systemic vasculitis with respiratory tract involvement:*
   Allergic granulomatous angitis
   Wegener's granulomatosis

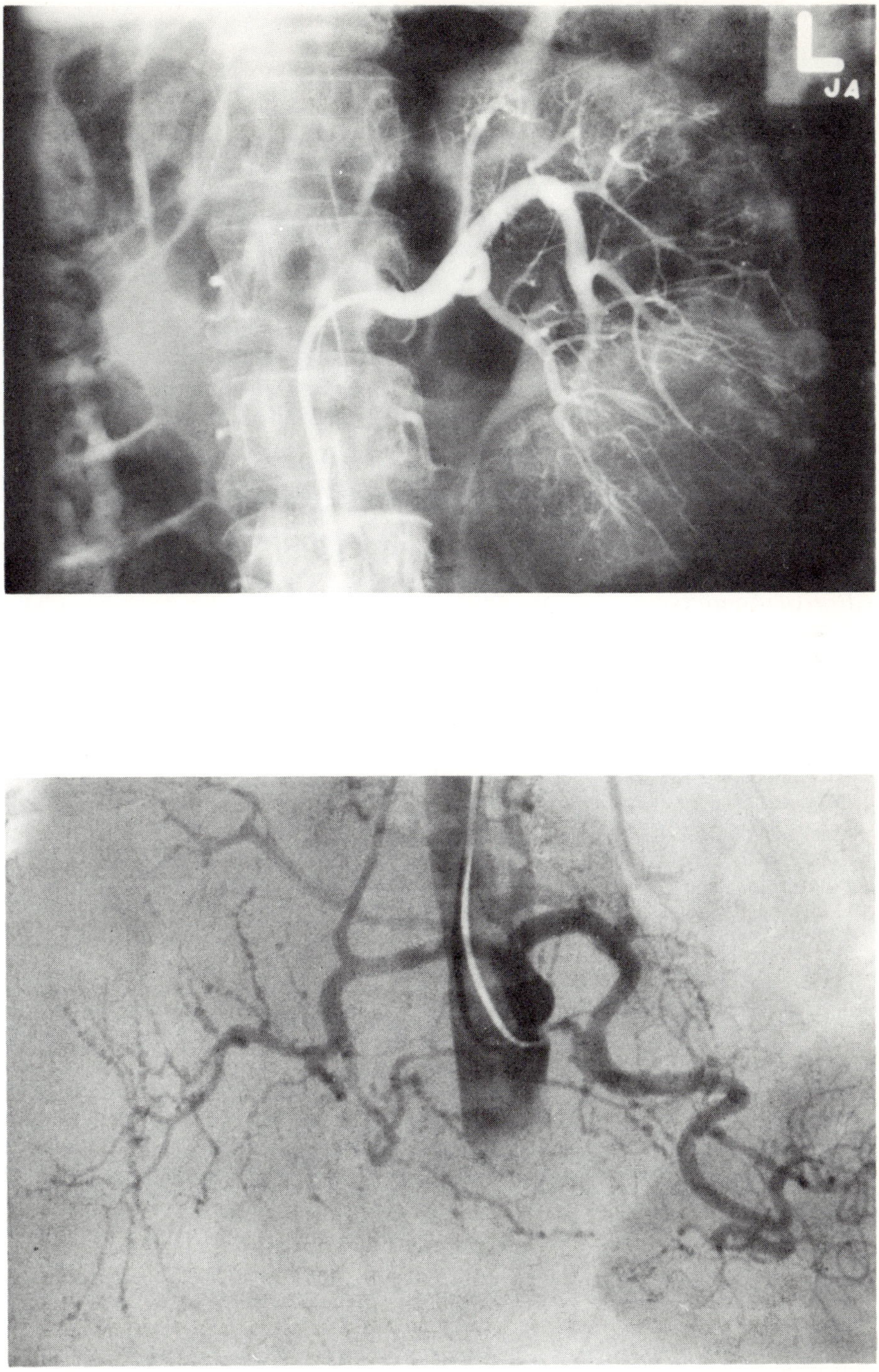

Figure 2: *Renal artery angiograms demonstrating polyarteritis nodosa. Note the small arterial aneurysms appearing as pools or beads of contrast dye. (From the* Learning File *of the Center for Devices and Radiological Health, FDA, case GU502.*

D. Hereditary Nephritis: Alport's Syndrome

1. *Clinical Features*

The syndrome of recurrent hematuria, proteinuria, progressive azotemia and deafness in young males is highly suggestive of Alport's syndrome. The family history is usually positive. Platelet abnormalities are found in 30–50% of patients.[57,58] Hematuria may be observed at any stage of the illness and bears no relationship to the prognosis.

2. *Pathology*

Glomerular hypercellularity and focal sclerosis are commonly seen on the biopsy. Electron microscopy shows splitting and lamination of lamina densa.[57–59]

E. Pyelonephritis and Urinary Tract Infection

1. *Clinical Aspects*

a. General Considerations: The approach to patients with acute infections of the genitourinary tract should (1) establish the diagnosis of urinary tract infection by documenting significant bacteriuria; (2) find the location of the infection within the urinary tract; (3) determine whether predisposing, reversible factors coexist; and (4) assess the risk of sepsis. The extent of clinical evaluation and intensity of the treatment are determined by the clinical presentation and the history of recurrences in the individual patient.[60]

b. Clinical Syndromes: Cystitis will most commonly cause nocturia and suprapubic discomfort. Bacteriuria is observed in only 50–70% of cases. Pyuria and bacteriuria may be observed with simple cystitis. Hematuria is mostly observed with coexisting renal involvement. Fever, generalized malaise, and leukocytosis may occur but are infrequent without associated pyelonephritis. In some situations (prostatism, indwelling catheters, etc.) recurrent cystitis can be cured if the predisposing factors are removed.

Acute pyelonephritis causes systemic signs and symptoms such as fever, chills, back pain, and costovertebral angle tenderness. Following therapy with antibiotics, pyuria and hematuria may disappear promptly, but bacteriuria may persist in nonobstructed patients.

2. *Pathogenesis*

Hematogenous seeding can occur with a variety of microorganisms including *Staphylococcus aureus*, *Salmonella*, and *Pseudomonas aeruginosa*. This mechanism, however, accounts for fewer than 5% of pyelonephritis cases. Bacterial endocarditis should be considered.

Ascending infection may occur, with the reservoir of urinary tract pathogens being the intestinal tract. Changes in the relative numbers of different bacteria in the stool and changes in the antibiotic susceptibility patterns of these organisms will have an impact on the pattern of urinary tract infections. This is a partial explanation for the differences between inpatient and outpatient urinary tract infections. Inpatients manifest higher incidence for non-*E. coli* and more antibiotic-resistant urinary tract infections than outpatients.

Several factors can favor introduction of bacteria into the bladder. Cystoscopy, catheterization of the urinary tract, or even gentle manual manipulation of the urethra results in the introduction of bacteria into the bladder. Sexual intercourse is a widely publicized culprit. Kunin et al. showed that the prevalence of bacteriuria in the general female population is 12.8 times higher than among nuns of similar age.[60]

Although urinary tract infection usually remains limited to the bladder, a significant proportion of bladder infections in women with a normal urinary tract anatomy extend via the ureters to the kidneys. This may result in a variety of renal lesions from mild pyelitis to involvement of entire lobules of the medulla and cortex, with full-blown acute pyelonephritis.

F. Renal Tuberculosis

Approximately 10% of the new cases of tuberculosis reported annually in the United States are extrapulmonary, and among these, the genitourinary tract is the leading site.[61] In most cases, renal tuberculosis remains silent for years while irreversible renal destruction takes place. Hence, when faced with unexplained sterile pyuria and/or hematuria, the clinician should rule out renal tuberculosis.[62]

Although genitourinary tuberculosis usually results from "silent bacillemia" accompanying pulmonary tuberculosis, concomitant pulmonary findings are found in only two-thirds of newly diagnosed cases of renal tuberculosis. Dysuria, hematuria, flank pain, and pyuria are the most frequent symptoms of active genitourinary tuberculosis. A positive PPD skin test is found in 93% of patients.[63]

Radiographic examinations, diagnostic only in advanced renal tuberculosis, demonstrate gross strictures, cavities, and calcifications. Otherwise, x-rays of early renal tuberculosis may be undistinguishable from chronic pyelonephritis.[63]

Treatment of renal tuberculosis is essentially medical, involving the use of antituberculosis drugs for 18 to 24 months.

G. Other Infections

There is a wide variety of other infectious agents capable of causing upper or lower urinary tract infection. They may be relatively common in certain clinical settings or rare in other settings. An extensive listing of various agents would be inappropriate. Included in such a list would be parasites and syphilis[64] (Fig. 3).

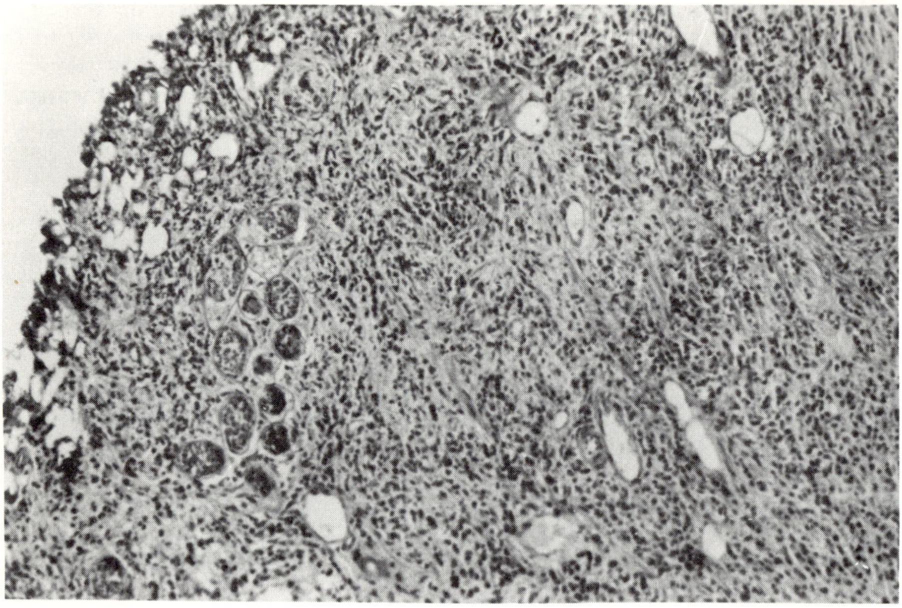

Figure 3: *A photomicrograph demonstrating bladder involvement by* Schistosomiasis (S. haematobium) *coincidental with transitional cell carcinoma. Embryonated ova are seen as cystic structures (100×).*

REFERENCES

1. Chang BS. Red cell morphology as a diagnostic aid in hematuria. *JAMA.* 252:1747–1749, 1984.
2. Birch DF, Fairley KF. Haematuria: Glomerular or non-glomerular? *Lancet.* 2:845–846, 1979.
3. Addis T. *Glomerular Nephritis: Diagnosis and Treatment.* New York, MacMillan, 1948, p. 42.
4. Fairley KF, Birch DF. Hematuria: A simple method for identifying glomerular bleeding. *Kidney Int.* 21:105–108, 1982.
5. Cameron JS, Turner DR, Ogg CS, Sharpstone P, Brown CB. The nephrotic syndrome in adults with "minimal change" lesions. *Q J Med.* 43:461–488, 1974.
6. Habib R, Kleiknecht G. The primary nephrotic syndrome in children. In: *Pathology Annual,* 6:417–474. Sommers SC, Ed. New York, Appleton-Century-Crofts, 1975.
7. Chamberlain MJ, Pringle A, Wrong OM. Oliguric renal failure in the nephrotic syndrome. *Q J Med.* 35:215–235, 1966.
8. Giangiacomo J, Cleary TG, Cole BR, Hoffsten P, Robson AM. Serum immunoglobulins in the nephrotic syndrome: A possible cause of minimal change nephrotic syndrome. *N Engl J Med.* 293:8–12, 1975.
9. Thomson PD, Barratt TM, Stokes CR, Turner MW, Soothill JF. HLA antigens and atopic features in steroid-responsive nephrotic syndrome of childhood. *Lancet.* 2: 765–768, 1976.
10. Sherman RL, Susin M, Weksler ME, Becker EL. Lipoid nephrosis in Hodgkin's disease. *Am J Med.* 52:699–706, 1972.
11. Heptinstall RH. Pathology of the Kidney. 2nd Ed. Boston, Little, Brown & Co., 1974.

12. Grishman E, Churg J. Pathology of nephrotic syndrome with minimal or minor glomerular changes. In: *Glomerulonephritis: Morphology, Natural History and Treatment*. Kincaid-Smith P, Mathew TH, Becker El, Eds. New York, John Wiley and Sons, 1972, pp. 165–181.
13. Ooi BS, Chen BT, Tan KK, Khoo OT. Longitudinal studies of lipoid nephrosis. *Arch Intern Med*. 130:883–886, 1972.
14. Jao W, Pollak VE, Norris S, Levy P, Pirani CL. Lipoid nephrosis: An approach to the clinicopathologic analysis and dismemberment of idiopathic nephrotic syndrome with minimal glomerular changes. *Medicine*. 52:445–468, 1973.
15. Grupe WE, Makker SP, Ingelfinger JR. Chlorambucil treatment of frequently relapsing nephrotic syndrome. *N Engl J Med*. 295:746–749, 1976.
16. Kida H, Iida H, Dohi K, Nakamoto Y, Mizumura Y, Takeuchi J. Period of freedom from relapse as an indication of cure in minimal change nephrotic syndrome in adults. *Nephron*. 19:153–157, 1977.
17. Habir R. Focal glomerular sclerosis. *Kidney Int*. 4:355–361, 1973.
18. Siegel NJ, Kashgarian M, Spargo B, Hayslett JP. Minimal change and focal sclerotic lesions in lipoid nephrosis. *Nephron*. 13:125–137, 1974.
19. Berger J, Hinglais N. Les depots intercapillaires d'IgA-IgG. *J Urol Nephrol* (Paris). 74:694–695, 1968.
20. Levy M, Beaufils H, Gubler MC, Habib R. Idiopathic recurrent macroscopic hematuria and mesangial IgA-IgG deposits in children (Berger's disease). *Clin Nephrol*. 1:63–69, 1973.
21. Lowance DC, Mullins JD, McPhaul JJ, Jr.: IgA associated glomerulonephritis. *Int Rev. Exp Pathol*. 17:143–172, 1977.
22. Whitworth JA, Leibowitz S, Kennedy MC, Cameron JS, Chantler C. IgA and glomerular disease. *Clin Nephrol*. 5:33–36, 1976.
23. Baart de la Faille-Kuyper E, Kater L, Kuijten RH, Kooiker CJ, Wagenaar SS, van der Zouwen P, and Dorhout Mees EJ. Occurrence of vascular IgA deposits in clinically normal skin of patients with renal disease. *Kidney Int*. 9:424–429, 1976.
24. Droz D. Natural history of primary glomerulonephritis with mesangial deposits of IgA. *Contrib Nephrol*. 2:150–157, 1976.
25. Hayslett JP, Krassner LS, Bensch KG, Kashgarian M, Epstein FH. Progression of "lipoid nephrosis" to renal insufficiency. *N Engl J Med*. 281:181–187, 1969.
26. Pierides AM, Malasit P, Morley AR, Wilkinson R, Uldall PR, Kerr DNS. Idiopathic membranous nephropathy. *Q J Med*. 46:163–168, 1977.
27. Row PG, Cameron JS, Turner DR, Evans DJ, White RHR, Ogg CS, Chantler C, Brown CB. Membranous nephropathy: Long-term follow-up and association with neoplasia. *Q J Med*. 44:207–239, 1975.
28. Rosen S. Membranous glomerulonephritis: Current status. *Human Pathol*. 2:209–231, 1971.
29. Coggins CH. The effect of short-term prednisone treatment in adult nephrotics with minimal change (MC) and membranous (M) histology. *Kidney Int*. 12:463, 1977. (Abstr.)
30. Okuda R, Watanabe Y, Yamanoto Y, West CD. The origin of membranoproliferative nephritis. Evidence against an origin from acute poststreptococcal nephritis. *Am J Dis Child*. 119:291–295, 1970.
31. Dreher WH, Zimmerman SW, Simpson DP. Hyperchloremia associated with membranoproliferative glomerulonephritis. *Nephron*. 18:321–325, 1977.
32. Burkholder PM, Hyman LR, Krueger RP. Characterization of mixed membranous and proliferative glomerulonephritis: Recognition of three varieties. In: *Glomerulonephritis: Morphology, Natural History and Treatment*. Kincaid-Smith P, Mathew TH, Becker EL, Eds. New York, John Wiley and Sons, 1972, pp. 557–589.
33. Habib R, Kleinknecht C, Gubler MC, Levy M. Idiopathic membranoproliferative glomerulonephritis in children: Report of 105 cases. *Clin Nephrol*. 1:194–214, 1973.
34. Habib R, Gubler MC, Loirat C, Ben Maiz H, Levy M. Dense deposit disease: A variant of membranoproliferative glomerulonephritis. *Kidney Int*. 7:204–215, 1975.

35. Rosen S: Crescenteric glomerulonephritis: Occurrence, mechanisms and prognosis. In: *Pathology Annual,* 10:37–64, Sommers SC, Ed. New York, Appleton-Century-Crofts, 1975.
36. Hamburger J. Les glomerulonephrites malignes. In: *Entretiens de Bichat.* Vol. 1, Paris, Expansion Scientifique Francaise, 1956.
37. Pollack VE, Mendoza N. Rapidly progressive glomerulonephritis. *Med Clin North Am.* 55:1397–1415, 1971.
38. Glassock RJ. A clinical and immunopathologic dissection of rapidly progressive glomerulonephritis. *Nephron.* 22:253–264, 1978.
39. Lockwood CM, Rees AJ, Pearson JA, Evans D, Peters DK, Wilson CB. Immunosuppression and plasma-exchange in the treatment of Goodpasture's syndrome. *Lancet:* 711–715, 1976.
40. Lockwood CM, Rees AJ, Pinching AJ, Pussell B, Sweny PL, Uff J, Peters DK. Plasma-exchange and immunosuppression in the treatment of fulminating immune-complex crescentic nephritis. *Lancet.* 1:63–67, 1977.
41. Bennett WM, Bardana EJ, Houghton DC, Pirofsky B, Striker GD. Silent renal involvement in systemic lupus erythematosis. *Int Arch Allergy Appl Immunol.* 55:420–428, 1977.
42. Mahajan SK, Ordonez NG, Feitelson PJ, Lim VS, Spargo BH, Katz AI. Lupus nephropathy without clinical renal involvement. *Medicine.* 56:493–502, 1977.
43. Dubois EL. *Lupus Erythematosus.* 2nd Ed. New York, McGraw Hill, 1974.
44. Agnello V. Immunopathogenesis of lupus nephritis. In: *Advances in Nephrology,* 6:119–136. Hamburger J, Crosnier J, Maxwell MH, Eds. Chicago, Year Book Medical Publishers, 1976.
45. Estes D, Christian CL. The natural history of systemic lupus erythematosis by prospective analysis. *Medicine* (Baltimore), 50:85–95, 1971.
46. Baldwin DS, Gluck MC, Schacht RG, Gallo G. The long-term course of poststreptococcal glomerulonephritis. *Ann Intern Med.* 80:342–358, 1974.
47. Ginzler E, Nicastri AD, Chen CK, Friedman EA, Diamond HS, Kaplan DS. Progression of mesangial and focal to diffuse lupus nephritis. *N Engl J. Med.* 291:693–696, 1974.
48. Donadio JV, Holly KF, Ferguson RH, Ilstrup DM. Progressive lupus glomerulonephritis: Treatment with prednisone and combined prednisone and cyclophosphamide. *Mayo Clinic Proceed.* 51:484–494, 1976.
49. Donadio JV. Treatment of lupus nephritis. *Nephron.* 19:186–189, 1977.
50. Donadio JV, Burgess JH, Holly KF. Membranous lupus nephropathy: A clinicopathologic study. *Medicine* (Baltimore). 56:527–536, 1977.
51. Pollack VE. Treatment of lupus nephritis. In: *Advances in Nephrology.* 6:137–161. Hamburger J, Crosnier J, Maxwell MH, Eds. Chicago, Year Book Medical Publishers, 1976.
52. Allen DM, Diamond LK, Howell DA. Anaphylactoid purpura in children (Schonlein-Henoch Syndrome): review with a follow-up of renal complications. *Am J Dis Child.* 99:833–854, 1960.
53. Counahan R, Cameron JS. Henoch-Schonlein nephritis. *Contrib Nephrol.* 7:143–165, 1977.
54. Hurley RM, Drummond KN. Anaphylactoid purpura nephritis. Clinicopathological correlations. *J Pediatr.* 81:904–911, 1972.
55. Zeek PM. Periarteritis nodosa and other forms of necrotizing angitis. *N Engl J. Med.* 248:764–772, 1953.
56. Conn DL, McDuffie FC, Holley KE, Schroeter AL. Immunologic mechanisms in systemic vasculitis. *Mayo Clin Proc.* 51:511–518, 1976.
57. Perkoff GT, Nugent CA, Jr., Dolowitz DA, Stephens FE, Carnes WH, Tyler FH. A follow-up study of hereditary chronic nephritis. *Arch Intern Med.* 102:733–746, 1958.
58. Whalen RE, Huang S, Peschel E, McIntosh HD. Hereditary nephropathy, deafness and renal foam cells. *Am J Med.* 31:171–186, 1961.

59. Spear GS, Slusser RJ. Alport's syndrome: Emphasizing electron microscopic studies of the glomerulus. *Am J Pathol.* 69:213–220, 1972.
60. Kunin CA. In: Detection, Prevention and Management of Urinary Tract Infections. 3rd Ed. Philadelphia, Lea & Febiger, 1979.
61. Greenberger ME, Wershub LP, Auerbach O. The incidence of renal tuberculosis: In 500 autopsies for pulmonary and extrapulmonary tuberculosis. *JAMA.* 104:726–754, 1935.
62. Borthwick WM. Present position of urinary tuberculosis. *Br J Urol.* 42:642–655, 1970.
63. Heptinstall RH. In: *Pathology of the Kidney.* 2nd Ed. Boston, Little, Brown & Co., 1974.
64. Ng RCK, Seto DSJ. Hematuria: A suggested work-up strategy. *Postgrad Med.* 75:139–144, 1984.

Chapter 5

Fibrinolysis

Birger Astedt, M.D., and Inga Marie Nilsson, M.D.

I. Fibrinolysis

In renal disease, fibrinolytic problems are often involved. For example, hemorrhage is common in uremia, and intracapillary and intraglomerular fibrin deposits occur in glomerulonephritis that have to be dissolved by the fibrinolytic defense system.

For the understanding of the etiology of these complications and to give a theoretical background for their diagnosis and therapy, a review of the fibrinolytic system first will be given and then applied to clinical problems in renal disease.

A. The Fibrinolytic System

Fibrinolysis is a Latin-Greek hybrid word meaning "fiber dissolution." The term was coined by Dastre in 1893. Fibrinolysis is defined as the enzymatic breakdown of fibrinogen and fibrin.

The fibrinolytic system has significance in many aspects of health and disease. It constitutes an important defense system in the prevention of *thrombosis*. Fibrin deposits, which might occur, on the vessel endothelium are readily dissolved by the fibrinolytic defense system. The action of the fibrinolytic system on the thrombi already formed has been termed *thrombolysis*. In inflammatory processes, fibrin is formed, protecting surrounding tissue. This fibrin is then removed by the fibrinolytic system. In *tissue repair*, fibrin is a necessary matrix upon which there is a proliferation of vessels; the residual fibrin has then to be removed by the fibrinolytic system. The significance of fibrinolysis in *tumor growth* with formation of neoplastic vessels is similar to that in tissue repair.

A survey of the components of the fibrinolytic system is given in Figure 1. In

From Bern MM (ed.) *Urinary Tract Bleeding: Diagnosis and Control by Medical, Radiologic, and Surgical Techniques.* Mount Kisco, NY, Futura Publishing Co., Inc., 1985.

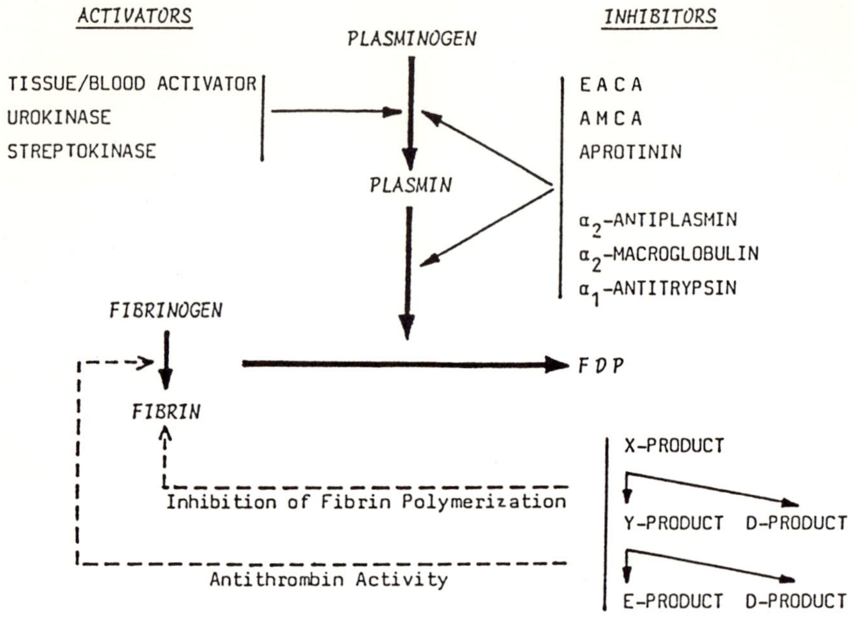

Figure 1: *The fibrinolytic system.*

the blood plasma there is an inactive enzyme precursor, *plasminogen*. When activated by an *activator*, this precursor is converted into the active proteolytic enzyme *plasmin*, which breaks down fibrinogen and fibrin into *fibrinogen-fibrin degradation products* (FDP) of different molecular sizes. There are *inhibitors* of plasminogen activation as well as of plasmin.

1. Plasminogen-Plasmin

Plasminogen, the inactive precursor of plasmin, is a β-globulin with molecular weight of about 90,000 daltons. Its concentration in healthy adults is about 200 μg/ml plasma or 2.2 μmol/L. Plasminogen concentrations can be determined immunologically or by a functional clot-dependent method. The concentration of plasminogen is often given relative to that in a normal standard pool of plasma, but absolute values are also given. The source of the production of plasminogen is still debatable. Most likely it is synthesized in liver cells.[1,2] The synthesis of plasminogen is rapid, as is apparent from its quick recovery after treatment with streptokinase, wherein it goes from practically nil to normal within 12–24 hours.[3,4] Plasminogen has a certain affinity for fibrinogen and fibrin. Most preparations of fibrinogen are therefore contaminated with plasminogen.

Human plasminogen is a single polypeptide chain. The N-terminal amino acid in the molecule is glutamic acid. When this native glu-plasminogen is converted to plasmin by the action of activators, a single arginine-valine bond in the plasminogen molecule is split, resulting in a two-chain plasmin molecule consisting of a heavy chain with a molecular weight of 65,000 daltons and a light chain with a molecular weight of 25,000 daltons, which are held together by two disulphide bonds. This plasmin has been called glu-plasmin, since the N-terminal amino acid in the heavy chain is glutamic acid. Glu-plasmin is able to split a polypeptide of about 7,000 daltons from a glu-plasminogen molecule, resulting in a plasminogen molecule with lysine as the N-terminal amino acid. This lys-plasminogen is then more susceptible to cleavage by an activator. This dual mechanism of activation of plasminogen thus means there is an accelerated process in the activation of the precursor plasminogen into the active enzyme plasmin.

Members of a few families have been reported to have a low plasminogen level, but no symptoms of disease were observed. Some individuals with an abnormal plasminogen have had increased tendency to thrombosis.[5,6] From a practical clinical point of view, plasminogen constitutes an immense source of proteolytic activity and will always be present in sufficient amounts.

2. Plasminogen Activators

The conversion of plasminogen into plasmin is affected by two naturally occurring activators: tissue/blood activator and urine activator (urokinase). The tissue plasminogen activators are present in most organs, but especially in the uterus, kidneys, prostate, thyroid, lungs, and heart. Plasminogen activators are serine-proteinases that activate plasminogen by cleavage of an arginine-valine bond in the plasminogen molecule.[7,8] The activity of plasminogen activators can be determined on plasminogen-containing fibrin plates by calculating the area of the lytic zones.[9] Plasminogen activator in tissues can be localized and semiquantified by the histochemical fibrin slide technique. Here cryostate sections are covered by a plasminogen-contaminated fibrin film. Presence of plasminogen activator results in lytic zones in the blue-stained fibrin film, the area of which can be calculated.[10]

a. Tissue/Blood Activator: Tissue/blood activator is synthesized in the vessel wall, most likely in the endothelium.[11–13] It is liberated from the vessel wall into the bloodstream following physical exercise, venous occlusion, or stimulation with certain pharmacologicals, e.g. adrenalin and vasopressin analogues. Its physiological significance is to remove early fibrin deposits that might occur on the vessel endothelium thereby preventing thrombosis. The majority of patients with recurrent thrombotic diseases have a low content of plasminogen activator in their vessel walls with an impaired ability to release the activators.[14] These defects in the tissue/blood plasminogen activator is also of importance in inflammatory diseases and in tissue repair.

Tissue/blood plasminogen activator is synthesized as a single polypeptide chain of a molecular weight of about 70,000 daltons. Proteolytic cleavage results in a two-chain form, a heavier chain of 40,000 and a lighter chain of 30,000 daltons, held together by one interchain disulphide bond. The active site is localized in the lighter chain.

Some melanoma cell lines have been found to produce a plasminogen activator similar or identical to the tissue/blood plasminogen activator. Cultures of such melanoma cells have allowed the gathering of larger amounts of plasminogen activator, making it possible to raise an antiserum against the plasminogen activator. A new immunoradiometric method has been designed for determining the tissue/blood plasminogen activator, which detects tissue/blood activator in a concentration of 1 μg/L or even less.[15]

b. Urokinase: This is produced by certain kidney cells and secreted in the urine.[16,17] In tissue culture, it has been found also to be released from cells of other organs.[15] The physiological significance of urokinase is mainly to dissolve fibrin in clots, which might occur in the urinary excretory pathways.

Urokinase exists in different molecular forms, having different molecular weights.[18–21] The high molecular form exists as a single chain and a two-chain form held together by disulfide bonds. By reduction, the high molecular weight form of 54,000 daltons is separated into a heavy chain of 33,000 daltons and a light chain of 21,000–18,000 daltons. The heavy chain, which contains the active enzymatic site, constitutes a low molecular form of urokinase. A very high molecular weight urokinase of about 90,000–100,000 daltons seems to be an aggregation of the low molecular forms along with protein fragments of various size.[21]

The enzymatic activity of urokinase can be determined on plasminogen-containing fibrin plates, or by radioimmunoassay.[22] Urokinase does not cross-react with the tissue/blood plasminogen activator.[23] The concentration of urokinase in urine is about 50–100 μg/L. It is still debated if minor, hardly detectable amounts are present in plasma.

3. Inhibitors of Fibrinolysis

The proteinase inhibitors of the fibrinolytic system are α_1-antiplasmin, α_2-macroglobulin, C_1-esterase inhibitor, antithrombin III, α_1-antichymotrypsin and inter-α-trypsin inhibitor.

a. α_2-Antiplasmin: One of the most important inhibitors of fibrinolysis is α_2-antiplasmin, which was identified by three independent groups.[24–26] The α_2-antiplasmin is a single-chain polypeptide with a molecular weight of about 65,000–70,000 daltons. It is an α_2-globulin and immunologically different from the other inhibitors mentioned above. The concentration of α_2-antiplasmin in plasma and serum is about 1–1.5 μmol/L. It is a fast-acting plasmin inhibitor and forms a 1:1 stoichiometric complex with plasmin. This complex then has no proteolytic activity. The α_2-antiplasmin also forms a complex with plasminogen. It is thought that about 30% of the α_2-antiplasmin in the circulation is complexed with plasminogen.[27] The complex with plasmin is extremely stable but that of plasminogen is labile. The binding of α_2-antiplasmin to plasmin and plasminogen is dependent on lysine binding sites in the enzyme molecules but also to plasmin at the active site.

Plasmin formed in the circulating bloodstream has a short life-span because it is rapidly complexed and inactivated by α_2-antiplasmin. The tissue/blood activator binds to fibrin and activates the fibrin-bound plasminogen. The plasmin formed, which is bound to fibrin through its lysine binding site, is probably protected from rapid inactivation by α_2-antiplasmin.[28] This mechanism is thus of importance for the lysis of fibrin deposits and thrombi.

b. α_2-Macroglobulin: This is a proteinase inhibitor with a molecular weight of about 725,000 daltons. Its concentration in plasma is about 4 μmol/L. It is slowly synthesized. The α_2-macroglobulin reacts slowly and reversibly with plasmin, and complexes with urokinase. The active site of urokinase is not necessary for complex formation with α_2-macroglobulin.

c. α_1-Antitrypsin: This also inhibits urokinase by the formation of an irreversible enzyme inhibitor complex.

d. Antithrombin III: This is the most important coagulation inhibitor in plasma. It also forms an irreversible enzyme-inhibitor complex with urokinase.

e. Specific Plasminogen Activator Inhibitors: After preparation of this chapter, interest has been focused to a fast-acting specific plasminogen activator inhibitor that has been shown to be synthesized by endothelial cells. It has a molecular weight of about 50,000 and forms complexes with urokinase as well as the tissue plasminogen activator.[80] It does not inhibit plasmin. In a study of patients with recurrent thrombosis, increased concentration of a specific plasminogen activator inhibitor has been found in the majority of the patients.[81] Recently, a specific plasminogen activator inhibitor, immunologically different from the endothelial inhibitor, has been isolated from pregnancy plasma. It has a molecular weight of 70,000 and cross-reacts with an inhibitor derived from placenta. It forms complexes with urokinase as well as with tissue plasminogen activator and has no inhibitory effect on plasmin.[82] The physiological significance of this inhibitor is probably to secure hemostasis during pregnancy.

4. *Fibrinogen-Fibrin Degradation Products (FDP)*

FDP form when fibrinogen and fibrin are broken down by plasmin. In a series of reactions, fibrinogen and fibrin are split into fragments of various molecular sizes (Fig. 2).[29,30]

On degradation of fibrinogen (molecular weight [MW] 300,000) by plasmin, first fragment X (MW 240,000) is formed together with some small fragments A, B, and C (stage 1 of digestion). The larger fragment X is still slowly but completely clottable by thrombin. On further degradation of fragment X, fragments Y (MW 155,000) and D (MW 83,000) are formed (stage 2 digestion). Fragment Y is unclottable by thrombin. The further degradation of fragment Y results in the formation of fragments D and E (MW 50,000) (stage 3 of digestion).[31]

Fragment X and Y are together termed the "high molecular weight split (HMWS) products." D and E are called the "end split products." The fragments X and Y, as well as D and E have antigenic determinants identical to fibrinogen. The small fragments A, B, and C, do not cross-react with fibrinogen. Fragments D and E contain distinct antigenic determinants of the parent fibrinogen molecule.[32] Fragment E is probably derived from the N-terminal disulphide knot of fibrinogen.

Antiserum has been raised against fibrinogen and D and E fragments. This has made typing of the FDP possible.[33] Furthermore, neoantigens specific for fibrinogen D fragment have been found,[34,35] which makes it possible to distin-

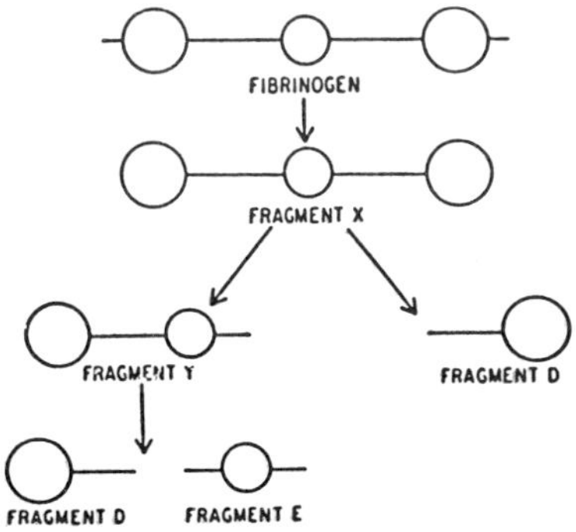

Figure 2: *Fibrinogen degradation products, based on a report by Marder VJ, et al.*[29,30]

guish between D fragments derived from fibrinogen and fragments derived from fibrin.

HMWS products, i.e. X and Y fragments, are the degradation products most commonly found in the blood in various clinical disorders. They may occur separately, but they often form complexes with soluble monomers of fibrinogen and fibrin.[36] On formation of a fibrin clot, about 70% of fragment X, 50% of HMWS (X + Y), and 10% of D and E fragments are retained in the clot. FDP have many effects on blood coagulation. D and E fragments have mainly a weak antithrombin effect.

For the determination of FDP, serum is used because plasma contains fibrinogen, which has the same antigenic determinants as FDP. Addition of an inhibitor of fibrinolysis, such as EACA or Trasylol®, prevents activation of plasminogen in the samples. Four methods are used.

The tanned red cell hemagglutination inhibition immunoassay (TRCHII)[37,38] is probably the assay most commonly used. Serum to be tested is incubated with the highly diluted antifibrinogen serum. Afterwards, fibrinogen-coated red blood cells are added. The consequent degree of inhibition of aggregation is a measure of the amount of FDP or fibrinogen-fibrin-related antigen in the sample. This method can measure concentrations down to about 0.5μg/ml.

In the staphylococcal clumping test, fibrinogen, fibrin monomers, and fragments X and Y can be aggregated by certain strains of *Staphylococcus aureus*.[39] The highest dilution of serum that produced aggregation is determined. This method enables measurement of FDP down to 0.5−1 μg/ml. No reaction is obtained with D or E products. A rapid latex agglutination inhibition method using latex particles coated with human fibrinogen is useful for screening purposes.[40,41]

An immunochemical method has been designed based on Laurell's technique.[42] A glass plate is covered with agarose gel containing specific antibodies to anti-D. Serum from the patient to be tested is placed in a hole punched in the gel. The test serum is forced into the gel with the aid of an electric current. If the samples contain degradation products, peaks appear in the gel resembling rockets in the electrophoretic direction. The height of these peaks depends on the concentration of the antigen. With this method, FDP can be measured down to a concentration of 5 μg/ml. Antiserum against fibrinogen and D and E fragments, respectively, has made further typing of FDP possible.[33]

B. Fibrinolysis in Renal Failure

1. Uremia

A bleeding tendency in uremia has long been known. Morgagni reported a woman who had "the odor of urine on her breath and was vomiting blood and bleeding from the nose." The main hemorrhagic complication associated with uremia is spontaneous *mucosal bleedings*, particularly from the nose and the gastrointestinal tract. Other serious hemorrhagic complications of uremia can include *hemorrhagic pericarditis* and *intracranial hemorrhage*. The bleeding tendency can be explained mainly by reduced platelet adhesiveness and aggregation (see Chapters 1 and 2.) Larsson[43] and McNicol et al.[44] found that the bleeding tendency was suppressed by a low fibrinolytic activity in the blood, which was explained by a marked increase of inhibitors of plasminogen activation. The inhibitors of plasminogen activation by urokinase (urokinase inhibitors) were also found to be increased in 95% of dialysed cases, in 78% of conservatively treated chronic cases, and in 82% of acute cases. The α_2-macroglobulin and slow-reacting plasmin inhibitors were normal in conservatively treated uremia patients, and normal or increased in patients with acute uremia.[45] In contrast, antiplasmin activity in acute renal failure can be increased,[46] and it can be reduced in patients with heavy proteinuria.[47]

Fibrinogen-fibrin degradation products in serum were significantly more common in patients with acute uremia than in conservatively treated chronic uremia patients. Thus, the low fibrinolytic activity in the blood and the tendency to deposition of fibrin in uremia is not due to inhibition of plasmin activity or to lack of plasminogen activators, but can be explained by the marked increase of inhibitors of plasminogen activation. FDP has also been demonstrated in the urine in those cases not having anuria.[43]

2. *Urinary Urokinase in Renal Disease*

Urokinase dissolves and removes fibrin deposits and blood clots that occur in the excretory pathways of the kidney. The concentration of urokinase when measured by immune assay in urine in healthy individuals is fairly constant, but varies widely with the diuresis (Table I). Some patients with renal disease have been studied with the new radioimmunoassays. In nephrotic syndrome and in mild glomerulonephritis where the glomerular filtration rate is not reduced, there is no reduction in urokinase secretion.

In disorders where the glomerular filtration rate is reduced, even if only moderately, the urokinase excretion is very low or undetectable (Table I). In one case of hemolytic uremic syndrome, urokinase did not reappear in the urine until the glomerular filtration rate had increased to 10 ml/min/m^2. Urokinase excretion in urine thus seems to be an indicator of the number of functioning nephrons. This indicates that determination of urokinase can be of diagnostic and prognostic value in kidney disease.

3. *Fibrinogen-Fibrin Products in Renal Disease*

FDP is a common finding in the urine in renal diseases. They originate from intracapillary and intraglomerular fibrin deposits degraded by the fibrinolytic activity of the blood, initiated by the tissue/blood activator. Damage of the glomerular basement membrane causes increased permeability, which then permits the entrance of fibrinogen and FDP into the excretory pathways. If the glomerular basement membrane permeability increases, larger FDPs or even fibrinogen can enter the urine. Thereafter, in Bowman's space and in the excretory pathways, fibrinogen and FDP are degraded further by the action of urokinase.

Intracapillary and intraglomerular fibrin deposits have been found in glomerulonephritis, eclampsia, and uremia.[48–52] In some cases with this lesion, FDP can also be detected in serum. Following renal transplantation, FDP might

Table I
Secretion of Urokinase in Urine in Health and Renal Disease

Subjects	Urokinase μg/24 h	Glomerular Filtration Rate ml/min/m^2
Controls		
10–20 yrs	$\bar{X}$ 61 (18–106)	Normal
3–10 yrs	$\bar{X}$ 34 (11–61)	Normal
Patients		
Nephrotic syndrome	27–90	>70
Glomerulonephritis	49	>70
Hypoplasia	<2	5
Polycystic disease	<2	30
Haemolytic uremic syndrome	0–3	0–10

appear in the urine and in the serum. Increased concentrations are found during episodes of rejection.[53,54]

In *glomerulonephritis*, FDP is the serum as well as in the urine has been found predominantly in the proliferative and in the acute forms. Less often, FDP are found in membranous and minimal glomerulonephritis. In 24 patients with different types of glomerulonephritis, FDP could not be demonstrated in serum and was seen in only one unconcentrated urine sample.[55] However, in 24-hour samples, FDP was found in 20 of 24 patients, (30–1,650 μg/24 hours) mainly of the high molecular type. Healthy control subjects had no FDP, even in concentrated urine.

FDP is more often demonstrable during chronic uremia in the urine than in the serum.[56,57] FDP was found in the serum in 37% and in unconcentrated urine in 39% of the patients. The amount of FDP varies with the activity of the disease,[43] and is mainly the high molecular weight types.[33]

In the *hemolytic-uremic syndrome*, FDP in the serum and urine is commonly found.[58,59] In our experience, following the concentrations of FDP in renal disease has been useful mainly for following the course of the disease and the effect of therapy.

Following *renal transplantation*, serum FDP has been demonstrated during the first postoperative week and during episodes of rejection.[33,48,53,54] The occurrence of FDP in the urine in such patients is now considered very informative. The occurrence of FDP in the urine later than 2 weeks after operation can be regarded as a sign of rejection,[50,53,54,60] while the absence of FDP in the urine does not preclude rejection.[61] In patients without signs of rejection, Ekberg and Pandolfi demonstrated FDP in unconcentrated urine in all patients up to 25 days after the transplantation (0.6–65 mg/24 hours) and for 2–3 weeks in serum (40–50 μg/ml).[50] In the concentrated 24-hour urine samples, FDP could be found up to 12 weeks postoperatively (1.5–20 mg/24 hours). In the acute rejection episodes, FDP was demonstrated in a very high concentration (15–220 mg/24 hours). The occurrence of FDP was the first sign of rejection in the unconcentrated urine samples of two of ten patients. Persistence of FDP later than 12 weeks indicated some complication such as glomerulonephritis in the transplant or chronic rejection. The fibrinogen degradation products were mainly of the high molecular weight forms.

4. *Renal Vein Thrombosis*

Renal vein thrombosis has for a long time been considered a cause of nephrotic syndrome. However, there is now evidence that renal vein thrombosis is a consequence or complication of the nephrotic syndrome.[62] There is also evidence that patients with nephrotic syndrome are at risk for thrombosis in other sites, i.e. pulmonary emboli, femoral thrombosis, mesenteric thrombosis, cerebral vein and inferior vena cava thrombosis. Patients with nephrotic syndrome may have a modest increase of the clotting factors[47] and a depressed level of antithrombin III, due to excretion of antithrombin III in the urine[63] (see Chapter 1). The risk of thromboembolic complication in nephrotic syndrome, especially renal vein thrombosis, indicates the need for anticoagulative treatment. Plasminogen is elevated in the nephrotic syndrome and antiplasmin is decreased. There may be an inhibitor to lysis, causing decreased euglobulin lysis and activation by urokinase.[47,64]

5. *Dialysis*

Patients receiving dialysis for chronic renal failure have altered fibrinolysis similar to those not receiving dialysis.[44,65,66] The endothelial cells of these patients release normal amounts of plasminogen activator,[67,68] with normal or reduced amounts of plasminogen,[66,44] but there is increased inhibition of activation.[44,65,69] These inhibitors appear to be retained amino acids,[70] which are cleared by hemodialysis.[69] On the other hand, peritoneal dialysis causes loss of the activators.[69] Dialysis membranes also seem to activate the fibrinolytic system.[71]

C. Inhibitors for Antifibrinolytic Therapy

In their systematic search for a substance with antifibrinolytic properties, Okamoto and co-workers found that epsilon aminocaproic acid (EACA) had the strongest antifibrinolytic effect.[72] EACA was then rapidly introduced as a valuable antifibrinolytic drug in various clinical bleeding disorders.[73] However, large amounts of EACA are needed to have a sufficient effect. A more potent fibrinolytic drug is 4-amino-methyl-cyclohexane-carboxylic acid (AMCHA), also termed tranexamic acid.[74] This drug is about 7−10 times more potent than EACA.[75,76] Another active agent is aprotinin (Trasylol®), a protease inhibitor, which is derived from bovine pancreas, parotid gland and lung, with a molecular weight of about 6,500 daltons.

These inhibitors of fibrinolysis, mainly AMCHA, have been very helpful in the treatment of various bleeding disorders due to primary or secondary fibrinolysis, and in hemorrhage due to local fibrinolysis, i.e. menorrhagia, hemorrhage at prostatectomy, hemorrhage in the digestive tract, and adjuvant treatment in patients with hemophilia and in obstetric bleeding. AMCHA is relatively contraindicated in cases with macroscopic hematuria because of risk of clot formation in the excretory pathways. The antifibrinolytic mechanism of AMCHA is complex. One mode of action is blockade of the lysine-binding sites in the plasminogen and plasmin molecule, thereby inhibiting the binding of plasminogen and plasmin to the fibrin substrate.

Furthermore, AMCHA inhibits the activation of plasminogen by urokinase and the blood/tissue activator. It also potentiates the inhibitory effect of natural inhibitors by dissociating the plasmin bound to fibrin, following which the liberated plasmin easily binds to the natural inhibitors, mainly α_2-antiplasmin.[77]

The antifibrinolytic effect of aprotinin is due to its action as a noncompetitive inhibitor of plasmin. It also inhibits urokinase and the tissue/blood activator by complex formation. Aprotinin is not secreted in the urine.

An important question is whether therapy with EACA and AMCHA predisposes to thrombosis and intravascular coagulation. There are isolated reports of arterial or venous thrombosis associated with antifibrinolytic therapy, but in most cases a disease known to predispose to thrombosis has also been present. Detailed studies using phlebography or ^{125}I-fibrinogen uptake have shown no change in the incidence of venous thrombosis attributable to treatment with EACA after prostatectomy. The incidence of thrombosis was not significantly different as detected by the ^{125}I-fibrinogen uptake test in 201 prostatectomy patients, of whom 100 had taken 1 gram AMCHA three times a day and 101 had taken a placebo.[78] An explanation for the nonthrombotic effect of AMCHA might be the fact that the content of plasminogen activator in the vessel wall is shown not to be depressed by administration of AMCHA.[79] Thus there is no conclusive evidence for a clinically detectable thrombotic effect of EACA or AMCHA.

REFERENCES

1. Johnson AJ, Skoza L, Tse AO. Studies on plasmin inhibition and plasminogen activation and its inhibition. *Thromb Diath Haemorrheol.* (Suppl) 32:105, 1969.
2. Bohmfalk JF, Fuller GM. Plasminogen is synthesized by primary cultures of rat hepatocytes. *Science.* 209:408–410, 1980.
3. Fletcher AP, Alkjaersig N, Sherry S. The maintenance of a sustained thrombolytic state in man. I. Induction and effects. *J Clin Invest* 38:1096–1110, 1959.
4. Robertson BR, Nilsson IM, Nylander G. Thrombolytic effect of streptokinase as evaluated by phlebography of deep venous thrombi of the leg. *Acta Chir Scand.* 136: 173–180, 1970.
5. Aoki N, Moroi M, Sakata Y, Yoshida NG, Matsuda M. Abnormal plasminogen: A hereditary molecular abnormality found in a patient with recurrent thrombosis. *J Clin Invest.* 61:1186–1195, 1978.
6. Kazama M, Tahara C, Suzuki Z, Gohchi K, Abe T. Abnormal plasminogen: A case of recurrent thrombosis. *Thromb Res.* 21:517–522, 1981.
7. Robbins KC, Summaria L, Hsieh B, Shah RJ. The peptide chains of human plasmin: Mechanism of activation of human plasminogen to plasmin. *J Biol Chem.* 242:2333–2342, 1967.
8. Heimburger N. Basic mechanism of action of streptokinase and urokinase. *Thromb Diath Haemorrheol.* (Suppl) 47:21, 1971.
9. Nilsson IM, Olow B. Fibrinolysis induced by streptokinase in man. *Acta Chir Scand.* 123:247–266, 1962.
10. Pandolfi M. Histochemistry and assay of plasminogen activators. *Rev Eur Etud Clin Biol.* 17:254–260, 1972.
11. Astedt B, Pandolfi M. On release and synthesis of fibrinolytic activators in human organ culture. *Rev Eur Etud Clin Biol.* 17:261, 1972.
12. Loskutoff DG, Edgington TS. Synthesis of a fibrinolytic activator and inhibitor by endothelial cells. *Proc Natl Acad Sci USA* 74:3903–3907, 1977.

13. Levin EG, Loskutoff DJ. Comparative studies of the fibrinolytic activity of cultured vascular cells. *Thromb Res.* 15:869–878, 1979.
14. Isaacson S, Nilsson IM. Defective fibrinolysis in blood and vein walls in recurrent "idiopathic" venous thrombosis. *Acta Chir Scand.* 138:313–319, 1972.
15. Holmberg L, Kristoffersson AC, Lecander I, Wallen P, Astedt B. Immunoradiometric quantification of tissue plasminogen activator secreted by fetal organs: Comparison with urokinase. *Scand J Clin Lab Invest.* 42:347–354, 1982.
16. Lesuk A, Terminiello L, Traver JH. Crystalline human urokinase: Some properties. *Science.* 147:880–882, 1965.
17. White WF, Barlow GH, Mozen MM. The isolation and characterization of plasminogen activators (urokinase) from human urine. *Biochemistry.* 5:2160–2169, 1966.
18. Doleschel W. Isolierung einer dritten humanen Urokinase. (^{S}o-Typ) *Wien Klin Wochenschr.* 87:282–284, 1975.
19. Holmberg L, Bladh B, Astedt B. Purification of urokinase by affinity chromatography. *Biochem Biophys Acta.* 445:215–222, 1976.
20. Somberano ME, Ong EB, Johnson AJ, Levy M, Schoellmann G. Purification and characterization of two forms of urokinase. *Biochem Biophys Acta.* 445:763–773, 1976.
21. Holmberg L, Astedt B. Urinary urokinase subunits and urokinase derived from normal and neoplastic endometrium. In: *Progress in Fibrinolysis.* Vol. V. Davidson JF, et al., Eds. Edinburgh, Churchill Livingstone, 1981, p. 31.
22. Astedt B, Holmberg L, Lecander I, Thorell J. Radioimmunoassay of urokinase for quantification of plasminogen activators released in ovarian tumour cultures. *Eur J Cancer.* 17:239–244, 1981.
23. Astedt B. No crossreaction between circulating plasminogen activator and urokinase. *Thromb Res.* 14:535–539, 1979.
24. Mullertz S, Clemmensen I. The primary inhibitor of plasmin in human plasma. *Biochem J.* 159:545–553, 1976.
25. Collen D. Identification and some properties of a new fast-reacting plasmin inhibitor in human plasma. *Eur J Biochem.* 69:209–216, 1976.
26. Moroi M, Aoki N. Isolation and characterization of Alpha-$_2$-plasmin inhibitor from human plasma. *J Biol Chem.* 251:5956–5965, 1976.
27. Collen D, Wiman B. The fast-acting plasmin inhibitor of human plasma. In: *Progress in Fibrinolysis.* Vol. IV. Davidson JF, et al., Eds. Edinburgh, Churchill Livingstone, 1979, p. 11.
28. Wiman B, Collen D. Molecular mechanism of physiological fibrinolysis. *Nature.* 272:549–550, 1978.
29. Marder VJ. Identification and purification of fibrinogen degradation products produced by plasmin: Consideration on the structure of fibrinogen. *Scand J Haematol.* (Suppl) 13:21–36, 1971.
30. Marder VJ, Francis CW, Doolittle RF. Fibrinogen structure and physiology. In: *Hemostasis and Thrombosis: Basic Principles and Clinical Practice.* Colman RW, Hirsh J, Marder VJ, et al., Eds. Philadelphia, Lippincott, 1982, pp. 145–163.
31. Marder VJ. Fibrinogen and fibrin degradation products. Physicochemical and physiological considerations. *Thromb Diath Haemorreol.* (Suppl) 47:85–98, 1971.
32. Nussenzweig V, Seligmann M. Analyse, par des methodes immunochimiques, de la degradation par la plasmine du fibrinogene humain et de la fibrine, a differents stades. *Rev Hematol.* 15:451–466, 1960.
33. Bouma BN, Hedner U, Nilsson IM. Typing of fibrinogen degradation products in urine in various clinical disorders. *Scand J Clin Lab Invest.* 27:331–335, 1971.
34. Plow EF, Edgington TS. Molecular events responsible for modulation of neoantigenic expression: The cleavage-associated neoantigen of fibrinogen. *Proc Natl Acad Sci USA.* 69:208–212, 1972.
35. Plow EF, Edgington TS. Discriminating neoantigenic differences between fibrinogen and fibrin derivatives. *Proc Natl Acad Sci USA.* 70:1169–1173, 1973.
36. Lipinski B, Wegrzynowicz Z, Budzynski AZ, Kopec M, Latallo ZS, Kowalski E. Soluble unclottable complexes formed in the presence of fibrinogen degradation

products (FDP) during the fibrinogen-fibrin conversion and their potential significance in pathology. *Thromb Diath Haemorrheol.* 17:65–77, 1967.
37. Merskey C, Kleiner GJ, Johnson AJ. Quantitative estimation of split products of fibrinogen in human serum, relation to diagnosis and treatment. *Blood* 28:1–18, 1966.
38. Merskey C, Lalezari P, Johnson AJ. Tanned red cell haemagglutination inhibition immunoassay for fibrinogen-fibrin-related antigen (fibrinolytic degradation products) in human serum. *Scand J Haematol.* (Suppl) 13:83–85, 1971.
39. Hawiger J, Niewiarowski S, Gurewich V, Thomas DP. Measurement of fibrinogen and fibrin degradation products in serum by staphylococcal clumping test. *J Lab Clin Med.* 75:93–108, 1970.
40. Allington MJ. Detection of fibrin(ogen) degradation products by a latex clumping method. *Scand J Haematol.* (Suppl) 13:115–119, 1971.
41. Svanberg L, Hedner U, Astedt B. Value of determination of F.D.P. during pregnancy by immunochemical and latex agglutination inhibition method. *Acta Obstet Gynecol Scand.* 53:81–83, 1974.
42. Nilehn J-E. Separation and estimation of "split products" of fibrinogen and fibrin in human serum. *Thromb Diath Haemorrheol.* 18:487–498, 1967.
43. Larsson SO. On coagulation and fibrinolysis in renal failure. *Scand J. Haematol.* (Suppl) 15, 1971.
44. McNicol GP, Barakat AA, Douglas AS. Plasma fibrinolytic activity in renal disease. *Scot Med J* 10:189–194, 1965.
45. Larsson SO, Hedner U, Nilsson IM. On coagulation and fibrinolysis in acute renal failure. *Acta Med Scand.* 189:443–451, 1971.
46. Kanfer A, Vandewalle A, Beaufils M, Delarue F, Sraer JD. Enhanced antiplasmin activity in acute renal failure. *Br Med J.* 4:195–202, 1975.
47. Thomson C, Forbes CD, Prentice CRM, Kennedy AC. Changes in blood coagulation and fibrinolysis in the nephrotic syndrome. *Q J Med.*(new series) 43:399–407, 1974.
48 McCluskey RT, Vassalli P, Gallo G, Baldwin DS. An immunofluorescent study of pathogenic mechanisms in glomerular diseases. *N Engl J Med* 274:695–701, 1966.
49. McKay DG. *Disseminated Intravascular Coagulation: An Intermediary Mechanism of Disease.* New York, Hoebner Medical Division Harper and Row, Publishers, 1965.
50. Ekberg M, Pandolfi M. Origin of urinary fibrin/fibrinogen degradation products in glomerulonephritis. *Br Med J* 2:17, 1975.
51. Hall CL, Blainey JD, Gaffney PJ. Origin or urinary fibrin-fibrinogen degradation products in renal glomurular disease. *Nephron* 23:6–9, 1979.
52. Kamitsuju H, Tani K, Taniguchi A, Masuyama H, Iida Y, Fakui H. Urinary fibrin-fibrinogen degradation products and intraglomerular fibrin-fibrinogen deposition in various renal diseases. *Thromb Res.* 21:285–294, 1981.
53. Braun WE, Merrill JP. Urine fibrinogen fragments in human renal allografts: A possible mechanism of renal injury. *N Engl J Med.* 278:1366–1371, 1968.
54. Carlsson S, Hedner U, Nilsson IM, Bergentz SE, Ljungqvist U. Kidney transplantation and fibrinolytic split products in serum and urine. *Transplantation.* 10:366–371, 1970.
55. Hedner, U, Ekberg M, Nilsson IM. Urinary fibrin/fibrinogen degradation products (FDP) and glomerulonephritis. *Acta Med Scand.* 195:81–85, 1974.
56. Rayner H, Parashevas F, Israels LG, Israels ED. Fibrinogen breakdown products: Identifcation and assay in serum and urine. *J Lab Clin Med.* 74:586–596, 1969.
57. Hedner, U, Nilsson IM. Clinical experience with determination of fibrinogen degradation products. *Acta Med Scand.* 189:471–477, 1971.
58. Luke RG, Siegel RR, Talberg W, Holland N. Heparin treatment for post partum renal failure with microangiopathic haemolytic anaemia. *Lancet.* II:750–752, 1970.
59. Katz J, Lurie A, Kaplan BS, Krawits S, Metz J. Coagulation findings in the hemolytic-uremic syndrom of infancy: Similarity to hyperactute renal allograft rejection. *J Pediatr.* 78:426–434, 1971.
60. Antoine B, Neveu T, Ward PD. Fibrinuria during renal transplantation. *Transplantation.* 8:98–109, 1969.

61. Schmitt E, Seyfarth M, Templin R, Schneider P, Klinkman H. Diagnostic value of urinary fibrin degradation products. *Nephron.* 25:25–29, 1980.
62. Llach F, Papper S, Massry SG. The clinical spectrum of renal vein thrombosis: Acute and chronic. *Am J Med* 69:819–827, 1980.
63. Kauffman Rh, Veltkamp JJ, Van Tilburg NH, Van Es LA. Acquired antithrombin III deficiency and thrombosis in the nephrotic syndrome. *Am J Med.* 65:607–613, 1978.
64. Barr RD, Ouna N, Rees PH. Blood coagulation, fibrinolysis and the mercurial nephrotic syndrome. *J Trop Med.* 79:235–236, 1976.
65. Edward N. Fibrinolysis in patients on regular hemodialysis. *Clin Nephrol.* 1:97–100, 1973.
66. Kostering H, Girndt J, Matthaei D, Naidu R, Quellhorsst E. Alterations of clotting factors and platelets during hemofiltration. *J Dialysis.* 1:607–617, 1977.
67. Nilsson IM, Pandolfi M. Assay of fibrinolytic activity of the vessel wall. *Prog Chem Fibrinol Thromb.* 2:1–13, 1976.
68. Remuzzi G, Bertani T, Livio M, Cavenaghi AE, Mysliwiec M, Marchesi D, Donati MB, de Gaetano G, Mecca G. Vascular factors in the pathogenesis of uraemic bleeding. In: *Proceedings of the European Dialysis and Transplant Assoc.* 15:449–455. Robinson BHB, Hawkins JH, Eds. Istanbul, June, 1978.
69. Canavese C, Stratta P, Pacitti A, Mangiarotti G, Riacca M, Oneglio R, Vercellone A. Impaired fibrinolysis in uremia: Partial and variable correction by four different dialysis regimes. *Clin Nephrol.* 17:82–89, 1982.
70. Nilsson IM. Unbalanced coagulation-fibrinolysis system in glomerulonephritis and kidney transplantation. In: *Endothelium Platelets, and Prostaglandins: Fresh Insights in Renal Disease.* (International symposium.) Remuzzi G, Mecca G, de Gaetano G, Eds. New York, Raven Press. Bergano, September, 1979, pp. 305–320.
71. Ollendorf P, Storm O, Rygg I, Arnfred. Activation of the thromboplastic and fibrinolytic system during extracorporeal circulation. *Acta Chir Scand.* 122:217–223, 1961.
72. Okamoto S, Nakajima T, Okamoto U, Watanabe H, Iguchi Y, Igawa T, Chien C-C, Hayashi T. A surprising effect of E-amino-caproic acid on the bleeding of dogs, produced with the activation of plasmin in the circulatory blood. *Keio J Med.* 8: 247–266, 1959.
73. Nilsson IM, Sjøerdsma A, Waldenstrom J. Antifibrinolytic activity and metabolism of ε-aminocaproic acid in man. *Lancet.* 1:1322–1326. 1960.
74. Okamoto S, Okamoto U. Amino-metyl-cyclohexane-carboxylic acid: AMCHA. A new potent inhibitor of the fibrinolysis. *Keio J Med.* 11:105, 1962.
75. Andersson L, Nilsson IM, Nilehn J-E, Hedner U, Grandstrand B, Melander B. Experimental and clinical studies on AMCHA, the antifibrinolytically active isomer of p-aminomethyl cyclohexane carboxylic acid. *Scand J Haematol.* 2:230, 1965.
76. Dubber AH, McNicol GP, Douglas AS. Amino methyl cyclohexane carboxylic acid (AMCHA): A new synthetic fibrinolytic inhibitor. *Br J Haematol.* 11:237–245, 1965.
77. Thorsen S. Influence of fibrin on the effect of 6-aminohexanoic acid on fibrinolysis caused by tissue plasminogen activator or urokinase. In: *Progress in Chemical Fibrinolysis and Thrombolysis.* Vol 3, Davidson JF, Rowan RM, Samama MM, Eds. New York, Raven Press, 1978, p 269–283.
78. Hedlund PO. Postoperative venous thrombosis in benign prostatic disease. *Scand J Urol Nephrol.* (Suppl) 27, 1965.
79. Astedt B, Liedholm P, Wingerup L. The effect of tranexamic acid on the fibrinolytic activity of vein walls. *Ann Chir Gynaecol.* 67:203, 1978.
80. van Mourik JA, Lawrence DA, Loskutoff DJ. Purification of an inhibitor of plasminogen activator (antiactivator) synthesized by endothelial cells. *J Biol Chem.* In press.
81. Nilsson IM, Ljungnér H, Tengborn L. Two different mechanisms in patients with venous thrombosis and defective fibrinolysis. Low concentration of plasminogen activator or increased concentration of plasminogen activator inhibitor. *Br Med J.* In press.
82. Lecander I, Åstedt B. Isolation of a new specific plasminogen activator inhibitor from pregnancy plasma. *Br J Haematol.* In press.

Chapter 6

Antifibrinolytic Drug Therapy

Lester Persky, M.D.

I. Antifibrinolytic Drugs Available

Of the many potential inhibitors of the fibrinolytic system that have been investigated, only three have reached clinical trials. Two of these, epsilon aminocaproic acid (EACA) and 4-aminomethylcyclohexanecarboxylic acid (AMCHA), were discovered by Okamoto and his associates while searching for a synthetic plasmin inhibitor.[1–3] Melander and Okamoto, working independently, found that the *trans* form of AMCHA had antifibrinolytic activity.[4,5] Andersson and co-workers further investigated the clinical activity of this isomer, which they named tranexamic acid (AMCA).[6–7] AMCA has an antifibrinolytic activity six to ten times that of EACA and is now used more widely than EACA in countries other than the United States, where it is currently unavailable.[8–11] AMCA, when administered orally, causes nausea less frequently than does EACA. In the United States, only EACA (as AMICAR®, Lederle Laboratories, American Cyanamid Co.) is available as an antifibrinolytic agent.

The third, a naturally occurring protease inhibitor, available as Trasylol®, inhibits plasmin as well as its prime target, kallikrein. It is isolated from bovine pancreas, parotid, and lung.[4] Trasylol has not been used in urinary tract surgery because it does not impair the action of urokinase;[12,13] rather it is a noncompetitive inhibitor of plasmin, with which it forms a stoichiometric 1:1 inactive complex.[14] Furthermore, it does not pass into the urine due to its large molecular size, but is excreted as a number of smaller inactive, breakdown products.[15,16]

II. Clinical Indications for Use of Antifibrinolytic Agents

A. Upper Tract Bleeding

The urologist must often contend with severe and continued episodes of intraoperative and postoperative bleeding. Such excessive bleeding after surgery is due mainly to inadequate surgical hemostasis. There is no substitute for good surgical technique and an intact hemostatic system (see Chapter 9). The release into the urinary tract of the activator of plasminogen, urokinase, leads to enhanced fibrinolytic activity and the premature dissolution of hemostatic clots.[17,18] The efficacy of antifibrinolytic therapy depends on the identification of the underlying causes of postoperative bleeding.[19]

1. *Fibrinolysis*

Prentice,[10] in a recent review article, identified four main groups of disorders in which the normal physiologic balance between coagulation and fibrinolysis may be lost. They are:

- primary fibrinolysis of hyperplasminemia } hyperplasminemia
- secondary fibrinolysis as a consequence of disseminated intravascular coagulation (DIC) } hyperplasminemia
- local fibrinolysis within organs or tissues
- coagulation defects associated with normal fibrinolysis.

It is sometimes difficult to distinguish *clinically* between primary fibrinolysis and intravascular coagulation with secondary fibrinolytic response. For this, a detailed laboratory investigation is needed (see Chapter 5). Primary fibrinolysis can be controlled by the use of antifibrinolytic agents such as EACA.[20] Secondary fibrinolysis in DIC is a defense mechanism in response to intravascular coagulation, and its inhibition may lead to worsening of widespread thrombosis.[21–25] If required, in such cases it is recommended that antifibrinolytic agents be given concurrently with heparin.[25]

In 1961, McNicol et al. showed that urokinase, the plasminogen activator present in the tissues of the urinary tract and in urine, dissolves blood clots and sustains bleeding.[26] Other investigators confirmed this finding and studied the use of antifibrinolytic agents to control this type of urinary tract hemorrhage.[27,28] Surgery on tissues rich in plasminogen activator can cause primary fibrinolysis. This includes renal surgery, prostatectomy, and surgery for some malignancies.[20,29,30] In the operating room, when hemostatic problems appear, a survey of clotting can be begun by performing a whole-blood clotting time. The patient's blood is placed in a plain glass tube, and held in the hand as an improvised 37°C incubator. The presence of nonclotting blood or a defective clot indicates hemostatic abnormality, and more detailed tests for the coagulopathy or accelerated clot lysis should be carried out.[10] In the absence of adequate laboratory support, when the blood is incoagulable or the clot is defective, fibrinogen may be administered to the patient while support is being obtained. When accelerated clot lysis is present, a presumptive diagnosis of hyperplasminemia can be made and treatment can be initiated with fibrinogen, which is available in plasma, cryoprecipitate, or fibrinogen preparations. In these instances, the adding of EACA or AMCA can lead to dramatic and rapid clinical improvement.

We have found EACA to be a useful complement to surgery in the treatment of:

- immediate and delayed postoperative urinary hemorrhage
- bleeding due to genitourinary neoplasms, and
- hemorrhage occurring as a sequel to radiation.

2. *Sickle Cell Disease and Trait*

Intermittent and sometimes prolonged hematuria, referred to as "essential hematuria," is associated with sickle cell trait and sickle cell disease (see Chapter 3). This potentially life-threatening complication had been treated during the 1950s by unilateral nephrectomy, which was followed almost invariably by bleeding from the remaining kidney. Immergut and Stevenson first reported on the use of EACA to control prolonged hematuria associated with sickle cell trait in four cases using 4 gm/day for 3–7 days.[31] Allen reported on 29 patients with this type of bleeding and suggested that conservative treatment with EACA would be preferred.[32] Vega et al. reported on the use of EACA at 5 gm IV plus 10 gm IV over 12 hours, followed by an additional 10 gm over 12 hours, if needed, to stop the hematuria of sickle cell trait/disease.[33] In eight of the 11 patients treated, gross hematuria ceased within 72 hours. In the remaining three, recurrent hematuria occurred in the next 3–6 weeks. Repetition of the EACA treatment cleared the hematuria. No untoward side effects of the drug were reported.

Black et al. reviewed 44 episodes of prolonged hematuria in 40 patients with sickle cell trait/disease who were treated with EACA.[34] They reported that hematuria subsided in 2.2 ± 0.3 days in the treated group (24 episodes). In their study, therapy with EACA was not associated with an increase in thrombosis. However, since spontaneous clot formation in the renal collecting system is associated with any bleeding within the renal pelvis, and since EACA therapy can increase this likelihood, they cautioned that treatment should be limited to those patients with severe or prolonged hematuria.[25,35] This opinion was also expressed by Rizza in a 1980 review article on the use of inhibitors of fibrinolysis in the treatment of hemophiliacs.[36]

3. *Hemophilias*

In the hemophilias, hematuria is the third most common type of bleeding seen (see Chapter 1). McNicol, in 1961, was the first to report on the use of EACA to treat hematuria in a hemophiliac.[37] Since then it has become apparent that the secondary obstructing clots that develop within the urinary tract are sufficiently common that a therapy with EACA or AMCA is relatively contraindicated in hemophiliacs suffering from hematuria, whenever appropriate factor replacement therapy is available. Clot formation in these patients is a complication that is frequently present to a minor degree, but is sometimes severe enough to impair seriously the renal function.[38,39] Therefore, upper urinary tract bleeding in these patients should be managed conservatively and with factor replacement as long as and whenever possible.

4. *Renal Biopsies*

Patients who must undergo renal biopsy may have subsequent severe and protracted hematuria. Prolonged hematuria does not usually require surgical intervention except when bleeding is perirenal, and then exploration, possibly with nephrectomy, may be needed.[40] In reporting on the treatment of hemorrhage secondary to percutaneous nephropyelostomy treated by arterial embolization, Eckhauser et al.[41] gave an incidence of 5% for significant complications of this procedure.

Ambrus et al.,[15] Haygood et al.,[42] Silverberg et al.,[43] and Savdie et al.[44] reported on the use of EACA to inhibit urokinase and thus allow normal hemostasis to control the bleeding. Savdie and co-workers reported on six patients.[44] One young man with interstitial nephritis required 13 units of blood prior to EACA therapy. Other patients over 50 years old with end-stage renal disease required three to five units of blood prior to EACA therapy. In five of the six patients treated, there was a rapid response to EACA therapy with cessation of bleeding, and in all cases there was no further requirement for blood transfusions. Lissoos[45] reported on two cases of stab wounds that resulted in persistent hematuria. The patients refused surgery and were treated with EACA orally. In both cases bleeding stopped, and within 3 days the urine was clear and healing progressed without surgical intervention. Thus, the administration of EACA is useful in accelerating intrarenal hemostasis and may reduce the need for blood transfusions and operative intervention.

B. Lower Tract Bleeding

The clearest and least controversial use of antifibrinolytic agents is in the treatment of lower urinary tract bleeding when associated with local fibrinolysis. These patients can, in general, be placed in one of the following categories: vesical cancers, prostatic neoplasms, or radiation treatment.

Patients with vesical neoplasms can be grouped into three categories. First are those with tumors that are inoperable because of local and distant metastases who have undergone repeated fulgurations and resections.[46] In the second category are patients with fairly extensive superficial tumors who are treated endoscopically. The third category includes those patients with disabling medical complications and persistent bleeding due to severe refractory tumors.

Patients classed as having prostatic neoplasms are those who have residual inoperable tumors. Their histories may include repeated resections, widespread metastatic disease, hormonal manipulation, and radiation. They are not candidates for radical surgery. Hemoglobin levels and other indicators of systemic intravascular coagulation can be monitored on an outpatient basis.

Patients treated with radiotherapy for prostatic and bladder cancers often have intravesicular and rectal telangiectactic blood vessels, which are difficult to control if they bleed. Hemorrhage can be due to cyclophosphamide-induced cystitis. Some success has been achieved in using EACA to control these hemorrhages.

1. Bleeding From the Bladder

Patients who have been treated with radiation, endocrine manipulation, or fulguration for genitourinary neoplasms are vulnerable to recurrent episodic hematuria. The management of these patients presents the clinician with a therapeutic problem. In the majority of cases, surgery or further radiation is of no value. Cytotoxic drugs have been evaluated with mixed results.[47,48] It is not practical to hospitalize these patients each time they bleed. Nor is it desirable to subject patients, who are frequently over 70, frail, and poor risks, to repeated anesthesia and intervention surgery. Yet it is precisely because of their poor physical condition that the debilitating effects of even moderate essential hematuria are most serious. In many cases the bleeding is contributed to by the fibrinolytic activity initiated by urokinase flowing over the resection or fulguration sites.[10,26]

In these cases, bleeding can be controlled by the use of EACA. To inhibit urokinase activity in the urine, concentrations of EACA above 10^{-2} M are required, a level that is substantially higher than plasma concentrations of 13 mg/100 ml (10^{-3} M) required for control of systematic fibrinolytic activity.[26,49] However, since the drug is concentrated in the urine to 50–100 times that of plasma, dosages lower than those used in systematic fibrinolytic conditions can be used.

Dosage schedules that have been used successfully are given in Table I. This approach keeps the patients ambulatory and minimizes the cost of treatment. The patients can be thereafter placed on a self-regulated dosage program. Few toxic effects with oral EACA have been reported in ambulatory patients. We used it regularly for 4 years (1977–1981) and did not have a case of pulmonary embolism or excessive clotting. By avoiding the psychologically distressing sign of gross blood in the urine, this program also avoids needless apprehension and anxiety on the part of the patient and family.

2. *Bleeding From the Prostatic Bed*

McNicol et al. first suggested that bleeding after prostatectomy could be the result of clot lysis due to urokinase functioning in its normal role of maintaining

Table I
Use of Epsilon Aminocaproic Acid for Fibrinolytic Bleeding

Cause of Hematuria	Immediate Therapy	Maintenance Therapy*
Prostatectomy	5 gm IV (in solution 1 gm/hr for 5 hr 1 gm/2–4 for 24–48 hr	2–4 gm/4 hr orally for 5–7 days
Bladder cancer	Bladder irrigation with 2% solution for 48–72 hr	2 gm/4 hr orally for 10–14 days
Delayed bleeding after nephrectomy	5 gm IV (in solution) 1 gm/hr for 8 hr 1 gm/4 hr until urine is clear for 24 hr	2 gm/4 hr orally for 10–14 days
Urokinase activity (to inhibit tissue activators)[58]	50 mg/kg, 8 hourly, IV or oral 100 mg/kg, 3–4 times a day	
Radiation cystitis	2 gm/4 hr orally for 10–14 days	2 gm/4 hr orally for 10–14 days

*Dosage should be reduced in patients with reduced creatinine clearance. Adapted from Persky L, et al. Used with permission.

patency in the urinary tract by lysing fibrinous deposits.[26] These workers, plus Andersson, Nilsson, and their co-workers, investigated the use of EACA to reduce postoperative blood loss in prostatic resections.[51–54] They demonstrated that this blood loss could be reduced regardless of surgical technique. After a review in 1966 of 744 patients treated with EACA to control hemorrhage, Nilsson, et al. recommended using intra- and postoperative EACA for prostatectomy patients.[55] They noted that unlike the clots formed in the upper urinary tract, clots that formed in the bladder are readily removed through a catheter or by cystoscopy. They used 3 gm EACA three times a day.

Vinnicombe and Shuttleworth reported a controlled, double-blind study of retropubic prostatectomy in 515 patients, of whom 259 received 6 gm EACA intravenously at 0.5 gm per hour for 12 hours, beginning at the time of operation.[56] They found no evidence of increased embolism or other complications as compared to the 256 control patients. Blood loss was reduced from 658.3 gm hemoglobin in untreated patients to 230.5 gm hemoglobin in treated patients on the first day ($P<0.005$) and from 870.2 gm hemoglobin in untreated to 344.8 gm hemoglobin in treated patients on the fifth day ($P<0.01$).

In another double-blind study, Sack et al. found a significant reduction in postoperative bleeding among those treated with EACA.[57] This study involved 56 patients, of whom 20 underwent perineal and 36 underwent suprapubic prostatectomies. The dose of EACA used was 5 gm given intravenously every 6 hours in 500 ml of 5% dextrose solution given until bleeding stopped (up to 60 hours). Hedlund reported a double-blind study in which AMCA was given to 92 nonselected patients who underwent transvesical prostatectomy.[58] Treatment with both 3 gm and 1.5 gm AMCA per day, administered intravenously, resulted in a statistically significant reduction in bleeding. Side effects were few and were minimized when the drug was administered slowly. Gow studied 300 patients who underwent transurethral resection (TUR) for the treatment of prostatic hypertrophy (202 cases), sclerosis of the bladder neck (62 cases), and carcinoma (36 cases).[59] The average age of these patients was 71 years, and the range was 47–91 years. Fifty-one patients were over 80 years old. Epsilon aminocaproic acid at 1 gm per hour for 12 hours was administered intravenously to help control the bleeding. This report emphasized that the patients should be ambulatory the day after the operation and should be free to move without catheter or intravenous lines within 48 hours. Other reports of successful control of post-prostatectomy hemorrhage with AMCA are by Landmann (53 of 59 cases),[60] Ennemoser and Heidbrink (17 prostatectomies),[61] and Kaufmann[62] and Lassner.[63]

It is not our practice to employ EACA prophylactically at the beginning of a TUR. In this respect, it is important to stress the role of recovery room personnel in dealing with bleeding problems. They need to maintain good bladder irrigation and to monitor closely the flow and color of the irrigant solution for evidence of blood in the urine. Because they are well versed with the procedures and are attuned to the problems of clotting in the urinary tract they call promptly if any problem arises.

Lipsky and Hubmer reviewed their 4-year experience with the use of tranexamic acid for hemorrhage due to fibrinolysis in prostatectomy patients.[64] They do not consider its routine prophylactic use necessary, but do recommend prophylactic measures in patients with a history of hematuria or when large adenomas are being treated.

III. Pharmacology

A. Dose/Duration/Distribution

After intravenous administration of 10 gm EACA (or 100 mg EACA/kg bodyweight), an initial serum concentration of about 150 mg/100 ml was achieved within one-half hour. The serum concentration fell to 3.5 mg/100 ml within 3–4 hours. When 100 mg/kg bodyweight of EACA was given by mouth, the peak plasma concentration was 30 mg/100 ml at 2–3 hours after dosage. After 4 hours it was 16 mg/100 ml. After 6 hours, the concentration was similar to that found after intravenous injection.[65]

The amount of EACA excreted into the urine varies somewhat with the mode of administration.[65–67] EACA has been demonstrated to enter human red blood cells and tissues. Its concentration is apparently dependent on the extracellular concentration. Approximately 80–85% of an administered dose is recovered unaltered in the urine, indicating that for the most part it is not actively metabolized. Andersson et al. found that about 70% of an IV dose was excreted in the urine in 24 hours.[67] McNicol et al. reported a urinary recovery of 86 ± 8.7% of the administered dose. The 24-hour urinary recovery after oral administration was between 64% and 78%.[66] It has been suggested that recoveries of less than 100% could be due to delayed excretion or to metabolic breakdown.[65,66]

B. Intravesicular EACA

For treating patients in whom DIC may be present, the intravesicular use of EACA pioneered by Lassner may be used.[63] He used an isotonic solution of sodium chloride containing 2 gm/L of EACA and continuously irrigated the bladder via a double-flow catheter. Irrigation, rapid at first (300–500 ml/hour), was slowed gradually to 100 ml/hour as bleeding diminished. In a more recent study conducted by Lerner at the New York Medical College, EACA was used in seven patients as a postoperative bladder irrigant at 0.5% EACA in 1.5% glycine solution.[68] Irrigation was begun at 500–1,000 ml/hr and was slowed gradually to 100 ml/hr as bleeding diminished. Continuous irrigation was employed for 3 days. EACA was not detected in the patients' sera when assayed by a method sensitive to 5 μg/ml. In three additional patients administered EACA intraoperatively at the above-mentioned concentrations, the mean serum level detected was 34.7 μg/ml (range 21–60 μg/ml) (compared to 130 μg/ml needed for therapeutic inhibition of fibrinolysis).[68] No side effects were observed among any of these 10 patients. Thus, the minimal or zero absorption of the drug when administered intravesically reduces the likelihood of systemic side effects, especially when given to patients with DIC.

Clinical Pharmacology of AMCA (Table II)

Andersson and co-workers[6,16,67] studied the absorption and distribution of AMCA given intravenously and orally. After IV administration of 10 mg AMCA/kg of bodyweight, the serum concentrations were 18, 10, and 5 μg/ml after 1, 3, and 5 hours, respectively. When 10 mg/kg AMCA was given by mouth, the maximum serum concentration was 2 μg/ml after 3 hours. At 6 hours, the serum concentrations were approximately the same whether administration was by the oral or the intravenous route. When AMCA was given at 100 mg/kg by mouth, the serum levels were 8, 40, and 13 μg/ml at 2, 4, and 6 hours, respectively. It is apparent from these data that AMCA is not as efficiently absorbed from the gastrointestinal tract as is EACA. About 40% of an oral dose of 10–15 mg/kg is recovered in the urine in 24 hours.

Eriksson et al.[69] investigated the pharmacokinetics of a 1 gm dose of AMCA administered intravenously to normal volunteers. Following injection, the plasma concentrations dropped rapidly in the first hour followed by a slower elimination in which the half-life was 1.3 to 2 hours. Plasma levels at 2, 4, and 6 hours were approximately 20, 10, and 5 μg/ml, respectively; after 6 hours a half-life of 9–18 hours was reported. About half the dose was recovered unchanged in the urine in the first 3–4 hours, 90% to 95% within 24 hours, and 95% to 99% within 48–72 hours.[70] The delayed excretion was shown to be due to the distribution of AMCA into tissue compartments, making it unavailable for excretion.

AMCA is eliminated by glomerular filtration.[65] Impairment of renal function prolongs the biological half-life; in patients with serum creatinine levels of 500 μmol/L (5.6 mg/100 ml), the half-life was found to be 24–48 hours.

Andersson et al.[7] measured the fibrinolytic activity and concentrations of AMCA and EACA in serum and tissues obtained at surgery. They found that to obtain a 98% to 100% reduction of tissue activator, an AMCA concentration of 100 μg/ml or an EACA concentration of 1,000 μg/ml was required. For 86% inhibition, judged sufficient from clinical experience, the respective concentrations of AMCA and EACA were 10 μg/ml and 100 μg/ml. Effective antifibrinolytic levels of AMCA persisted longer in tissues than did those of EACA. Thus, after repeated intravenous (10 mg/kg, four to five times a day) or oral (20 mg/kg, three to four times a day) doses, adequate activity in tissues can be maintained for up to 17 hours without any further dosing.

IV. Complications

A. The Acute Side Effects

In humans, the acute side effects associated with these drugs include nausea (less often with oral AMCA than with oral EACA), intestinal cramps, diarrhea, dizziness, nasal stuffiness, conjunctival suffusion, headache, and skin rash. Myalgias, muscle weakness, abnormal muscle enzymes, and rarely myoglobinuria have been reported with high-dose EACA therapy.[71] These side effects rarely cause therapy to be discontinued. Hypotension is associated with both drugs, especially if infused rapidly.[58,72] This reaction appears to disappear after the first 24 hours.

An important question is whether treatment with AMCA or EACA predisposes the patient to thrombosis or disseminated intravascular coagulation. The true incidence of drug-induced thrombotic events is unclear, since many of the patients being treated may have acquired thrombotic diseases, such as thrombophlebitis or infarct, in the absence of antifibrinolytic treatment. Nilsson, in a report based on a 5-year clinical experience,[55] and again in a review published in 1980,[65] discusses use of EACA in 744 patients. Vinnicombe and Shuttleworth reviewed their double-blind multicenter study of 515 patients.[56] No evidence of increased thrombosis, embolism, or morbidity due to pulmonary embolism or myocardial infarction was found between the treated and the untreated groups. Hedlund[58] reported the incidence of deep venous thrombosis of the leg as detected by the very sensitive ^{125}I-fibrinogen uptake test in 201 prostatectomy patients, 100 of whom had received 1 gm of AMCA three times a day and 101 of whom received a placebo. There was no significant difference in thrombosis rate between the two groups. Sinclair et al. reported a double-blind placebo controlled study of patients undergoing prostatectomy for benign prostrate hypertrophy.[73] The ^{125}I technique was again used. They found no increase of deep vein thrombosis despite the fact that they used higher doses over a longer period (126 gm over 10 days) than had been used in other studies. Their conclusion was that in this group of patients undergoing prostatectomy with mean ages in the treated group of 67 years and in the control group of 70 years, there was no contraindication to the routine use of fibrinolytic inhibitors.

On the other hand, there is no doubt that EACA and AMCA perpetuate existing fibrin deposits. Ratnoff, in a review of the use of EACA, noted that serious thrombotic complications can occur.[74] While the antifibrinolytic agents alone do not cause clots to form, they do prevent their normal dissolution. Ratnoff, citing studies as contraindicating the use of these agents,[21–24] concluded that the thrombotic processes resulted from an underlying condition, e. g. prostatic carcinoma, or from a response to postsurgical trauma. (In selected conditions, heparin may actually be the preferred drug.[23]) Thus, patients in whom there is an underlying prethrombotic state or in whom there is active DIC should not receive these drugs. If care is exercised to exclude such patients, these drugs can be very useful to the patient and the surgeon.

B. The Long-Term Side Effects

No fetal abnormalities were seen in rats, rabbits, or mice given doses up to 5,000 μg of EACA kg/day.[75] When given in large doses to dogs and female rats, EACA resulted in a reversible 50% reduction of fertility.[76] Retinal changes were seen in dogs receiving AMCA for 1 year at doses approximately seven times greater than the maximum dose recommended for humans. However, no such changes were seen in dogs given three and one-half times the maximal oral dose given to humans when this dose was given over a period of 1 year, nor in rats given seven times the maximal dose over 22 months, nor in monkeys given 18 times the maximal intravenous dose for 14 days. No retinal changes have been reported in patients treated for months or years. Nevertheless, Nilsson recommends that patients being treated continuously over weeks should have their visual parameters checked.[65] Adenomas and adenocarcinomas were reported in rats after they were treated for 22 months, but not after 12 months of therapy, using oral treatment at 27 times the maximum dose of AMCA recommended for humans. No such tumors were seen in rats given six times the maximum human daily dose on a bodyweight basis.

Carroll and Tice reported that 0.3 – 1.4 gm of EACA/kg given intravenously to nephrectomised dogs produced hypokalemia.[77]

V. Conclusion

When hemorrhage is due to primary fibrinolysis, as after prostatectomy, the use of antifibrinolytic agents is indicated. An excellent review of antifibrinolytic therapy by Marder is available encompassing not only urologic conditions but also other clinical indications.[78] Studies over the years have established the safety and efficacy of antifibrinolytic agents in managing post-prostactectomy bleeding. Studies using EACA[37,53–57,65] or AMCA[58] demonstrated a reduction in postoperative bleeding with a low incidence of side effects. Later studies by Gow[59] with 300 patients, Sinclair[73] with 40 patients, and Osborne[79] with 965 patients confirm the findings of the earlier studies. Moreover, these studies suggest that operative technique and the patient's position on the operating table may have relevance to the occurrence of postoperative thrombosis. Where possible, transurethral resection is preferred to the retropubic or suprapubic resection. Sinclair noted in a double-blind trial of patients receiving EACA therapy after prostatectomy that 13 of 19 patients (68%) who had retropubic prostatectomies developed evidence of deep vein thrombosis (bilaterally in six cases), while seven of 21 patients (33%) who had transurethral resections had positive ^{125}I scans, (bilateral in three).[73] Mayo also demonstrated that the incidence of deep vein thrombosis was 51% after open retropubic prostatectomy and 10% following transurethral resection.[80]

Osborne, who treated 965 patients with EACA after transurethral prostatectomy, reported seven cases of pulmonary embolism and four cases of thrombophlebitis, as defined by clinical observation.[79] These patients were treated with anticoagulants with no subsequent mortality. This incidence of thromboembolic complications compares favorably with that reported in a series by Valk et al. of 2,223 transurethral prostatectomy patients given no EACA therapy.[81]

On those occasions where excessive fibrinolysis is secondary to diffuse intravascular coagulation, treatment with EACA or AMCA can be disastrous, precipitating widespread thrombosis.[21–25] O'Sullivan and Joyce[82] and Gralnick and Greipp[23] recommend that should DIC be demonstrated, adequate blood and plasma factors together with heparin should be administered, in conjunction with the help of an expert coagulationist.

As noted by Marder[78] and Prentice,[10] the use of antifibrinolytic agents or treatment of hematuria associated with upper genitourinary bleeding, such as occurs in hemophilia and the hemoglobinopathies, should be undertaken with

Table II
Use of Tranexamic Acid for Control of Hematuria

Condition	Immediate therapy	Maintenance
Conditions associated with local fibrinolysis (to inhibit tissue activators)	10–20 mg/kg, orally 3–4 times per day	Antifibrinolytic levels are maintained for 17 hours by this dosage
Inhibition of Urokinase	10 mg/kg, intravenously 20 mg/kg, orally 2–3 times a day	1–2 gm 2–3 times per day

caution and should be considered primarily for those in whom surgery is the alternative course.

REFERENCES

1. Okamoto S. British Patent Specifications 770693, 1957.
2. Okamoto S, Nakajima T, Okamoto U, Watanabe H, Iguchi Y, Igawa T, Chien CC, Hayashi T. A suppressing effect of epsilon amino-n-caproic acid on the bleeding of dogs, produced with the activation of plasmin in the circulatory blood. *Keio J Med.* 8:247–266, 1959.
3. Okamoto S, Okamoto U. Amino-methyl-cyclohexane-carboxylic acid: AMCHA. A new potent inhibitor of the fibrinolysis. *Keio J Med.* 11:105–115, 1962.
4. Melander B, Gliniecki G, Grandstrand B, Hanhoff G. Experimental studies on the antifibrinolytic activity of AMCHA. In: *Abstracts of the Xth International Congress of the Society of Haematology.* Stockholm, Aug 30–Sept. 4, 1964, G68.
5. Okamoto S, Kinjo K, Oshiba S, Mango M, Shimizu M, Sato S, Okamoto U. Behavior of tissue activators and the action of a series of potent inhibitors on fibrinolysis. In: *Abstracts of the Xth International Congress of the Society of Haematology.* Stockholm, Aug. 30–Sept. 4, 1964. G65.
6. Andersson L, Nilsson IM, Nilehn JE, Hedner U, Grandstrand B, Melander B. Experimental and clinical studies on AMCHA, the antifibrinolytically active isomer of p-aminomethyl cyclohexane carboxylic acid. *Scand J. Haematol.* 2:230–247, 1965.
7. Andersson L, Nilsson IM, Colleen S, Grandstrand B, Melander B. Role of urokinase and tissue activator in sustaining bleeding and the management thereof with EACA and AMCA. *Ann NY Acad Sci.* 146:642–658, 1968.
8. Dubber AHC, McNicol GP, Douglas AS, Melander B. Some properties of the antifibrinolytically active isomer of amino-methylcyclohexane carboxylic acid. *Lancet.* 2:1317–1319, 1964.
9. Dubber AHC, McNicol GP, Douglas AS. Amino methyl cyclohexane carboxylic acid (AMCHA), a new synthetic fibrinolytic inhibitor. *Br J Haematol.* 11:237–245, 1965.
10. Prentice CRM. Basis of antifibrinolytic therapy. *J Clin Pathol. Roy Coll Path.* 33(Suppl 14):35–40, 1980.
11. Amris CJ. Inhibition of fibrinolytic and thromboplastic activity by Trasylol. *Scand J. Haematol.* 3:19–32, 1966.
12. Lorand L, Condit EV. Ester hydrolysis by urokinase. *Biochemistry.* 4:265–270, 1965.
13. Walton PL. The hydrolysis of alpha-N-acetylglycyl-1-lysine methyl ester by urokinase. *Biochim Biophys Acta.* 132:104–114, 1967.
14. Dubber AH, McNicol GP, Uttley D, Douglas AS. In vitro and in vivo studies with Trasylol, an anticoagulant and a fibrinolytic inhibitor. *Br J Haematol.* 14:31–49, 1968.
15. Ambrus JL, Ambrus CM, Stutzman L, Schimert G, Niswander KR, Woodruff MW, Magoss IV. Treatment of fibrinolytic hemorrhage with proteinase inhibitors: A preliminary report. *Ann NY Acad Sci.* 146:625–641, 1968.
16. Andersson L. Fibrinolysis and its control. *S Afr Med J.* 46:182–185, 1972.
17. Albrechtsen OK. The fibrinolytic activity of human tissues. *Br J Haematol.* 3:284–291, 1957.
18. Williams JRB. The fibrinolytic activity of urine. *Br J Exp Pathol.* 32:530–537, 1951.
19. Andersson L. Antifibrinolytic therapy in genitourinary tract surgery. *J Clin Pathol. Roy Coll Pathol.* 33(Suppl 14):60–62, 1980.
20. Kwaan HC. Disorders of fibrinolysis. *Med Clin North Am.* 56:163–176, 1972.
21. Charytan C, Purtilo D. Glomerular capillary thrombosis and acute renal failure after epsilon amino caproic acid therapy. *N Engl J Med.* 280:1101–1104, 1969.

22. Gobbi F. Use and misuse of aminocaproic acid. *Lancet.* 2:472–473, 1967.
23. Gralnick HR, Greipp P. Thrombosis with epsilon aminocaproic acid therapy. *Am J Clin Pathol.* 56:151–154, 1971.
24. Naeye RL. Thrombotic state after a hemorrhage diathesis, a possible complication of therapy with epsilon aminocaproic acid. *Blood.* 19:694–701, 1962.
25. Stark SN, White JG, Langer L Jr, Krivit W: Epsilon amino caproic acid therapy as a cause of intrarenal obstruction in hematuria of haemophiliacs. *Scand J Haematol.* 2:99–107, 1965.
26. McNicol GP, Fletcher AP, Alkjaersig N, Sherry S. Impairment of hemostasis in the urinary tract: The role of urokinase. *J Lab Clin Med.* 53:34–46, 1961.
27. Nilsson IM. Local fibrinolysis as a mechanism for haemorrhage. *Thromb Diath Haemorrheol.* 34:623–633, 1975.
28. Prentice CR. Indications for antifibrinolytic therapy. *Thromb Diath Haemorrheol.* 34:634–643, 1975.
29. Imperati L. La fibrinolisi Post-Operatoria. *Rif Med.* 53:1694–1698, 1937.
30. Macfarlane RG. Fibrinolysis following operation. *Lancet.* 1:10–12, 1937.
31. Immergut MA, Stevenson T. The use of epsilon aminocaproic acid in the control of hematuria associated with hemaglobinopathies. *J Urol.* 93:110–111, 1965.
32. Allen TD. Sickle cell disease and hematuria: Report of 29 cases. J Urol. 91:177–183, 1964.
33. Vega R, Shanberg AM, Malloy TR. The use of epsilon aminocaproic acid in sickle cell trait hematuria. *J Urol.* 105:552–553, 1971.
34. Black WD, Hatch FE, Acchiardo S. Aminocaproic acid in prolonged hematuria of patients with sicklemia. *Arch Intern Med.* 136:678–681, 1976.
35. Lindgardh G, Andersson L. Clot retention in the kidneys as a probable cause of anuria during treatment of haematuria with epsilon-aminocaproic acid. *Acta Med Scand.* 180:469–473, 1966.
36. Rizza CR. Inhibitors of fibrinolysis in the treatment of haemophilia. *J Clin Pathol. Roy Coll Pathol.* 33 (Suppl 14):50–54, 1980.
37. McNicol GP, Fletcher AP, Alkjaersig N, Sherry S. The use of epsilon aminocaprioc acid, a potent inhibitor of fibrinolytic activity, in the management of postoperative hematuria. *J Urol.* 86:829–837, 1961.
38. Hilgartner MW. Intrarenal obstruction in haemophilia. *Lancet.* 1:486, 1966.
39. van Itterbeek H, Vermylen J, Verstraete M. High obstruction of urine flow as a complication of the treatment with fibrinolysis inhibitors of haematuria in haemophiliacs. *Acta Haematol.* 39:237–242, 1968.
40. Slotkin EA, Madsen PO. Complications of renal biopsy incidence in 5,000 reported cases. *J Urol.* 105:552–553, 1971.
41. Eckhauser ML, Haaga JR, Hampel N, Selman SH, Kedia KR, Wolkoff JS, Makker S, Persky L. Arterial embolization of renal allograft to control hemorrhage secondary to percutaneous nephropyelostomy. *J Urol.* 126:679–680, 1981.
42. Haygood TA, Atkins R, Kennedy JA, Cutter RE. Aminocaproic acid treatment of prolonged hematuria following renal biopsy. *Arch Intern Med.* 127:478–481, 1971.
43. Silverberg DS, Dossetor JB, Eid TC, Mant MJ, Miller JD. Arteriovenous fistula and prolonged hematuria after renal biopsy: Treatment with epsilon aminocaproic acid. *Can Med Assoc J.* 110:671–672, 1974.
44. Savdie E, Mahony JF, Storey BG. Control of bleeding after renal biopsy with epsilon aminocaproic acid. *Br J Urol.* 50:8–11, 1978.
45. Lissoos I. Epsilon-aminocaproic acid in the treatment of renal trauma. *S Afr Med J.* 46:1637–1638, 1972.
46. Sauvage R. Reoperation for massive hematuria after chemotherapy for bladder papillomatosis previously treated with surgery and cobalt therapy. *Acta Urol Belg.* 49:36–43, 1981.
47. Carter SK, Wasserman TH. The chemotherapy of urologic cancer. *Cancer.* 36:729–747, 1975.

48. Kedia KR, Gibbons C, Persky L. The management of advanced bladder carcinoma. *J. Urol.* 125:655–658, 1981.
49. McNicol GP, Fletcher AP, Alkjaersig N, Sherry S. The absorption, distribution, and excretion of epsilon aminocaproic acid following oral or intravenous administration to man. *J Lab Clin Med.* 59:15–24, 1962.
50. Persky L, Selman SH. Therapeutic application of epsilon aminocaproic acid in the urology patient. *Contemp Surg.* 17:23–35, 1980.
51. Andersson L. Treatment of so-called essential haematuria with fibrinolytic inhibitor (epsilon-aminocaproic acid). *Acta Chir Scand.* 124:355–364, 1962.
52. Andersson L. Fibrinolysis in patients with prostatic cancer. *Acta Chir Scand.* 126:172–183, 1963.
53. Andersson L. Fibrinolytic states in prostatic disease and their treatment with epsilon aminocaproic acid. *Acta Chir Scand.* 126:251–265, 1963.
54. Andersson L, Nilsson IM. Effect of 6-amino-n-caproic acid (6-ACA) on fibrinolysis and bleeding conditions in prostatic disease. *Acta Chir Scand.* 121:291–298, 1961.
55. Nilsson IM, Andersson L, Bjorkman SE. Epsilon-aminocaproic acid (EACA) as a therapeutic agent based on 5 year's clinical experience. *Acta Med Scand.* (Suppl 448):1-46 1966.
56. Vinnicombe J, Shuttleworth KE. Aminocaproic acid in the control of hemorrhage after prostatectomy: Safety of aminocaproic acid - a controlled trial. *Lancet.* 1:232–234, 1966.
57. Sack E, Spaet TH, Gentile RL, Hudson PB. Reduction of post prostatectomy bleeding by epsilon-aminocaproic acid. *N Engl J Med* 266:541–543, 1962.
58. Hedlund PO. Antifibrinolytic therapy with Cyklokapron in connection with prostatectomy: A double-blind study. *Scand J Urol Nephrol.* 3:177–182, 1969.
59. Gow JG. Transurethral resection: A study of three hundred cases. *The Practitioner.* 210:535–540, 1973.
60. Landmann E. Erfahrungen mit einem neuartigen Antifibrinolytikum in der Urologie. *Therapiewoche.* 18:1349–1352, 1968.
61. Ennemoser D, Heidbrink D. Antifibrinolytische Therapie bei Prostatektomien, Tonsillektomien und Adenotomien. *Med Welt.* 17:1028–1030, 1969.
62. Kaufmann J, Siefker K. Reduction of post prostatectomy bleeding by medication, (experience with the antifibrinolytic agent AMCHA). *Urologe.* 8:57–59, 1969.
63. Lassner J. The use of epsilon aminocaproic acid in prostaic surgery. *Anesth Analg.* (Paris) 22 (3):475–479, 1965 (Fr).
64. Lipsky H, Hubmer O. Fibrinolyseblutungen in der Urologie. *Zurolnephrol.* 62: 453–461, 1969.
65. Nilsson IM. Clinical Pharmacology of animocaproic and tranexamic acids. *J Clin Pathol. Roy Coll Pathol.* 33(Suppl 14):41–47, 1980.
66. McNicol GP, Fletcher AP, Alkjaersig N, Sherry S. Absorption, distribution, and excretion of aminocaproic acid following oral or intravenous administration to man. *J Lab Clin Med.* 58:15–24, 1962.
67. Andersson L, Nilsson IM, Colleen S, Grandstrand B, Melander B. Role of urokinase and tissue activator in sustaining bleeding and the management thereof with EACA and AMCA. *Ann NY Acad Sci.* 146:642–658, 1968.
68. Lerner R. American Urology Association, May, 1981.
69. Eriksson O, Kjellman H, Pilbrant A, Schannong M. Pharmacokinetics of tranexamic acid after intravenous administration to normal volunteers. *Eur J Clin Pharmacol.* 7:375–380, 1974.
70. Kjellman H. Comments by the manufacturer of Cyclokapron. In: *Haemostatic Drugs: A Critical Appraisal.* Verstraete M, Ed. The Hague, Martinus Nijhoff Medical Division, 1970, pp. 140–141.
71. Griffen JD, Ellman L. Epsilon aminocaproic acid (EACA): The clinical uses of epsilon aminocaproic acid. *Semin Thromb Hemostas.* 5:27–40, 1978.
72. Vermylen J, Verhaegen-Declercq ML, Verstraete M, Fierens F. A double-blind

study of the effect of tranexamic acid in essential menorrhagia. *Thromb Diathes Haemorrheol.* 20:583–587, 1968.
73. Sinclair J, Forbes CD, Prentice CRM, Scott R. The incidence of deep vein thrombosis in prostatectomized patients following the administration of the fibrinolytic inhibitor, aminocaproic acid (EACA). *Urol Res.* 4:129–131, 1976.
74. Ratnoff OD. Epsilon aminocaproic acid: A dangerous weapon (Editorial). *N Engl J Med.* 280:1124–1125, 1969. Cit. No. 4021263.
75. Kjellman H. Synthetic antifibrinolytics. In: *Haemorrhagic and Thrombotic Diseases.* Nilsson IM, Ed. London, John Wiley & Sons, 1974, pp. 140–141.
76. Eneroth G, Grant CA. Epsilon aminocaproic acid and reduction in fertility of male rats. *Acta Pharma Suec.* 3:115–122, 1966.
77. Carroll HJ, Tice D. The effects of epsilon aminocaproic acid upon potassium metabolism in the dog. *Metabolism.* 15:449–457, 1966.
78. Marder VJ, Butler FO, Barlow GH. Antifibrinolytic therapy. In: *Hemostasis and Thrombosis. Basic Principles and Clinical Practices.* Colman RW, Hirsh J, Marder VJ, Saltzman E, Eds. Lippincott, Philadelphia, 1982, pp. 640–653.
79. Osborne RW. Safety and efficacy of epsilon-aminocaproic acid in prostatectomy bleeding. *Curr Therap Res.* 31:839–845, 1982.
80. Mayo ME, Halil T, Browse NL. The incidence of deep vein thrombosis after prostatectomy. *Br J Urol.* 43:738–742, 1971.
81. Valk WL, Mebust WK, Melchior J, Foret JD. Present status of transurethral resection of the prostate for benign hypertrophy. *Urol Clin North Am.* 2:85–92, 1975.
82. O'Sullivan EF, Joyce JG. Abnormal bleeding after prostatectomy. *Med J. Aust.* 2: 1165–1169, 1972.

Chapter 7

Radiologic Manifestations of Urologic Hemorrhage

Edward S. Amis, Jr., M.D., and Richard C. Pfister, M.D.

I. Introduction

A. General Considerations

Urologic hemorrhage may manifest clinically in two forms: bleeding into the urinary collecting system, causing gross or microscopic hematuria, or bleeding into the retroperitoneum, occurring spontaneously from the adrenal gland or kidney, or following trauma to any of the urologic structures. The radiologic evaluation of patients with urologic bleeding differs depending on these presentations. The radiologic approach to both categories of patients, as well as the imaging findings, will be discussed in detail. The special instance of trauma to urologic structures will also be addressed.

B. Anatomic Considerations

Beyond the renal parenchyma, the urinary collecting system includes the calices, infundibula, renal pelvis, ureter, bladder, and urethra. Hematuria may result from parenchymal renal diseases, lesions of the kidney eroding into the collecting system, nonurologic retroperitoneal or intraperitoneal lesions eroding into these structures, disorders of the urothelium of the collecting system, stones formed within the collecting system, or trauma. Retroperitoneal hemorrhage may result spontaneously from rupture of adrenal or renal lesions, primary retroperitoneal diseases, or from trauma to the kidney or bladder.

To appreciate the radiologic changes that occur with urologic hemorrhage, especially with retroperitoneal bleeding, familiarity with basic retroperitoneal anatomy is essential (Fig. 1).

From Bern MM (ed.): *Urinary Tract Bleeding: Diagnosis and Control by Medical, Radiologic, and Surgical Techniques*. Mount Kisco, NY, Futura Publishing Co., Inc., 1985.

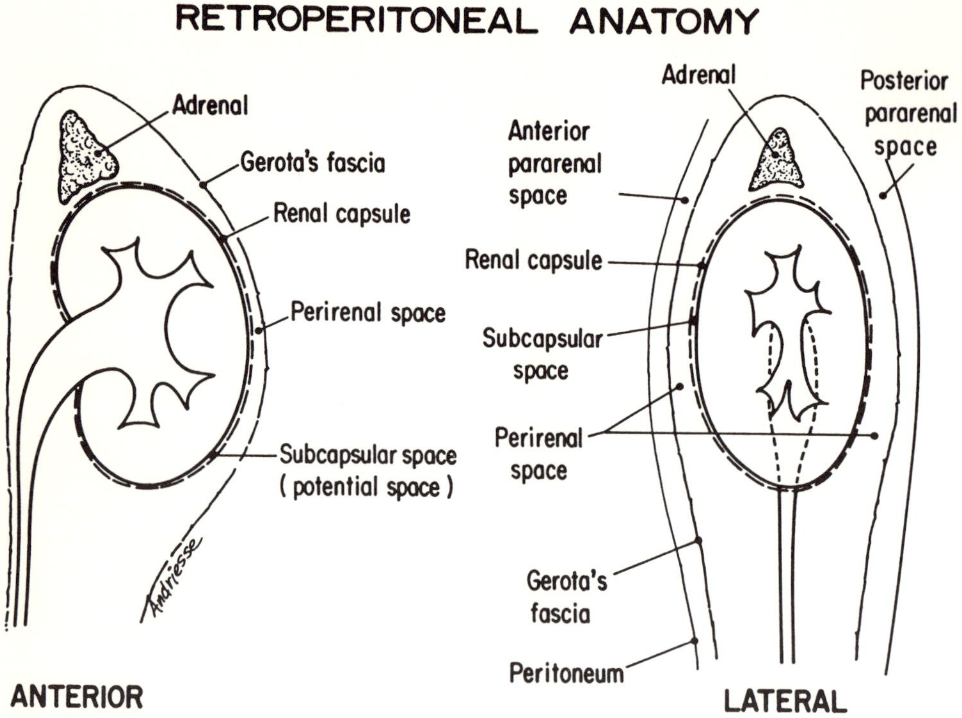

Figure 1: *Retroperitoneal anatomy (frontal and lateral views).*

The kidney is surrounded by a closely adherent, dense fibrotic capsule, the renal fascia of Gerota. It is separated from the renal capsule by a few millimeters to a few centimeters of perirenal fat.[1] Description of the anterior layer has been ascribed to Gerota[1] or Toldt,[2] and the posterior layer to Zuckerkandl.[2] These layers are fused cephalad and laterally, resulting in a cone that incorporates the adrenal in its most cephalad portion. A thin fascial plane also separates the adrenal from the kidney.[2] Renal hemorrhage may thus be contained by the renal capsule (subcapsular), or, if its integrity is breached, by the renal fascia (perirenal). Rarely, hemorrhage may localize anterior or posterior to the renal fascia (pararenal) or rupture intraperitoneally. As the cone of renal fascia is open inferiorly, perirenal hemorrhage may track caudad, resulting in ureteral compression or displacement. Each of these events results in a different radiologic appearance.

Extra-adrenal hemorrhage is usually into the perirenal space, and also may occasionally extend intraperitoneally. It is often difficult to determine the source of bleeding in some of these cases.

Normal Variants

In evaluating the patient with urologic hemorrhage, it is necessary to recognize the rather frequent developmental or acquired variants of the renal parenchyma and collecting systems which can mimic pathologic entities. With regard to the renal parenchyma, these variants have been called pseudotumors or cortical nodules. Developmental cortical nodules occur in the subcapsular region (fetal lobation, dromedary hump), the hilar lip (superior or inferior medial cushions, supra- or infrahilar bumps), and in the medullary region they occur as septa of Bertin.[3] They represent real or simulated masses in the kidney, which radiologically resemble neoplasm, but consist of normal renal tissue.[4] Acquired cortical nodules result from focal compensatory hypertrophy of residual normal renal tissue in kidneys scarred by chronic inflammatory disease or ischemia.[3] The diagnosis of these variants can usually be determined with a high degree of assurance by high quality nephrotomography as they will exhibit the same degree of opacification as the surrounding parenchyma.

Should further delineation be necessary, radionuclide imaging is highly accurate in differentiating pathologic renal masses from nodules of functioning normal tissue[5] (Fig. 2 a,b,c). Parenchymal labeling with radiopharmaceuticals occurs only in functioning renal tissue (nephrons). Pathologic masses will thus produce "cold" areas on renal scanning. Radiopharmaceuticals useful in labeling renal parenchyma include Tc-99m-dimercaptosuccinic acid (DMSA), Tc-99m-penicillamine, and to a lesser degree Tc-99-m-glucoheptonate (GHA), the latter being in more common use.[6] Rare cases have been reported in which tumors have concentrated the radiopharmaceutical, but this has only occurred with agents other than glucoheptonate.[6]

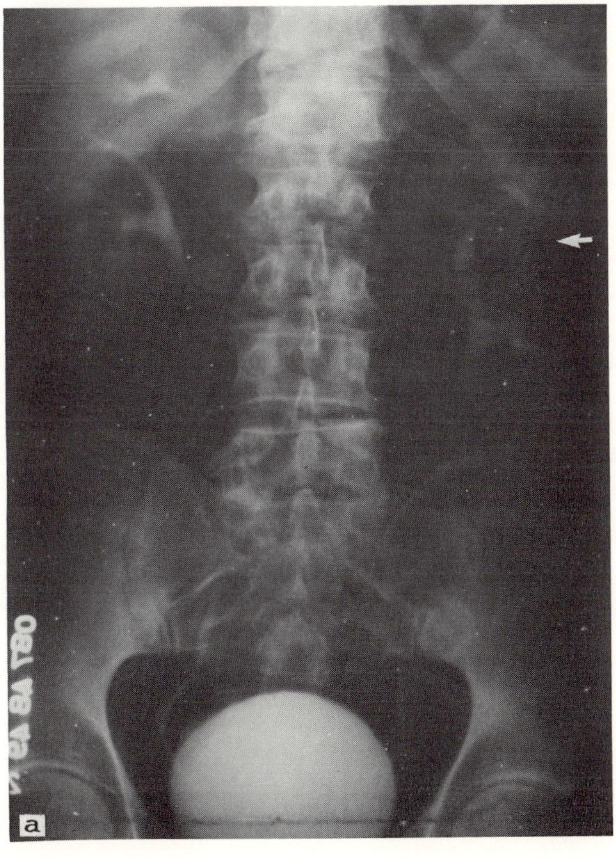

Figure 2: *Renal pseudotumor (column of Bertin)* **a.** *Mass effect seen in midportion of left kidney (arrow) on urogram. Note that radiographic density of mass is the same as that of the other parenchyma, indicating functional tissue. (Continued)*

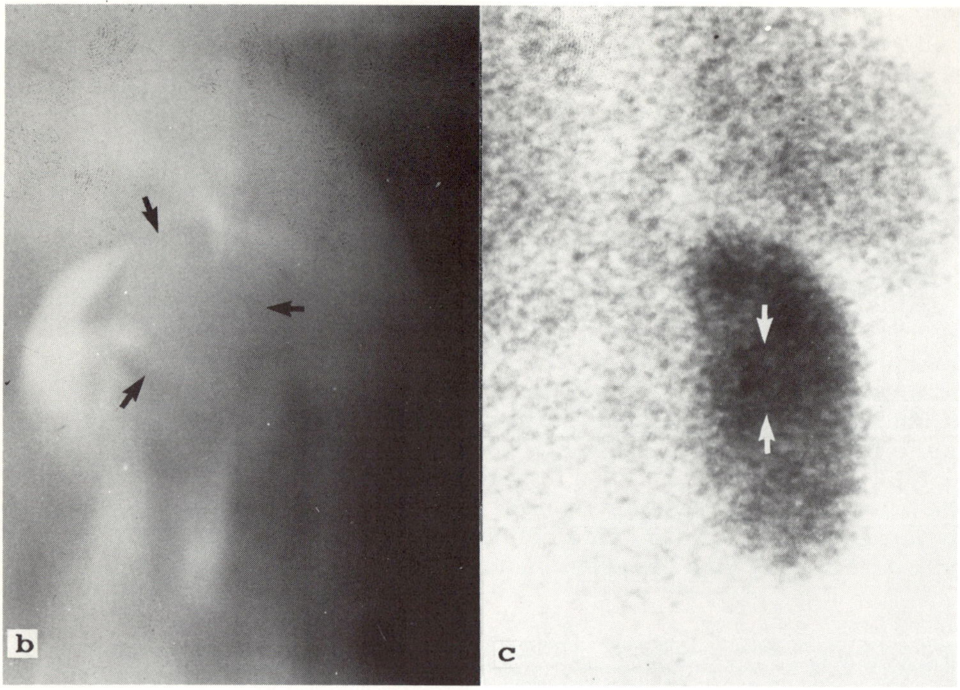

Figure 2: **b.** *Nephrotomogram confirms reasonably well-defined mass (arrows).* **c.** *GHA renal scan confirms that "mass" is indeed normal renal tissue due to its ability to concentrate the radiopharmaceutical (arrows) in normal tissue.*

In the collecting system, several entities can imitate pathologic lesions that cause hematuria. The most common of these is the impression of blood vessels on the infundibula or renal pelvis. These may be discrete and very bothersome. The diagnosis can be established easily, however, by use of abdominal compression during excretory urography or by retrograde pyelography. Both techniques result in distention of the upper collecting structures and obliteration of the vascular impression. Overlapping infundibula may also simulate a filling defect. This problem can be resolved with oblique views.

Though a benign variant, the aberrant papilla produces a real filling defect in an infundibulum or in the renal pelvis. This otherwise normal papilla projects directly into the lumen of the collecting system without the benefit of a normal, flared minor calyx.[7] The diagnosis can be strongly suspected when the defect has a smooth, conical shape that appears round or oval with peripheral forniceal contrast density when seen en face[8] (Fig. 3 a,b).

Finally, a blood clot alone may appear as a pathologic filling defect, and usually indicates a lesion elsewhere in the urinary tract. Clots obviously can occur in the presence of acute or recent gross hematuria and are smaller or absent on subsequent sequential studies.

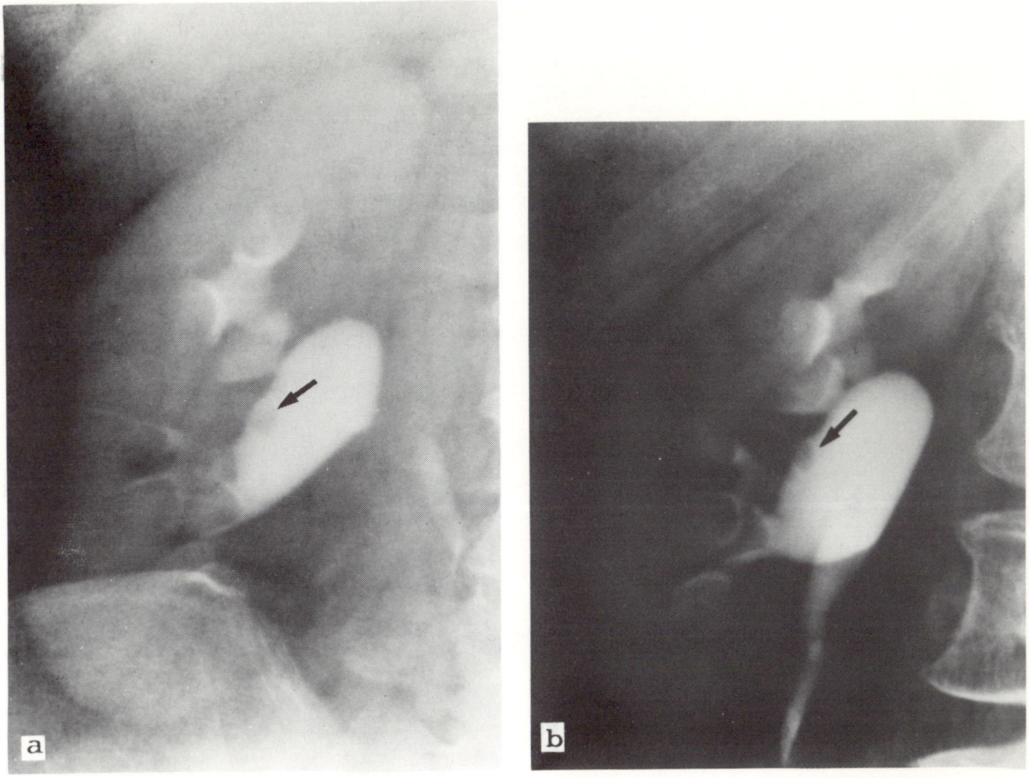

Figure 3: *Aberrant renal papilla.* **a.** *Frontal view: negative filling defect seen in lateral portion of renal pelvis (arrow).* **b.** *Oblique view: confirms normal papilla projecting into renal pelvis without minor calyx (arrow).*

II. Evaluation of Hematuria

A. General Considerations

There is no more important warning of urologic disease than painless hematuria (Fig. 4). While gross bleeding is the more obvious and frightening of the two, both micro- and macroscopic hematuria should be considered to be equally serious signs.[9] Both demand urologic and radiologic evaluation.

Urinalysis in most urology clinics is performed by a two-glass technique. Urination is begun in one glass and completed in a second. Hematuria that clears after the first glass is labeled *initial hematuria*, and indicates an anterior urethral lesion such as tumor, urethritis, stricture, or possibly foreign bodies. Hematuria confined to the second glass is called *terminal hematuria*. Its origin is usually the posterior urethra, bladder neck or trigone, and indicates lesions such as transitional cell carcinoma near the vesical neck and prostatitis. Hematuria that is equal in both glasses, termed *total hematuria*, indicates a source in the bladder or above.

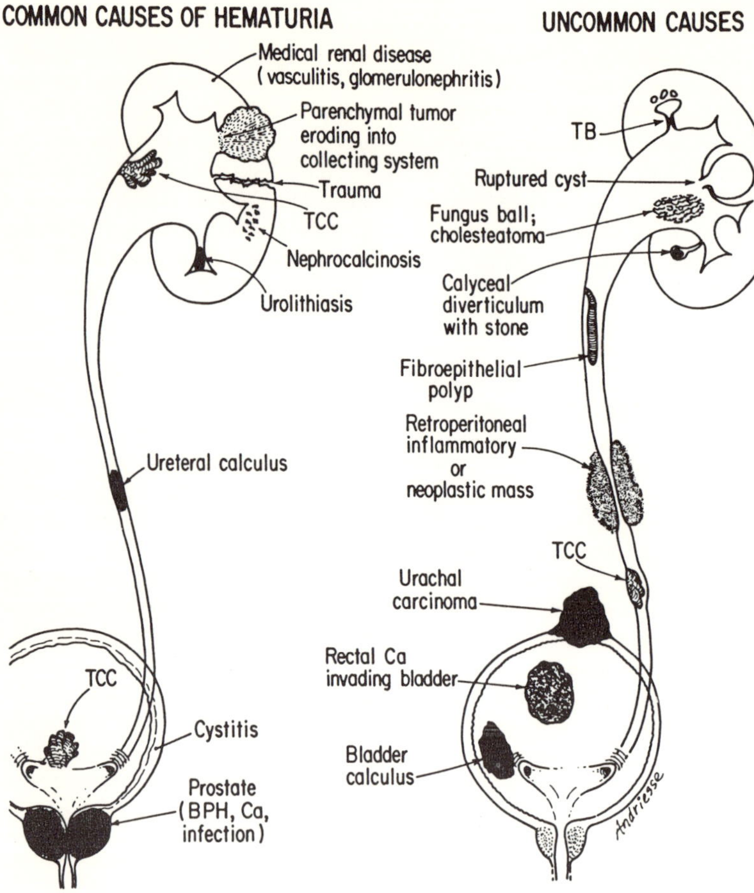

Figure 4: *Common and uncommon causes of hematuria.*

Lee and Davis[10] divided lesions responsible for gross hematuria in 1,000 patients into three groups: (1) intrinsic urinary lesions, (2) lesions of adjacent organs, and (3) complications of medical or systemic diseases. They found that males were more commonly affected than were females by a ratio of 2:1, that 20% were otherwise asymptomatic, and that no cause for the bleeding could be found in 8% (essential hematuria). Of highest import was that 22% were found to have carcinoma in the urinary tract.

The most common cause of hematuria found was cystitis, though prostatitis also was frequently associated with bleeding. Radiologic studies are usually normal in both of these disease processes, and the diagnosis is established by clinical evaluation and by cystoscopy.

Jonsson and Owman[11] reviewed 466 patients with micro- and macrohematuria and reported that no etiology for the bleeding could be found in 11.8%, correlating well with the previously mentioned study. The most common source of bleeding in their study was urinary calculi, which were often asymptomatic and nonobstructing. Lower urinary tract diseases, such as cystitis, urethritis, benign prostatic hypertrophy, carcinoma of the prostate, and bladder carcinomas were the second most common source. Furthermore, 6.4% of patients had dual sources of hematuria in their upper and lower urinary tracts.

It is of little consequence to ponder the most common cause of hematuria. Also, only a relatively small number of causes result in radiologically positive findings after exclusion of nonspecific signs such as filling defects due to clots or ureteral obstruction secondary to clots. What is significant is that malignant disease is the etiology in many patients. In conjunction with cystoscopy, intravenous urography including a plain film of the abdomen and nephrotomography remains the most useful examination in evaluating patients with hematuria.

B. Imaging Modalities

1. Plain Film of the Abdomen

The plain film of the abdomen, while occasionally useful for visualizing the renal outlines and soft tissue masses, is primarily useful for detection of abnormal lucencies, such as fat or gas, and abnormal densities, such as calculi or calcifications within mass lesions.

Gas in the renal parenchyma indicates emphysematous pyelonephritis. Gas within the collecting system suggests either infection with gas-forming organisms, such as coliform bacteria, or fistula formation from adjacent malignant or inflammatory bowel disease. Fat lucency may be due to angiomyolipoma or other fat-containing neoplasms such as lipoma or liposarcoma.

The large majority of urinary calculi (urolithiasis) are radiopaque. In a large survey, radiolucent uric acid stones comprised only 8% of all renal stones seen in the United States.[12] The remaining stones are composed of calcium salts, cystine, or magnesium ammonium phosphate (struvite, "infection stones").[13] Seventy percent contain calcium and thus are radiographically dense.[13] Cystine stones are not as radiodense, but can usually be well seen on high quality plain films.

Nephrocalcinosis denotes calcification in the cortical or medullary renal parenchyma, as opposed to urolithiasis, which denotes calculi within the collecting system. Lalli[14] reported a differential for nephrocalcinosis. In the cortex, calcifications may be due to cortical necrosis (shock, acute tubular necrosis, nephrotoxins), hyperoxaluria (Fig. 5), chronic glomerulonephritis, tuberculosis, and other less common entities. In the medulla, the majority of calcifications can be linked to distal renal tubular acidosis (Fig. 6), medullary sponge kidney, and hypercalcemic states such as hyperparathyroidism. Medullary sponge kidney may present as bilateral, unilateral, or segmental medullary calcifications, while the metabolic entities usually involve the kidneys bilaterally and somewhat symmetrically.

A localized calcification within the kidney is more ominous and should always suggest the possibility of renal neoplasm. Daniel et al.[15] reviewed 2,709 renal masses at the Mayo Clinic over a 10-year period and found calcifications in 111. Approximately 10% of renal cell carcinomas exhibited calcification. Nonperipheral, coalescent calcifications were associated with malignancy in 87% of cases (Fig. 7 a,b). Only 1–2% of renal cysts exhibited calcifications of the walls. While "rim-like" or "ring-like" calcifications suggest a benign cyst, the risk of malignancy is actually very high at 20%[16] (Fig. 8 a,b). The Mayo study further found that renal transitional cell carcinoma showed calcifications in 2.2% of

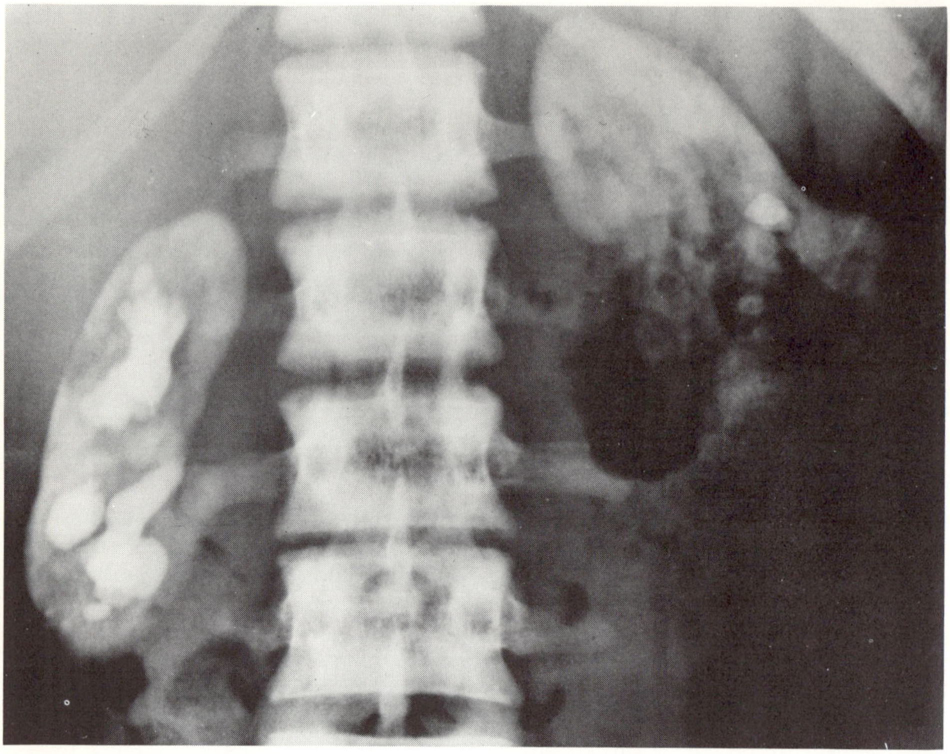

Figure 5: *Plain film of hyperoxalosis. Dense cortical nephrocalcinosis as well as staghorn calculi (urolithiasis) are well demonstrated in the right kidney.*

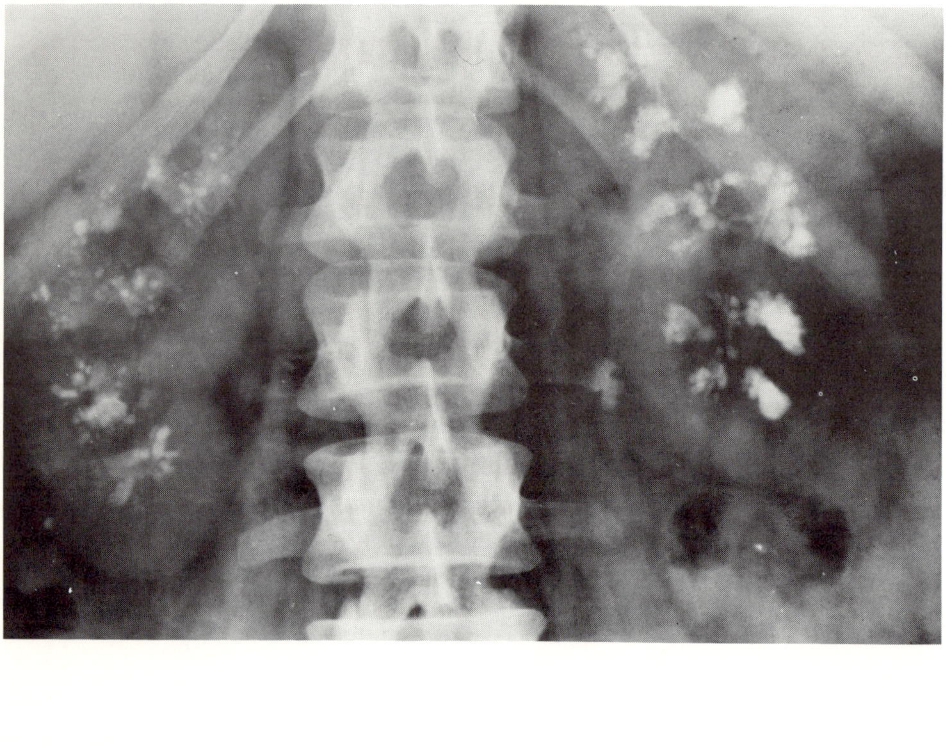

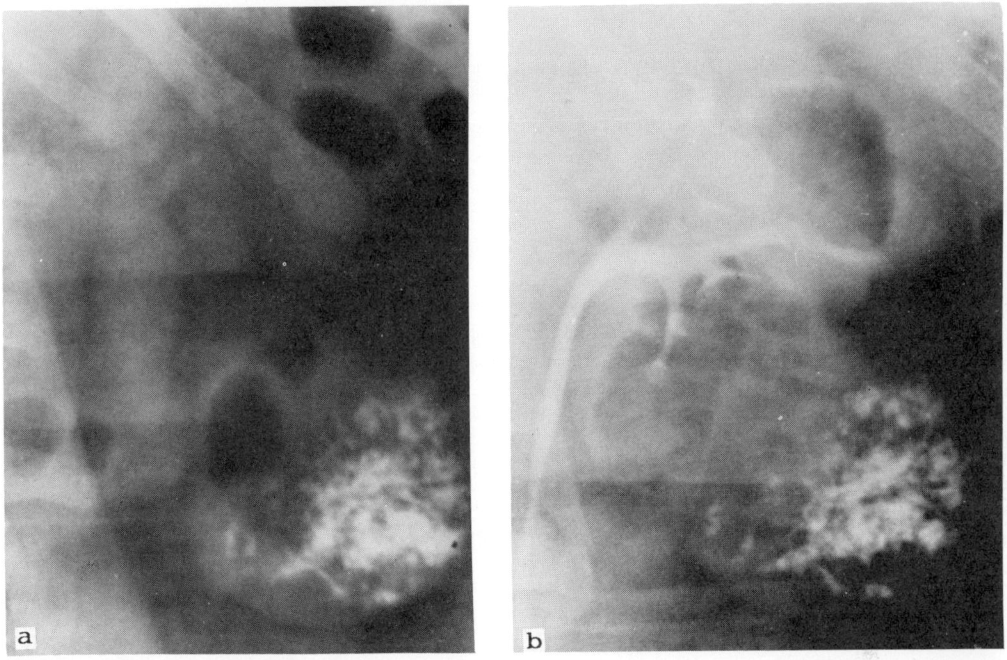

Figure 7: *Renal cell carcinoma.* **a.** *Plain film reveals coalescent calcifications in region of lower pole of left kidney.*
b. *20-minute film from urogram confirms location of calcifications in large renal mass.*

cases, metastatic lesions to the kidney (thyroid, Hodgkin's) in 9.1% of cases, multicystic dysplastic kidney in 30% of cases, xanthogranulomatous pyelonephritis in 75% of cases, and noted that Wilms' tumors exhibit calcifications in 5–17% of cases.

Mencini[17] reported a multitude of other lesions known to show renal calcifications. These include renal adenoma, angiomyolipoma, dermoid, fibroma, renal osteosarcoma, spindle cell sarcoma, renal abscess, hydatid cysts, schistosomiasis, tuberculosis, renal artery aneurysm, angiomatous malformations (hemangioendothelioma, hemangiopericytoma), and intrarenal hematomas.

While the list is long, and any of the above entities can be the source of hematuria, it is important to stress that a localized calcification within the kidney, whether coalescent or "rim-like," should be considered indicative of renal cell carcinoma until proven otherwise.

Granular or nodular calcification in the region of the bladder should suggest the possibility of malignancy (Fig. 9 a,b). Miller and Pfister[19] reported that radiographically detectable calcification occurs in approximately 0.5% of transitional and squamous cell carcinomas of the bladder.

Aside from calculi within the bladder, calcifications may also be visualized in or adjacent to the bladder wall. Pollack et al.[18] reported on the multiple

---

Figure 6: *Plain film of distal renal tubular acidosis. Note medullary location of nephrocalcinosis.*

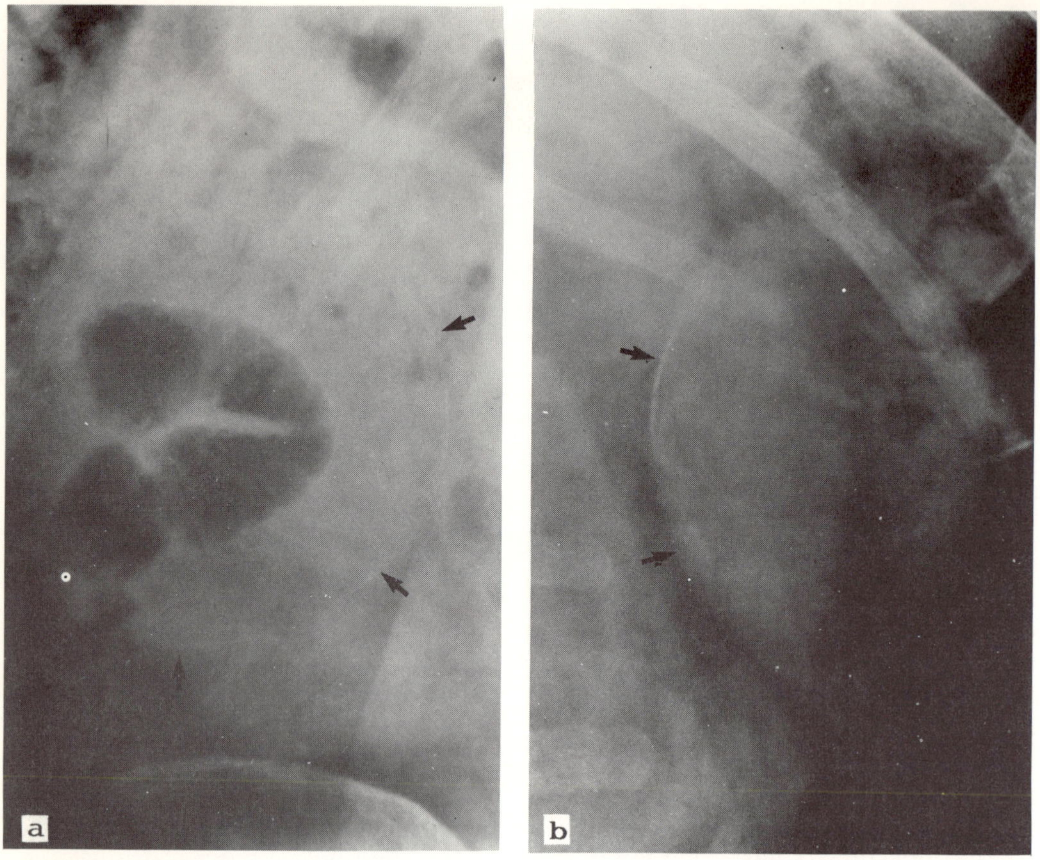

Figure 8: *"Rim-like" calcifications.* **a.** *Simple cyst (arrows).* **b.** *Renal cell carcinoma (arrows). (Note that nature of the mass cannot be determined by the peripheral location of the calcification.)*

etiologies of bladder calcification. Mural calcifications suggest either schistosomiasis (common) or tuberculosis (rare). Sheets of calcification are consistent with encrustation cystitis, amyloidosis, cyclophosphamide cystitis, or large transitional cell carcinomas. We have seen similar calcific sheets over a large benign prostate with intravesicular protrusion.

2. *Intravenous Urography*

With the introduction of organic media for excretory urography, and especially with the advent of bolus or infusion high dose techniques, excretory urography has become the foundation of urographic diagnosis. Generally, for an adult, 30 grams or more of iodine is delivered.[20] Radiographic contrast media is freely filtered by the glomerulus and is concentrated by the reabsorption of water in the tubules.[21] This results in an initial nephrogram followed by the subsequent pyelogram phase. This allows evaluation of both the renal parenchyma and the collecting system.

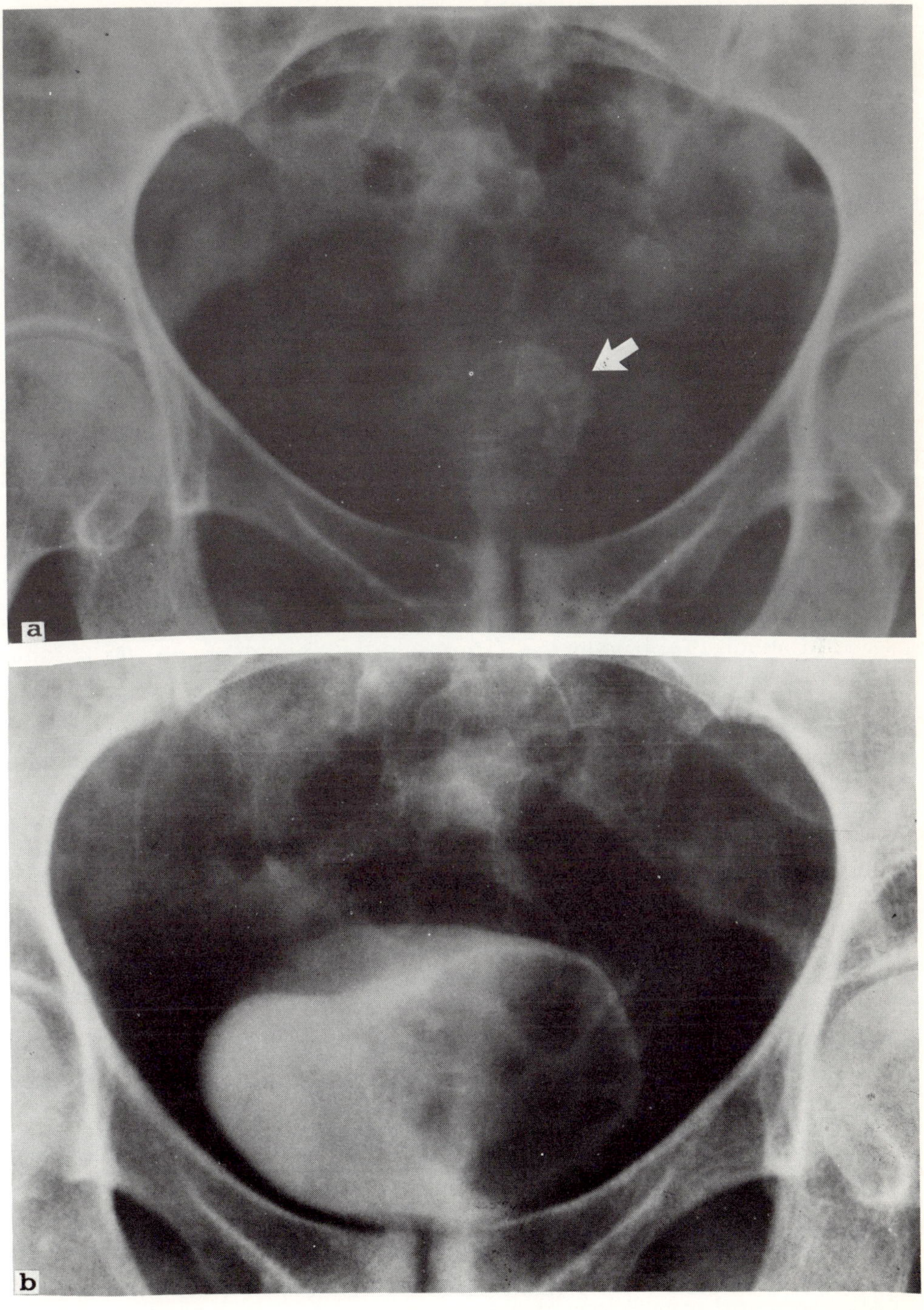

Figure 9: *Calcification in bladder tumor.* **a.** *Plain film reveals flocculent calcification in suprapubic region (arrow).* **b.** *Bladder phase of urogram confirms intravesical location of calcific mass (transitional cell carcinoma).*

Though first described in 1954,[22] nephrotomography, which improves visualization of the renal margins and parenchyma, has become a standard part of the excretory urogram only in the past decade. It is clearly indicated in the evaluation of patients with hematuria or suspected retroperitoneal hemorrhage.[23]

Among the few contraindications to excretory urography, the most important is chronic renal insufficiency due to medical parenchymal disease, notably diabetic nephropathy. The existing renal failure in such patients may be exacerbated by the contrast media. Furthermore, visualization will be suboptimal and the study will become nondiagnostic in the presence of moderate azotemia (creatinine 6–8 mg/dl). If it is necessary to perform nephrotomography in such patients, a moderate dose near 0.4 gm I/kg in a well-hydrated patient has been recommended.[24]

Overall, the incidence of adverse reactions to contrast material is 5%; in patients with a history of allergies, it rises to 10–12%; and in patients having suffered a reaction to a previous contrast study, it is 15–16%.[25] Pretesting and premedication have been reported to have essentially no value for preventing the reactions.[25] Should an adverse reaction occur, symptomatic or supportive treatment most often controls the situation.[26]

Normal renal fascia is rarely identified on urography. Should there be thickening and hypervascularity of the fascia in response to a variety of conditions, such as focal renal infarct, renal calculi, acute renal infections, or intra- and perirenal masses, it may be visualized by nephrotomography.[27]

Hematuria will be found to be due to upper urinary tract inflammatory disease in about 4% of patients.[10] These entities include acute and chronic pyelonephritis, bacterial nephritis (which may be focal cellulitis, the so-called lobar nephronia), acute and chronic glomerulonephritis, tuberculosis, and fungal diseases. The urogram is frequently normal in patients with either acute pyelonephritis or glomerulonephritis. If abnormal, the findings are often nonspecific and consist of a slight delay or decrease in visualization of the kidneys. The kidneys may be slightly enlarged. While pyelonephritis is usually unilateral, glomerulonephritis is usually a bilateral disease, which aids in the diagnosis. End-stage chronic glomerulonephritis results in bilateral, poorly visualized small kidneys.

In chronic pyelonephritis, the findings are more diagnostic, with focal parenchymal scarring occurring adjacent to a distorted or "clubbed" calyx. Scarring may occur anywhere in the kidney, but is more common in the upper pole. There may be compensatory hypertrophy of the adjacent normal parenchyma. As the disease progresses, there is often global wasting of the parenchyma with most or all of the calices abnormally deformed. Hematuria is rare in association with chronic pyelonephritis, and even though this entity may be found, other causes for the bleeding should be excluded.

Tuberculosis can present with parenchymal calcifications, papillary necrosis, hydrocalyx due to infundibular stricturing (Fig. 10), or hydronephrosis secondary to ureteral stricture. While any one of these findings is not specific for the diagnosis of tuberculosis, the occurrence of multiple findings should suggest the diagnosis.

Vascular accidents cause hematuria. Unfortunately, the urographic findings are frequently nonspecific. The degree of visualization of the kidney involved depends on the degree and chronicity of the venous or arterial obstruction, and the diagnosis is suspected on the basis of the clinical history. In patients with acute vascular compromise, whether due to renal vein thrombosis or renal

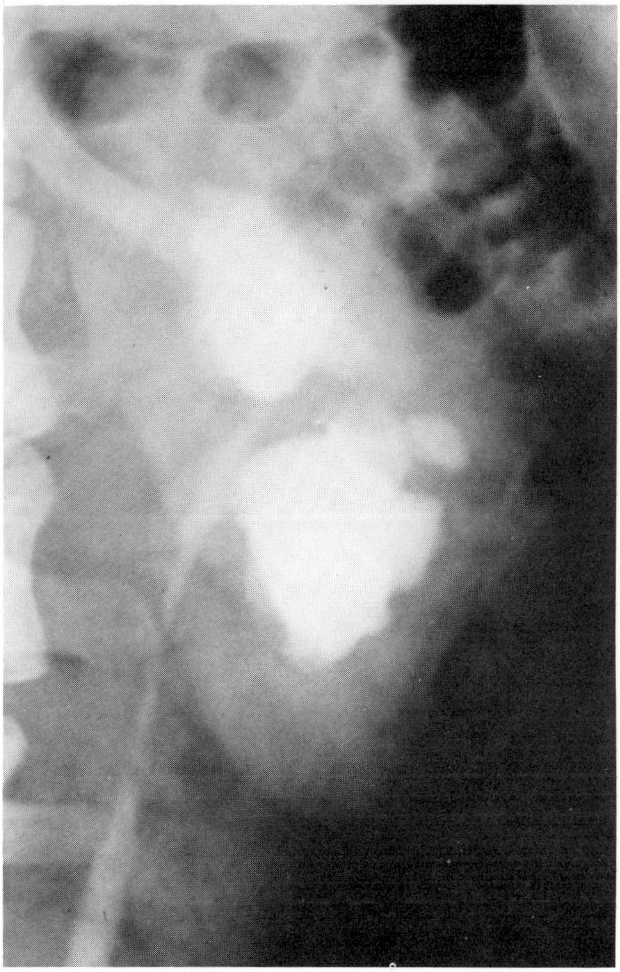

Figure 10: *Tuberculosis of kidney with multiple infundibular strictures and resultant hydrocalyces.*

arterial embolization, a subcapsular cortical nephrogram 2–4 mm thick may be seen on high dose nephrotomography. This has been called the renal subcapsular rim sign[18] and is felt to represent perfusion of the intact subcapsular cortex by collateral capsular circulation.

Renal masses that may cause hematuria are accurately detected by urography, particularly when nephrotomography is used. They cause protrusions beyond the normal renal outline, or, if wholly intrarenal, by mass effect upon the collecting system with resultant stretching and splaying of the infundibula. Simple cysts have characteristic nephrotomographic findings including homogeneous radiolucency, a paper-thin wall, and clear demarcation from the adjacent opacified parenchyma. Tumors, on the other hand, exhibit a mottled or solid appearance (Fig. 11 a,b). Tumor should be suspected in all renal mass lesions not rigidly meeting all the criteria for a simple cyst.

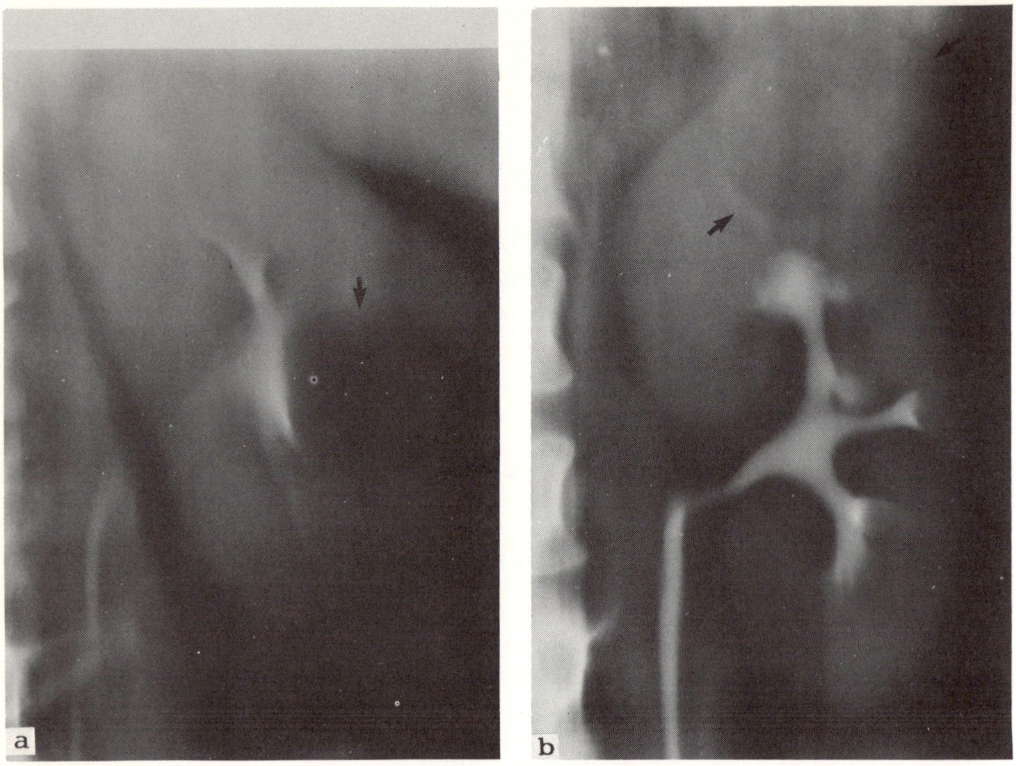

Figure 11: *Nephrotomographic characteristics of cyst vs. tumor.*
a. *Simple renal cyst. Note homogeneous radiolucency, absence of wall, and sharp parenchymal demarcation (arrows).* **b.** *Renal cell carcinoma. Note lucent necrotic center and thick wall (arrows).*

Necrotic or hemorrhagic tumors and renal abscesses may appear lucent in their central portion, but their wall is thick or irregular. Fat density can be seen in fatty tumors including liposarcomas. While hematuria is commonly found with renal tumors, it is rare with cysts and may indicate spontaneous rupture of the cyst into the collecting system.[29] Predisposing factors for cyst rupture include infection, polycystic kidneys, and bleeding diathesis, including that of anticoagulant therapy. The ruptured cyst can be seen to fill with contrast by both excretory urography and retrograde studies.

Another renal mass that can be detected by urography is the intrarenal hematoma, which is usually associated with trauma, collagen vascular disease, bleeding diathesis, or anticoagulant therapy.[30] Even anticoagulation within the therapeutic range can produce massive hematuria and intrarenal bleeding. Preexisting lesions are more likely to bleed than is a healthy kidney. Retroperitoneal hemorrhage secondary to anticoagulation will be discussed in a subsequent section.

The ureters should be visualized throughout their length in patients with hematuria. This can be aided by viewing various segments of the ureters on the standard sequence of films performed during excretory urography. Application of a compression band over the bony pelvis will further aid the visualization of

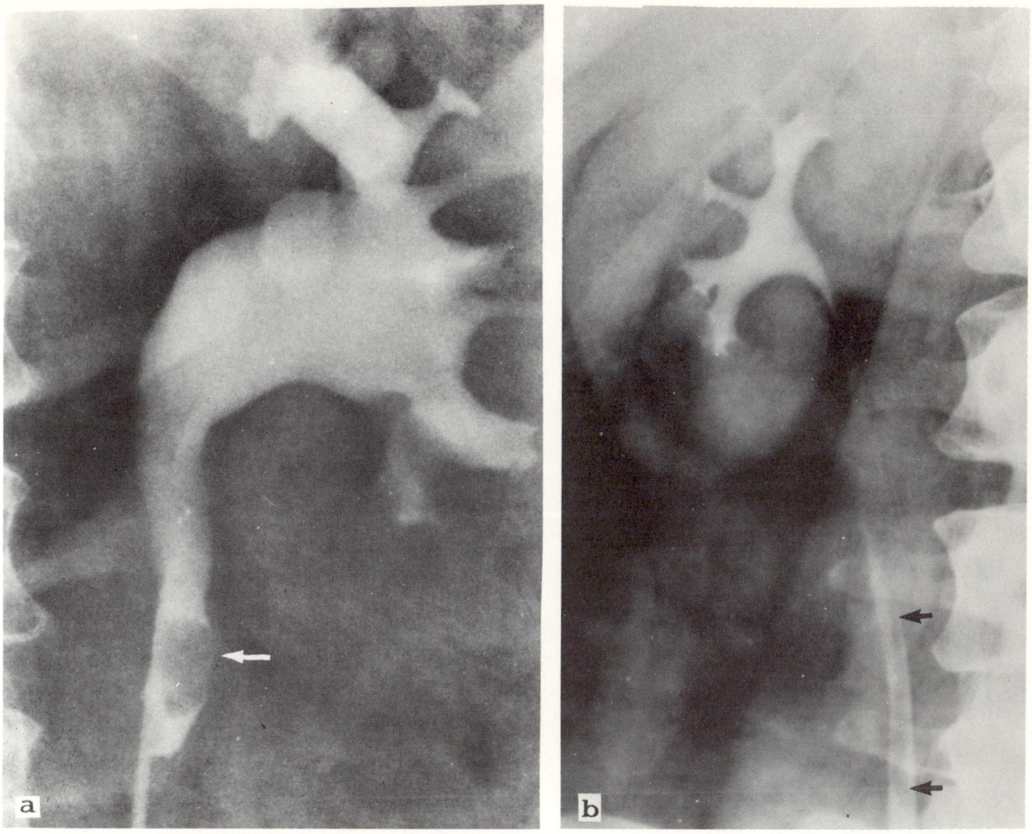

Figure 12: *Lesions of ureter causing hematuria.*
a. *Ureteral calculus (arrow).* **b.** *Fibroepithelial polyp with long stalk (arrows). (Continued.)*

the upper ureters. If a film is obtained immediately after release of the compression, the distal ureters usually will be well perfused and visualized due to contrast washing down from above.

Urinary obstruction of whatever degree can be detected by the excretory urogram. This often corresponds to the source of hematuria. The level of the obstruction may be at the infundibulum, ureteropelvic junction, or at any location in the ureter. Infundibular obstruction may be due to calculi, transitional cell carcinoma, or stricturing lesions such as tuberculosis. Vascular compression of an infundibulum may cause fullness of its adjacent calyx. Obstruction (at the ureteropelvic junction) is usually due to stones, crossing vessels, or congenital deficiency or derangement of the smooth muscles preventing normal peristaltic movement of the urine bolus. Intrinsic causes of ureteral obstruction and possibly bleeding include calculi, transitional cell carcinoma, and rarely, benign fibroepithelial polyps or ureteral valves (Fig. 12 a–d). Less likely to be associated with hematuria are the multiple causes of extrinsic ureteral compression, the protoype of which is retroperitoneal fibrosis. Inflammatory bowel disease including appendiceal abscess and regional enteritis may occasionally envelop the ureter, resulting in narrowing and hematuria. Most commonly, however, metastases will surround and obstruct the ureters.

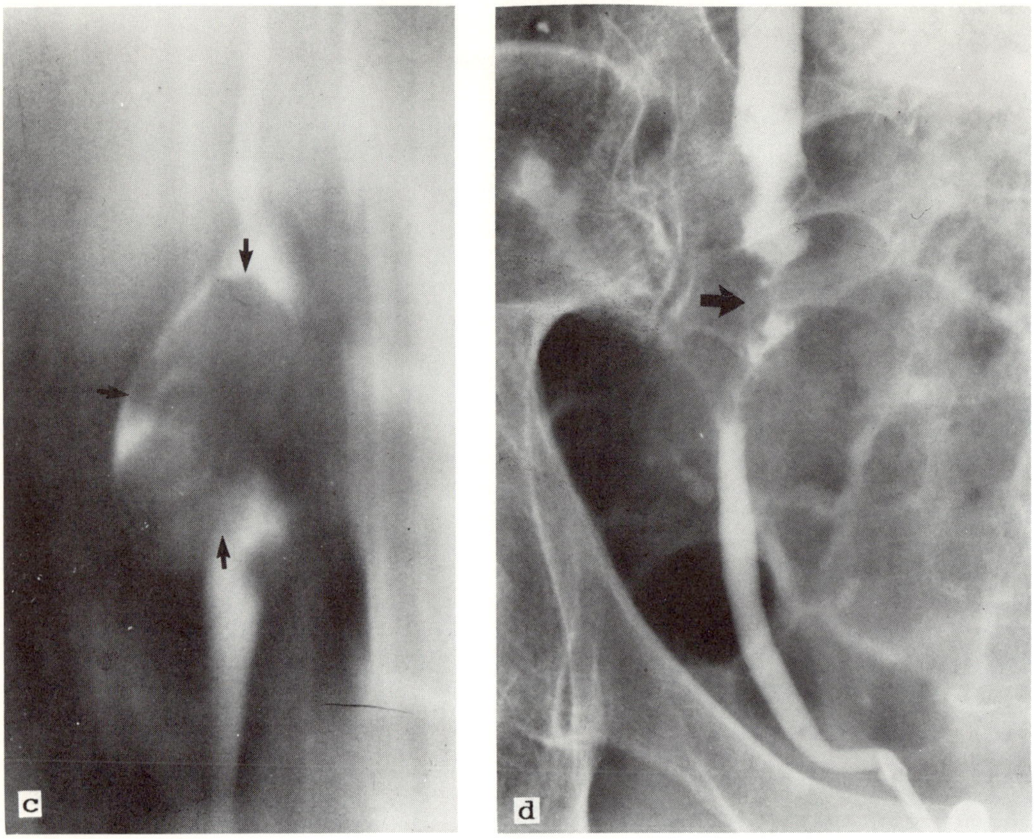

Figure 12: **c.** *Intraluminal transitional cell carcinoma (arrows).* **d.** *Infiltrating transitional cell carcinoma.*

If the point of an intrinsic obstruction of the collecting system correlates with a calcific density seen on the plain film, the diagnosis of obstructive urolithiasis can be established with certainty. If, however, no calcification is identified, the diagnosis becomes more difficult. There are multiple possible etiologies for filling defects in the intrarenal collecting system, whether obstructive or not. Transitional cell carcinoma (Fig. 13) should always be strongly suspected, while other lesions such as fungus balls (diabetics), epithelial debris from leukoplakia or cholesteatoma, sloughed papillae, radiolucent stones, and blood clots (Fig. 14) are excluded. To this end, computed tomography (CT) is very useful in determining tissue density and is very accurate in identifying radiolucent calculi, while retrograde or antegrade brushing of a lesion for cytologic study may help establish the diagnosis of carcinoma. These modalities will be discussed in detail later.

Blood clots occur in patients who currently have, or recently have had gross hematuria. They can be expected to resolve or significantly change their configuration on follow-up studies. Patients with gross hematuria may also have submucosal hemorrhage involving the renal collecting system. This can present as

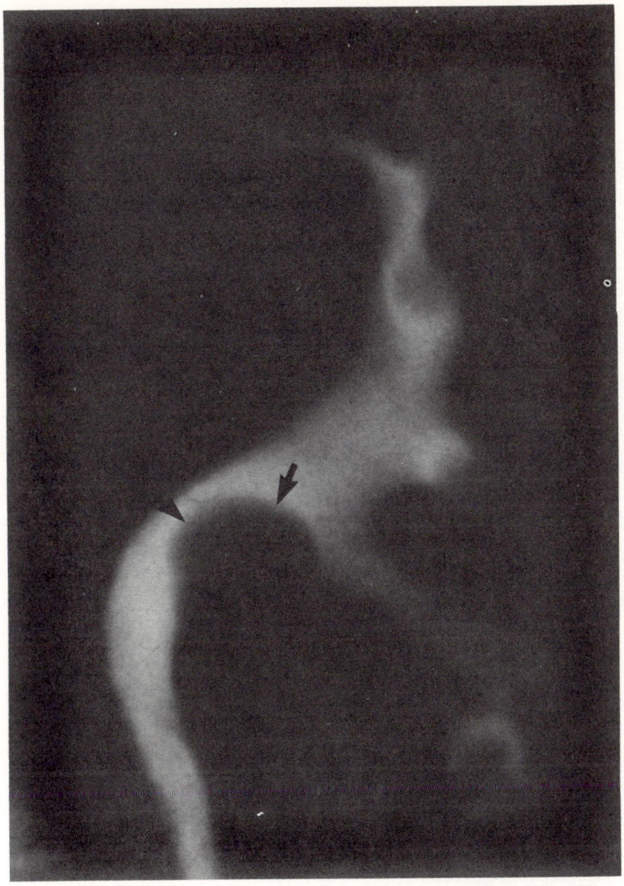

Figure 13: *Transitional cell carcinoma of renal pelvis (arrows).*

discrete filling defects, which can be confused with uroepithelial tumors, vascular impressions, or submucosal edema. They often bear a radiologic similarity to pyeloureteritis cystica,[31,32] a nonspecific response to chronic urinary tract infection, presenting as multiple, discrete rounded filling defects involving the renal pelvis and/or ureter. A similar finding in the bladder is termed *cystitis cystica*.

The bladder should be evaluated for displacement, inner wall irregularities, and filling defects on both full and post-voiding bladder films during the urogram. Tubular filling defects in the bladder in a patient with gross hematuria ("spaghetti sign") is indicative of blood clots emanating from the ureter.[33] Clots resulting from lower tract bleeding are more globular in appearance (Fig. 15). Localized defects with a papillary or a fronded appearance are highly suggestive of transitional cell carcinoma (Fig. 16). The single most valuable film for identifying bladder tumors is the post-voiding film. Using this projection, Hillman et al.[34] diagnosed 14 of 20 biopsy-proven tumors. The large majority of bladder tumors are transitional cell carcinoma (92%), and arise from the posterior and lateral walls (70%) or the trigone (20%).[35] Lesions occurring in the dome of the

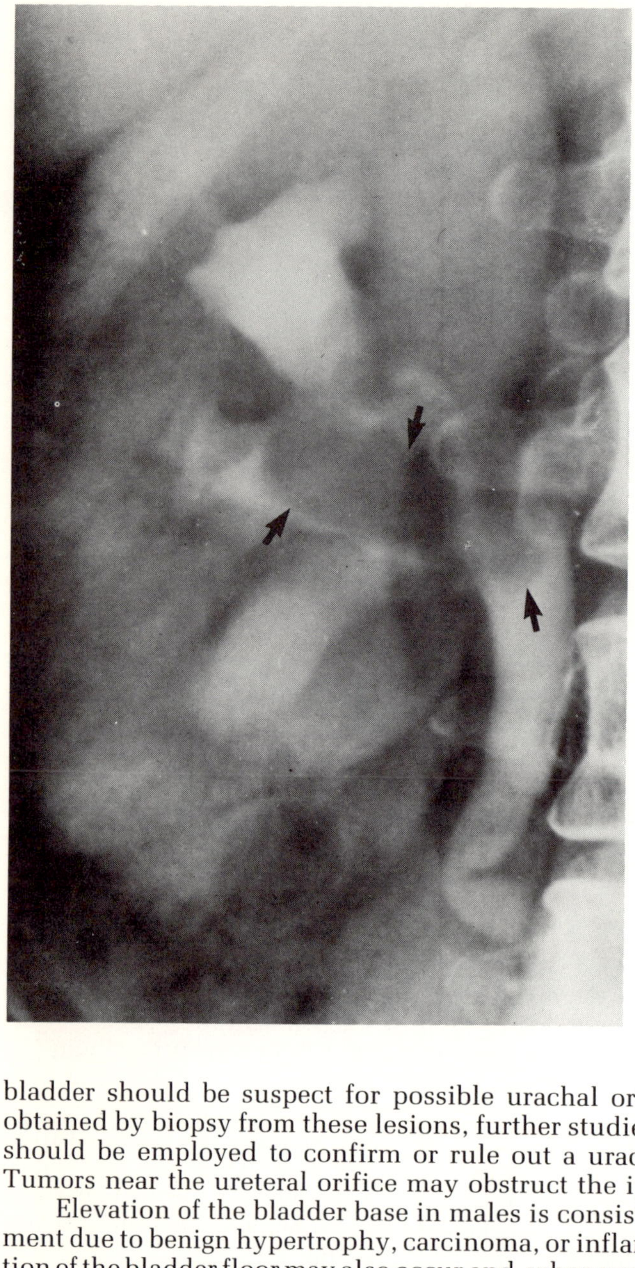

Figure 14: *Blood clot in renal pelvis (arrow) (anticoagulant etiology).*

bladder should be suspect for possible urachal origin. If adenocarcinoma is obtained by biopsy from these lesions, further studies such as ultrasound or CT should be employed to confirm or rule out a urachal mass[36] (Fig. 17 a,b,c). Tumors near the ureteral orifice may obstruct the ipsilateral ureter.

Elevation of the bladder base in males is consistent with prostatic enlargement due to benign hypertrophy, carcinoma, or inflammation. In females, elevation of the bladder floor may also occur and, when present, suggests bladder floor or urethral tumors, periurethritis, or urethral diverticulum.[37] These, of course, can be associated with hematuria. Circumferential compression or lateral displacement of the bladder may occur as a result of adenopathy of the iliac chain or pelvic hematoma following traumatic pelvic fracture. Trauma may also result in an intramural bladder hematoma with discrete mass effect.[38]

In summary, virtually any pathologic entity involving the urinary tract may cause hematuria. Intravenous urography is an excellent screening examination for such patients as it is highly accurate in detecting abnormalities in the kidneys

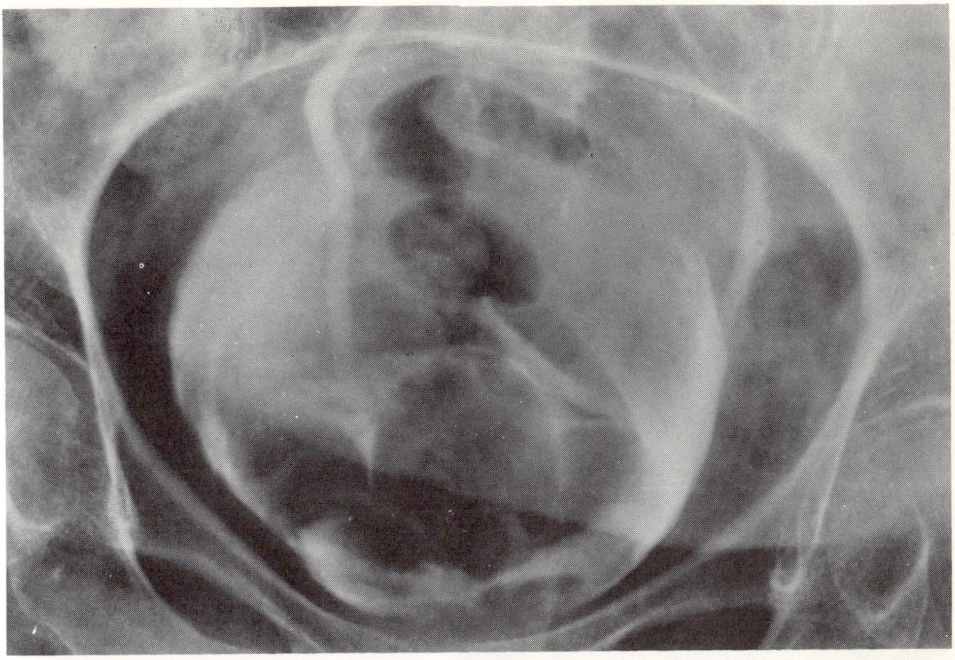

Figure 15: *Large amorphous clot in bladder secondary to hemorrhagic cystitis.*

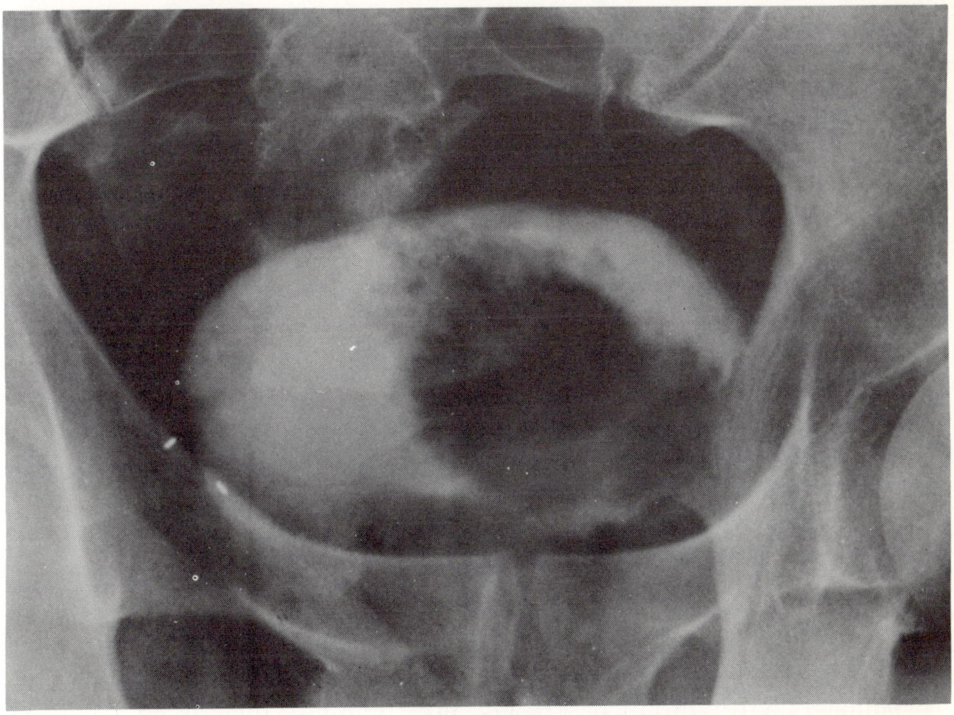

Figure 16: *Large transitional cell carcinoma of bladder with typical "fronded" appearance.*

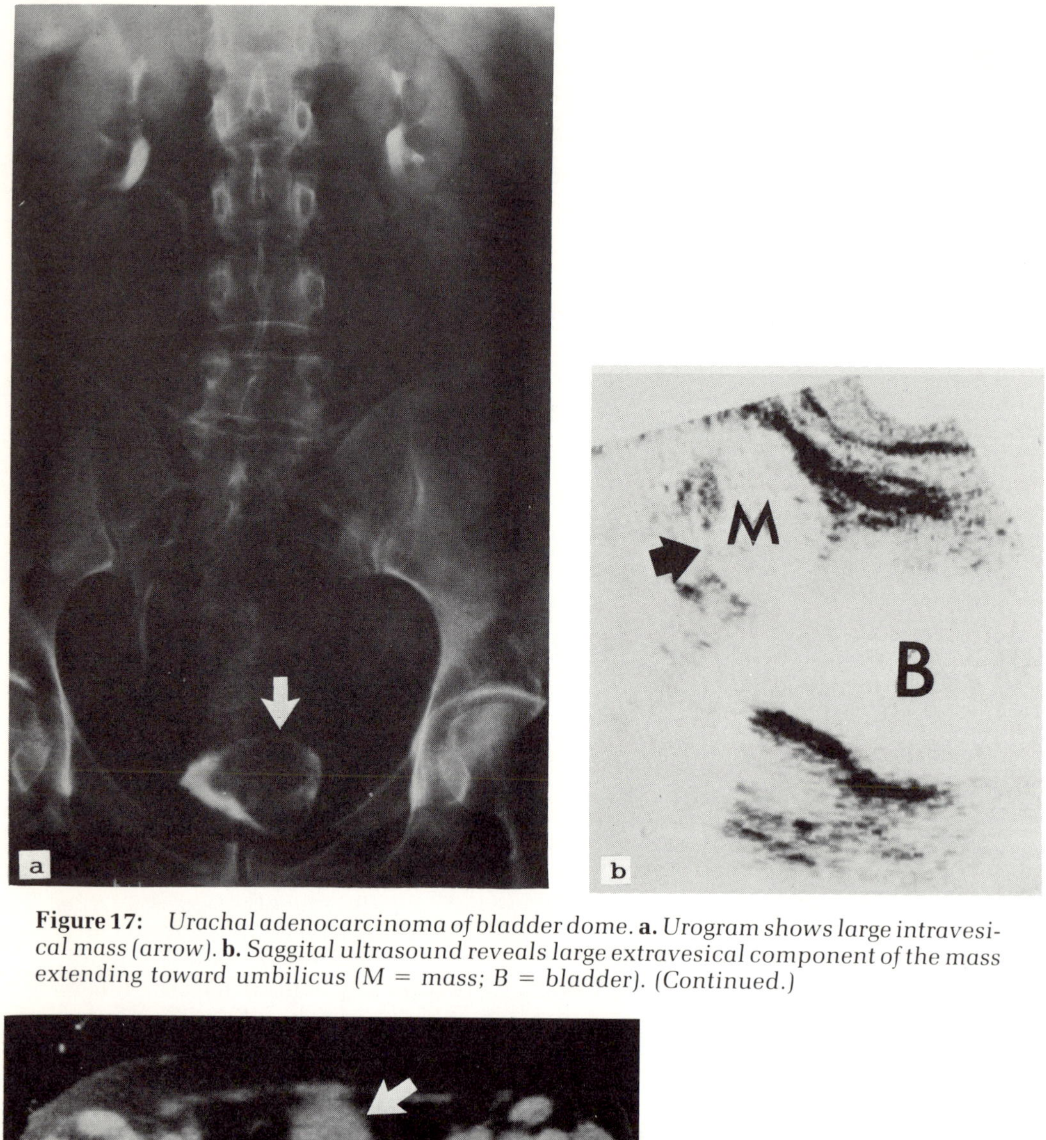

Figure 17: *Urachal adenocarcinoma of bladder dome.* **a.** *Urogram shows large intravesical mass (arrow).* **b.** *Saggital ultrasound reveals large extravesical component of the mass extending toward umbilicus (M = mass; B = bladder). (Continued.)*

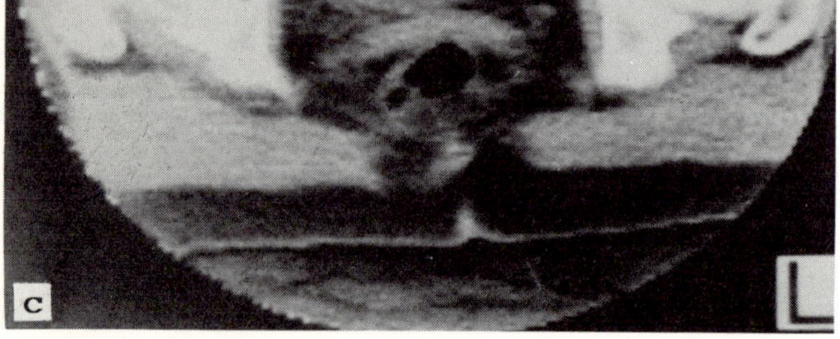

Figure 17: c. *CT study confirms anterior extravesical extension of mass (arrow).*

and ureters. Further radiologic modalities are often required to better delineate the nature of renal masses, areas of obstruction, and filling defects within the collecting system. Should bleeding persist in the light of a normal urogram, other studies, possibly including retrograde pyelography or angiography, may be indicated to diagnose occult lesions. Cystoscopy must be employed to evaluate the bladder urothelium.

3. Retrograde Pyelography

The ureter, renal pelvis, and intrarenal collecting system are visualized by retrograde ureteropyelography performed by the urologist under cystoscopic guidance. In this technique, the ureteral orifice is occluded by a bulb-tipped catheter while contrast is injected. Retrograde pyelography involves passage of a round-tipped catheter into the renal pelvis followed by injection of contrast. The usual indication for retrograde studies is inadequate visualization of the collecting system by excretory urography. Simultaneously, urine samples from each renal pelvis can be collected for cytological studies or infection localization.

Retrograde studies are also advocated in patients with a history of contrast reaction since, under normal conditions, less than 1% of the small amount of contrast material injected appears in the systemic circulation.[39]

There is a reported 4–5% incidence of infection introduced into the urinary tract by retrograde studies.[40] The relative contraindication to the study is obstruction, which, because of stasis of urine, might exacerbate an iatrogenically introduced infection.[41]

Filling defects in the collecting system as well as suspicious irregularities or narrowing can be confirmed with retrograde pyelography. A more specific radiographic finding is pyelocancerous backflow, which was first described by McAninch and Mostafa[42] in 1971. This occurs during antegrade pyelography also and involves extravasation of contrast into the renal parenchyma in a mottled and irregular pattern (Fig. 18). Originally thought to be pathognomonic for renal cell carcinoma eroding into the collecting system, it has since been described with other destructive parenchymal lesions such as intrarenal hematoma[43] and transitional cell carcinoma.[44]

4. Ultrasonography

During the past decade, ultrasonography has developed as an indispensable tool for the evaluation of the kidney and the retroperitoneum. The technique can help in the diagnosis of hematuria. With the advent of gray scale ultrasonography, resolution has improved to the point that occasionally small renal lesions are seen that are not seen by nephrotomography.[45]

The major indications for renal ultrasonography include the evaluation of filling defects within the collecting system, the distinction of cystic from solid renal masses, and the determination of obstruction versus medical renal disease as the etiology of azotemia. Pathologic changes within the kidney have been classified as types I and II.[46] In type I, there is enhancement of the cortico-

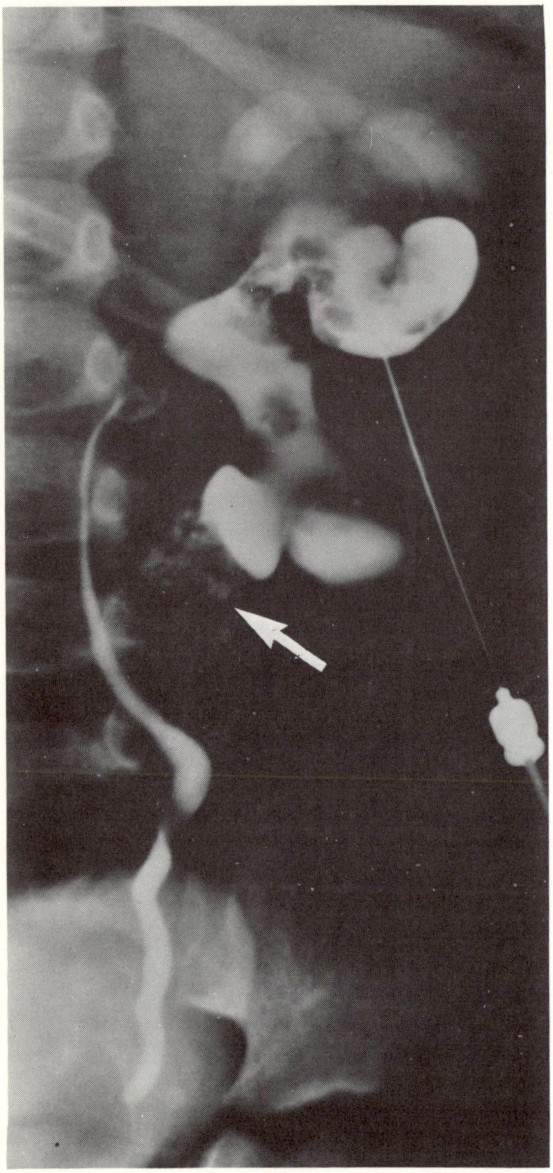

Figure 18: *Pyelocancerous backflow from lower pole calyx into infected Wilms' tumor seen during antegrade pyelography (arrow).*

medullary definition as an indicator of diffuse parenchymal disease. In type II, focal or diffuse disruption of parenchymal anatomy occurs. Focal disruption indicates mass, while diffuse disruption may indicate processes such as infantile polycystic kidney, pyelonephritis, or traumatic alterations.

Radiolucent renal calculi are among the most common renal pelvic filling defects. They may be composed of uric acid, xanthine, or mucoid matrix.[47] All urinary stones, whether radiolucent or radiopaque, exhibit the same sonographic findings, including a dense echo pattern associated with marked sound attenuation resulting in an acoustic shadowing effect distal to the calculus.

Clots and tumors do not produce acoustic shadowing. An appearance similar to that of a stone may be produced by intrarenal gas, which should be identifiable on the plain film.[48]

While the diagnosis of renal cyst can usually be established by high quality nephrotomography, there are still occasional mass lesions where the cystic or solid nature is in doubt. In many institutions, ultrasonography is performed on all mass lesions discovered by excretory urography. The ultrasonic characteristics of simple cyst are the absence of internal echoes, a clearly defined far wall, and the presence of distal acoustic enhancement. When these criteria are rigidly met, the diagnostic accuracy approaches 100%, though a cyst-like appearance by ultrasound has been reported in rare cases of hydrocalyx, xanthogranulomatous pyelonephritis, intrarenal hematoma, transitional cell carcinoma, lymphoma, and in renal cell carcinoma with central necrosis or hemorrhage.[49]

Should a renal mass be solid, ultrasonography is usually able to indicate the diagnosis. In cases of renal cell carcinoma, tumor extension into the ipsilateral renal vein and inferior vena cava occurs in 9–33% of patients.[50] This can often be detected by ultrasonography, thus confirming the diagnosis of malignancy. Furthermore, retroperitoneal node involvement and hepatic metastases may also be identified.

The majority of angiomyolipomas will exhibit a characteristic echodense pattern that should suggest the diagnosis.[51] This prominent echo pattern is a result of the fat content and disordered structure of the tumor. However, 5% of renal cell carcinomas will display a similar echodense pattern.[52]

Cronan et al.[53] evaluated ultrasonography of the bladder as a possible screening examination for bladder malignancy in patients with hematuria. Unfortunately, only four of 11 tumors subsequently proven by cystoscopy were seen prospectively.

5. Computed Tomography

Computed tomography has become an almost indispensable modality for evaluating hemorrhage in the urinary tract and retroperitoneum. For accurate interpretation of CT scans, one must be familiar with attenuation values of various tissues before and after the administration of contrast. Noncontrasted renal parenchyma measures about 30 HU (Hounsfield units), while following enhancement, the attenuation rises to 80–120 HU. Fat has low attenuation, usually in the range of −50 to −100 HU. Fresh blood measures 40–60 HU and will diminish with time as the clot liquefies and solid elements are absorbed. Most tumors, with the exception of those undergoing hemorrhage or necrosis and those with fatty elements, have roughly the same attenuation as renal parenchyma when seen on noncontrast scans. The urine-filled collecting system or fluid-filled cysts classically measure −5 to +5 HU. Urine excreted following intravenous contrast enhances dramatically, but there is no enhancement of fluid within simple renal cysts.

CT is far more sensitive than nephrotomography in detecting thickening of the renal fascia, though this is a nonspecific finding.[54] CT is useful in evaluating the peripelvic region of the kidney, an area occasionally somewhat vague on sonograms due to the multiplicity of tissue interfaces present (fat, fibrous tissue, vascular structures, lymphatics, and collecting structures). Recently, it seems to be replacing sonography as the method of choice for evaluating renal pelvic filling defects. CT is also helpful in diagnosing pseudotumors should a question remain after radionuclide scanning, as these masses are composed of normal renal tissue and have the same attenuation values pre- and post-contrast as the remainder of the renal parenchyma.

CT provides an accurate method for detecting and localizing renal calcifications which might have been vaguely seen (or not at all) on plain films. Even noncalcified stones appear much denser than the surrounding soft tissues on CT scans (Fig. 19 a,b). Federle et al.[56] reported five uric acid stones that appeared "pure white" by CT, with attenuation values ranging from 346 to 400 HU. Further, they detected stones as small as 2–3 mm in diameter. Their results were confirmed by Segal et al.[57] Thin overlapping sections at scan intervals of 5 mm are recommended to evaluate suspicious areas. Caution is advised in interpreting high attenuation values as consistent with a stone if contrast has been given within several days prior to the scan, as CT is highly sensitive to even minute amounts of residual contrast that may have coated or impregnated a soft tissue lesion.[58]

Renal pelvic clot can be appreciated by CT. Pollack et al.[59] reported attenuation values for renal pelvic clot as 55 HU, and transitional cell carcinoma as

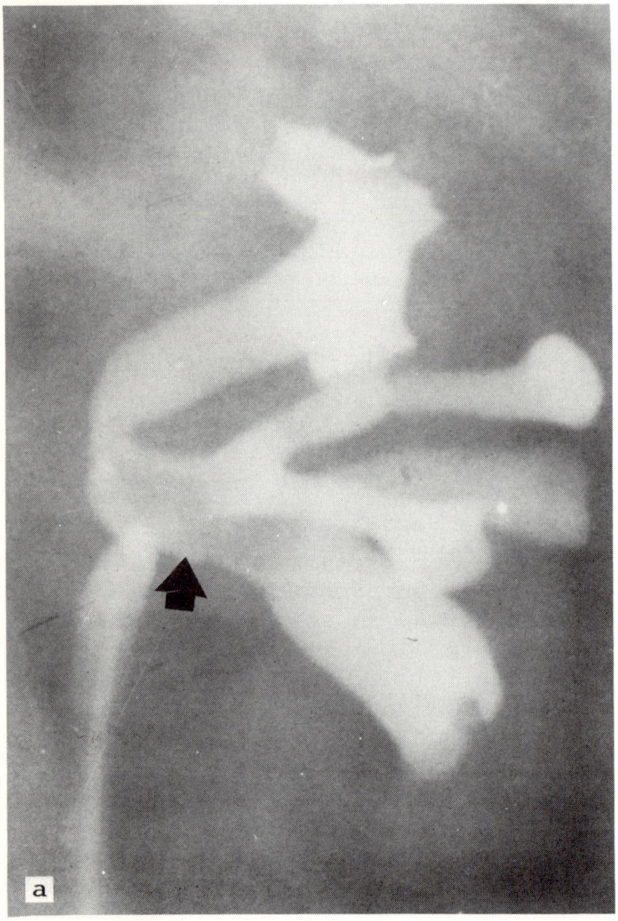

Figure 19: *Uric acid calculus in renal pelvis.*
a. *Retrograde pyelogram delineates negative filling defect in the renal pelvis (arrow) (plain film was normal). (Continued.)*

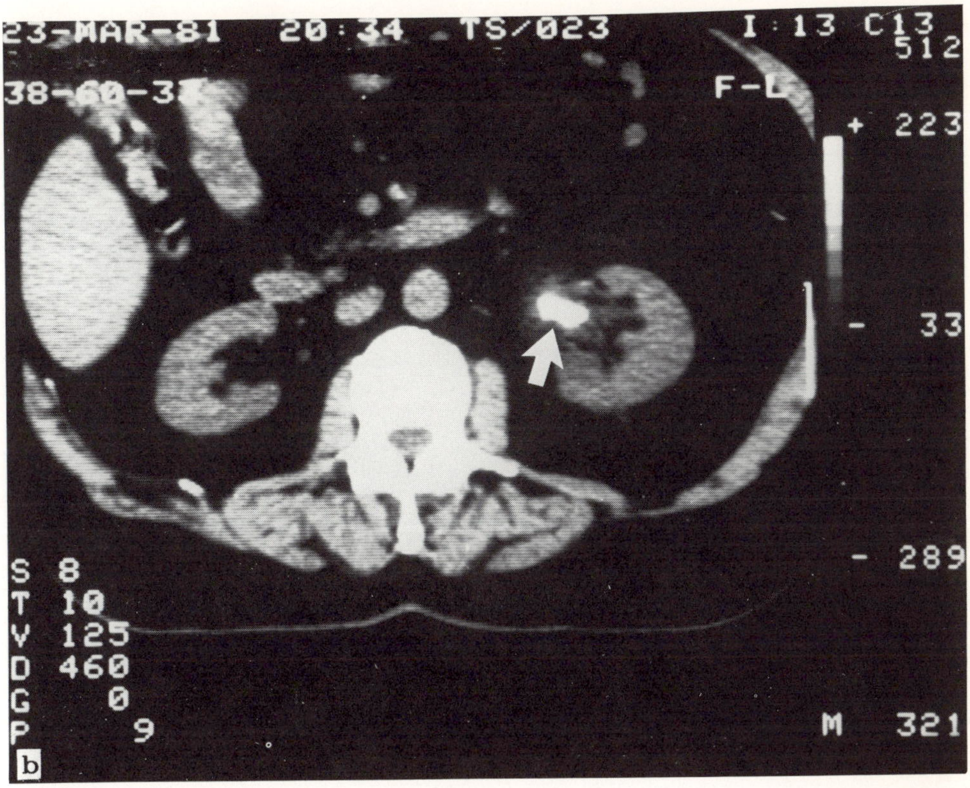

Figure 19: **b.** *CT section through lesion without contrast revealed high attenuation values (321 HU), indicative of stone density (arrow).*

30–40 HU. Unfortunately, absolute values of this slight difference may be unreliable. These entities present as negative defects in the contrasted collecting system (Fig. 20 a,b,c). With time, the clot usually resolves upon repeat CT study.

In evaluating renal cyst and renal mass lesions, CT excels. The criteria for diagnosing a simple cyst by CT are the same as those by nephrotomography, plus the additional requirement that it not enhance following contrast administration (Fig. 21 a,b). McClennan et al.[60] report 100% accuracy in the CT diagnosis of 56 cysts subsequently subjected to cyst puncture for confirmation. In a larger series, however, it is unlikely that any diagnostic modality can maintain a perfect record.

Renal cell carcinoma, on the other hand, has a far different appearance. It is often irregular or lobated, displaying a thick wall with indistinct parenchymal interface and inhomogeneous soft tissue attenuation.[61] Following contrast, the tumor may be seen to enhance by 10–30 HU due to vascular perfusion, which is not as pronounced an enhancement as occurs in normal renal parenchyma.[62] Isodense neoplasms do occur. Weyman et al.[63] reported that CT was more accurate and sensitive than angiography in detecting perinephric tumor extension, more sensitive in ascertaining lymph node involvement, and equally accurate in displaying ipsilateral renal vein and inferior vena caval involvement by tumor thrombus extension.

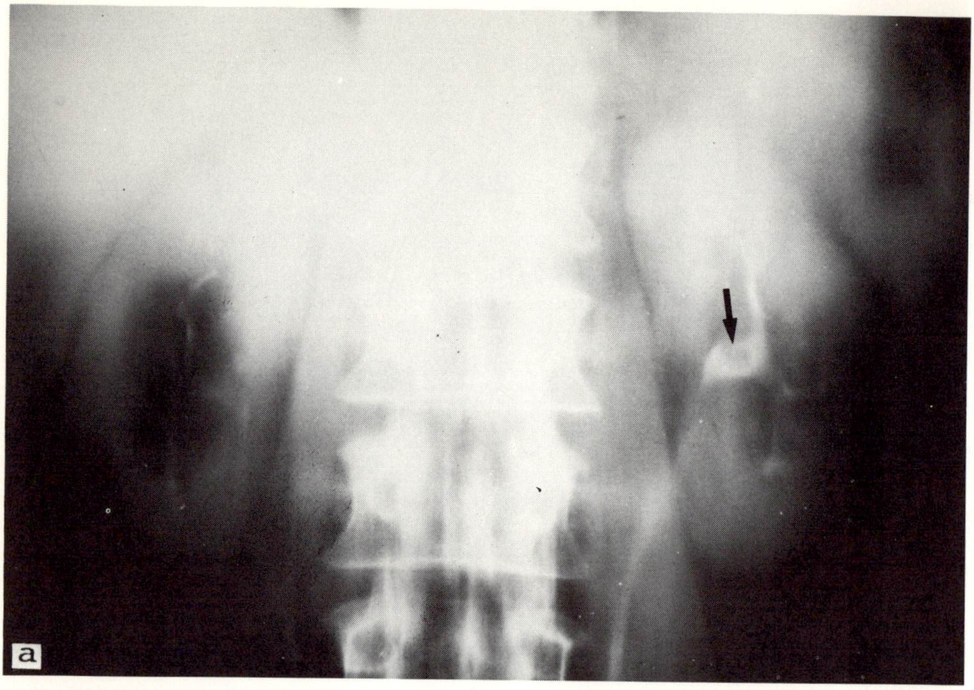

Figure 20: *Transitional cell carcinoma of renal pelvis.*
a. *Nephrotomogram shows small negative defect in renal pelvis (arrow) (unchanged on study 6 weeks later).*

Angiomyolipoma due to the presence of fatty tissue has a rather specific appearance on CT, as it does on ultrasonography. This is helpful as it has been concluded, in review of 34 cases, that angiography is not a definitive diagnostic procedure for this neoplasm.[64] It is highly beneficial if the diagnosis can be accurately determined preoperatively, since this benign lesion requires only partial nephrectomy rather than radical nephrectomy.

The correct radiologic diagnosis of angiomyolipoma requires the identification of fat within the tumor.[65] Bosniak[66] reported an accurate diagnosis preoperatively in all of 11 proven cases. In each case, fat with an attenuation value lower than −50 HU was present in at least one part of the tumor. Sherman et al.[67] advise caution, because in those angiomyolipomas that are composed primarily of smooth muscle,or in which hemorrhage has occurred, the CT appearance may be indistinguishable from other solid renal tumors.

Other renal tumors exhibiting enhancement due to hypervascularity, aside from renal cell carcinoma, include sarcomas and adenomas. Hypovascular lesions by CT include papillary renal cell carcinoma, transitional cell carcinoma, metastatic lesions, and lymphomatous infiltration of the kidney.[68]

In the bladder, CT is useful for evaluating the higher stages of transitional cell carcinoma.[69] A bladder filled with low contrast material, such as carbon dioxide or dilute urographic media, is optimal for staging since it allows visualization of the intraluminal tumor projection and thus defines the areas to be scrutinized for extravesical extension. CT is also able to demonstrate the ana-

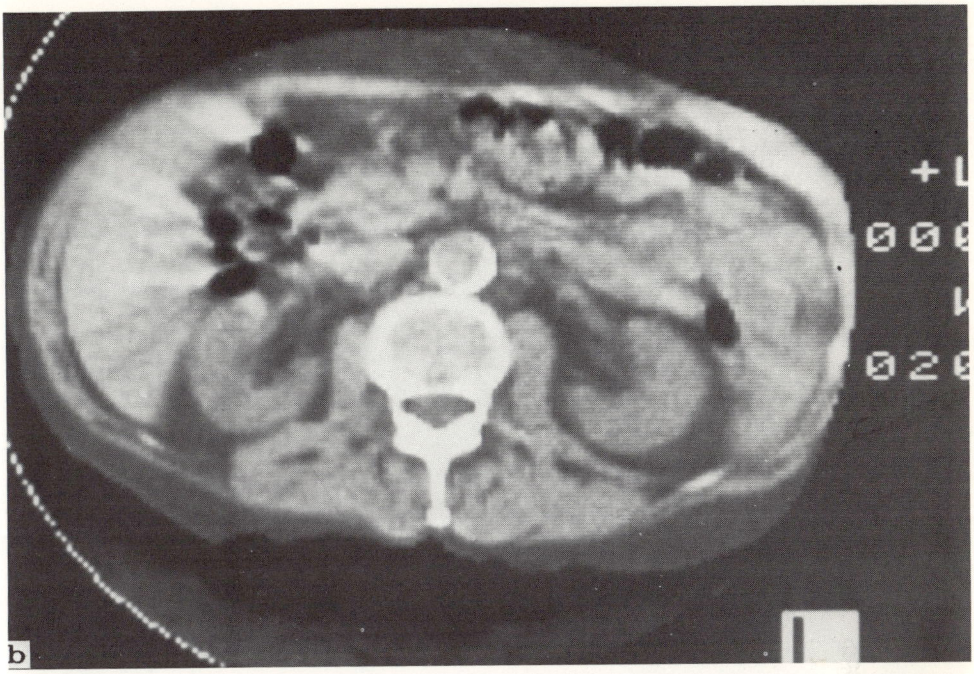

Figure 20: **b.** *Noncontrasted CT section through this region reveals no evidence of stone density.*

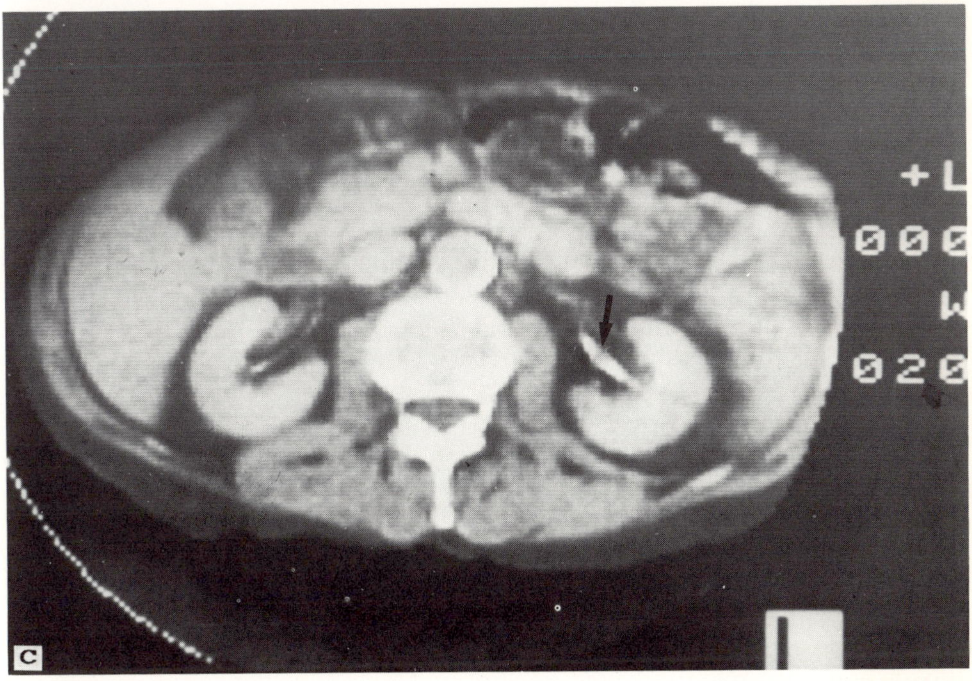

Figure 20: **c.** *Contrasted CT section confirms small defect in contrast column (arrow).*

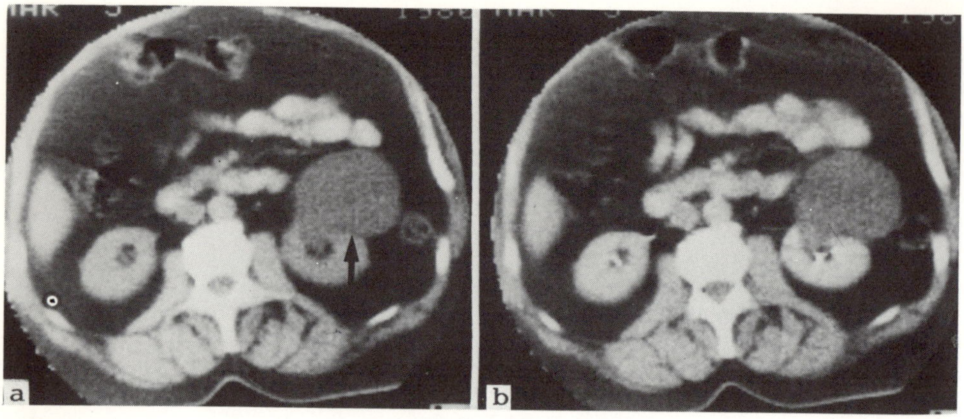

Figure 21: *CT evaluation of simple renal cyst.* **a.** *Precontrast section through cyst (arrow) showing all criteria needed to confirm diagnosis: homogenous lucency, thin wall, clear demarcation from parenchyma.*
b. *Post-contrast section reveals no enhancement of cyst.*

tomic relation of the mass of urachal carcinoma to the dome of the bladder[70] (Fig. 17c). Lymph nodes that are enlarged may be detected. These findings can change decisions regarding therapy.

6. Radionuclide Renal Scintigraphy

Radionuclide studies are most beneficial (in the evaluation of hematuria) for assessing trauma patients (as will be discussed in the subsequent section on retroperitoneal hemorrhage) and in distinguishing pseudotumors from pathologic masses (as already discussed). Other renal etiologies of hematuria that exhibit a reasonably specific radionuclide pattern are segmental infarction and renal vein thrombosis. Lisbona et al.[71] reported nine cases of presumed renal infarcts in which the Tc-99m-glucoheptonate scan revealed photon-deficient areas. The scintigraphic pattern in acute renal vein thrombosis is marked delay in flow, an enlarged kidney, and delayed accumulation of the radionuclide in the kidney.[72,73]

7. Loopography

Patients with small or large bowel urinary conduit for whatever reason, but especially following radical surgery for malignancy, may present with hematuria. Urography usually provides adequate visualization of the upper tracts, but the loop is often incompletely filled. To better visualize the conduit, retrograde loopography via a Foley catheter occluding the lumen is indicated.[74,75] Filling defects seen within the conduit that may be associated with the hematuria include calculi and recurrent or metastatic carcinoma (cervical or transitional cell) (Fig. 22).

8. Urethrography and Cystography

While the urethra, like the bladder, is best evaluated for hematuria by cystoscopy, retrograde urethrography occasionally can be used to visualize the

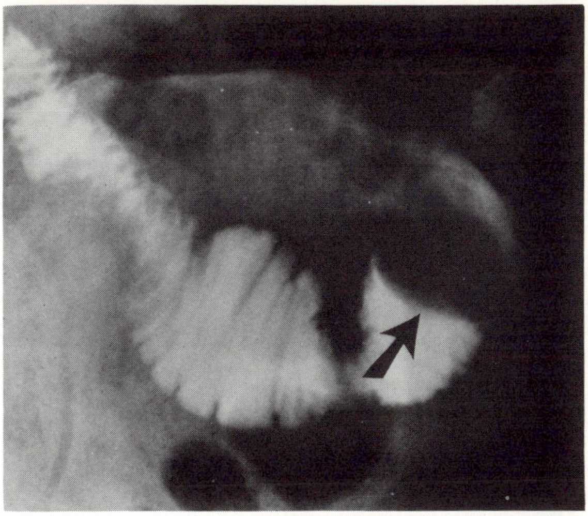

Figure 22: *Metastatic transitional cell carcinoma in ileal conduit in patient having undergone previous radical cystectomy. Note large negative defect (arrow) in loop on detailed urogram view.*

extent of an impassable lesion such as stricture, carcinoma, benign polyps, or condyloma accuminata.[76] Urethrography is also indicated in the evaluation of urethral trauma, especially in pelvic fractures, since 15% of these fractures are associated with posterior-urethral injuries.[77] Patients with pelvic fractures often have an indwelling Foley catheter inserted in the emergency room. Occasionally in such cases, the catheter may be draining well, but still it is desirable to visualize the integrity of the urethra. This can be accomplished by the double-catheter technique,[78] in which a small caliber catheter is passed alongside the Foley and contrast is injected at various levels of the urethra.

Cystography is a benefit in the evaluation of hematuria in those patients having suffered trauma to the lower abdomen or pelvic fractures. These patients are frequently not amenable to endoscopic exam of the bladder. Also, urography cannot always demonstrate a laceration of the wall due to low intravesical pressure. Retrograde filling of the bladder with contrast material, on the other hand, readily allows visualization of intra- or extraperitoneal extravasation. Oblique views or a post-drainage film are necessary to exclude retrovesical extravasation.

9. Percutaneous Procedures

Diagnostic percutaneous procedures for hematuria are reserved for cases in which the diagnosis cannot be accurately ascertained by less invasive modalities, or for situations in which conventional modalities yield conflicting results. As an example, antegrade pyelography may be necessary to demonstrate pathological lesions of the upper urinary tract when the excretory urogram is suboptimal and attempts at retrograde studies failed[79] (Fig. 23 a,b). Though not in common use, 11-17 F flexible fiberoptic scopes are now available which are able to traverse a well-developed nephrostomy tract for direct visualization of the intrarenal collecting system.[80]

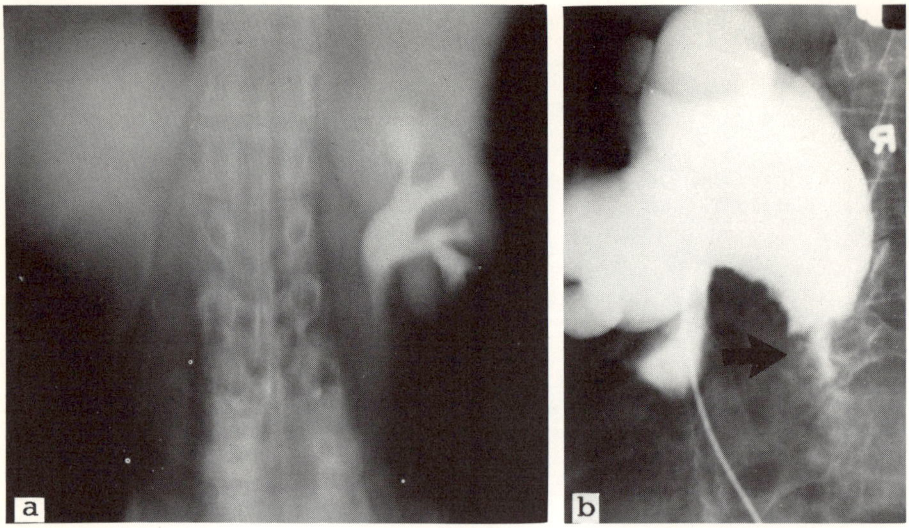

Figure 23: *Transitional cell carcinoma obstructing ureteropelvic junction.* **a.** *Nephrotomogram shows hydronephrotic right kidney.*
b. *Percutaneous antegrade pyelogram demonstrates the infiltrating, obstructing nature of the tumor (arrow). (From: Newhouse JH, Pfister RC. Antegrade pyelography. In:* **Interventional Radiology.** *Athanasoulis CA, Pfister RC, Greene RE, et al., Eds. Philadelphia, WB Saunders Co., 1982, p. 445.)*

Retrograde brushing of ureteral, renal pelvic, and caliceal lesions was first described in 1973 as an adjunct to urine cytology, which has false negative rates up to 67%.[81] The percutaneous route for brushing has been perfected,[82] which allows proper positioning in the region of a suspicious lesion facilitated by fluoroscopic control and contrast injection.

Renal cyst puncture is currently reserved for cases in which the diagnosis remains in doubt after evaluation by ultrasound and CT. In such cases, the mass appears primarily cystic, but with fine low-level diffuse echoes on ultrasonography, or the CT may reveal elevated attentuation values (Fig. 24 a,b,c). Aspiration of such lesions is often bloody, thus raising an additional diagnostic dilemma. Jackman and Stevens[83] found the incidence of hemorrhagic cysts to be 5.8% of all simple cysts. Etiologies of hemorrhagic cyst include trauma, cavernous hemangioma in the cyst wall, and spontaneous rupture of a vessel in the cyst wall.[84] Harris et al.[85] recommend surgical exploration for all hemorrhagic cysts, citing a 20–35% incidence of carcinoma since sometimes the "hemorrhagic cyst" (in reality) is a necrotic tumor with central hemorrhage.

Percutaneous needle aspiration may be used for sampling of solid tissue as well as fluid aspiration. In many cases a specific tissue diagnosis can be established[86] (Fig. 25 a,b). In this role, a thin needle biopsy can circumvent open surgical exploration in establishing a histologic diagnosis. Antegrade pyelography and needle aspiration of fluid-filled or soft tissue masses may be performed via fluoroscopic, ultrasound, or CT guidance. The choice is at the discretion of the radiologist and may be influenced by the size and location of the lesion.

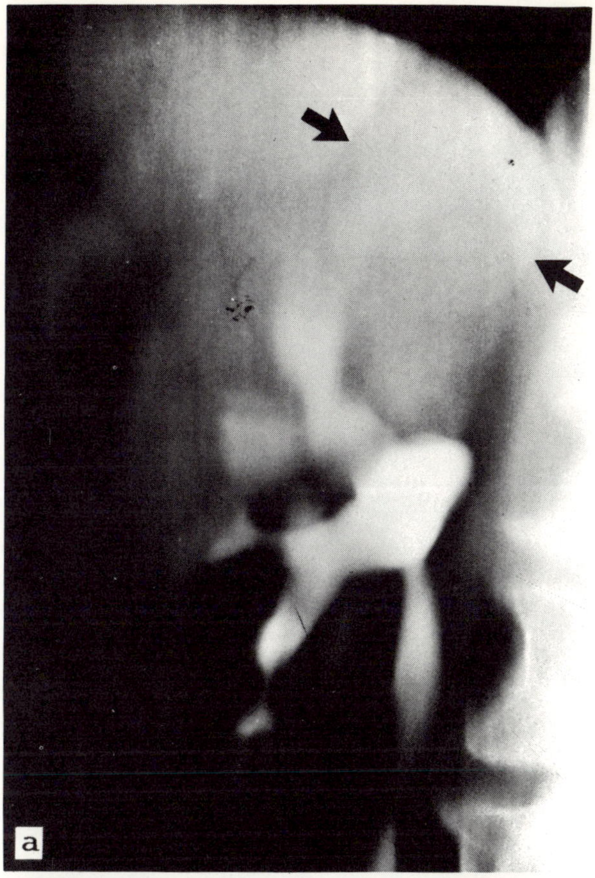

Figure 24: *Hemorrhagic renal cyst.* **a.** *Nephrotomogram shows upper pole mass, which has a relatively dense appearance (arrows). (Continued.)*

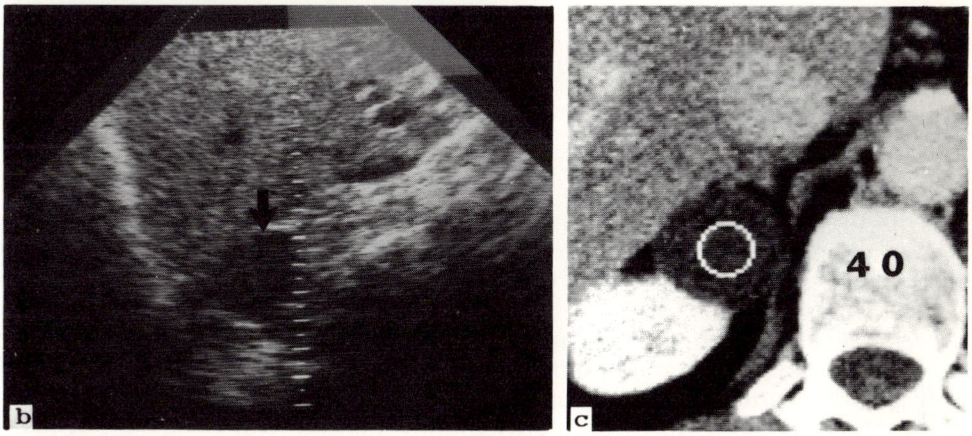

Figure 24: **b.** *Ultrasound reveals low-level echoes within lesion (arrow).* **c.** *CT section through mass exhibits attenuation values far too high for cyst (region of interest 40 HU). Needle puncture confirmed hemorrhagic fluid, and surgery revealed benign hemorrhagic cyst.*

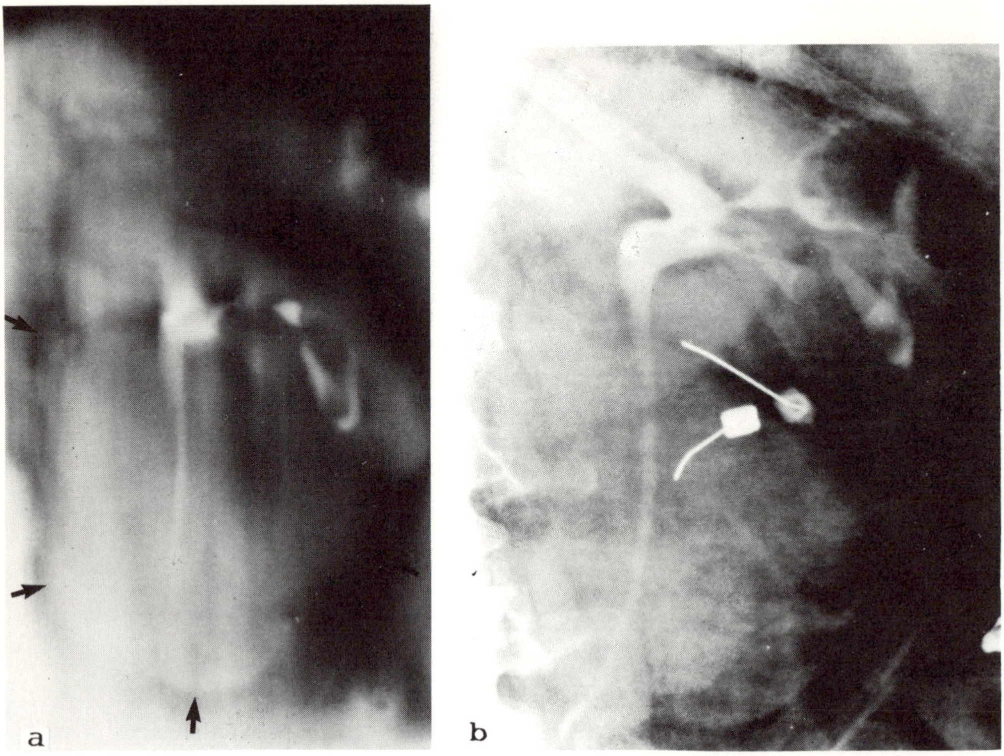

Figure 25: *Needle biopsy confirmation of renal cell carcinoma.*
a. *Nephrotomography reveals large solid mass (arrows) displacing left kidney upward and laterally.*
b. *Percutaneous needle aspiration biopsies of mass established the pathologic diagnosis.*

III. Evaluation of Retroperitoneal Hemorrhage

A. General Considerations

Retroperitoneal hemorrhage may be spontaneous or traumatic in origin. Wunderlich first described perirenal hemorrhage in 1856,[87] and this condition is occasionally called Wunderlich's disease. In cases of trauma the cause is usually obvious, while spontaneous bleeding is by definition without antecedent external cause.

The most common cause of massive retroperitoneal hemorrhage, other than trauma, is rupture of an abdominal aortic aneurysm.[88] Other sources of bleeding are the kidney and adrenal, as well as the renal, perirenal, and lumbar vessels. While renal bleeding most commonly manifests itself as hematuria,[89] it occasionally presents purely as intrarenal, subcapsular, perirenal, pararenal, or intraperitoneal hemorrhage. Hematuria may be missing due to the peripheral location of the renal lesion. Of 78 cases in the English literature reviewed in 1975, 43% of patients with spontaneous retroperitoneal hemorrhage due to renal causes exhibited microscopic or gross hematuria.[90] McCallum and Munro[91] reported that spontaneous hemorrhage from renal cell carcinomas created hematuria in 80% of cases.

Spontaneous intrarenal hematoma is unusual and, when present, is usually due to excessive anticoagulation therapy.[88] The radiographic finding is that of an intrarenal mass. Localized renal infarcts, vasculitis, and trauma can cause intrarenal hematomas. Hematomas in the pararenal spaces[92] are more common, and again trauma and anticoagulation therapy are the most frequently encountered causes.

Most frequently, hemorrhage occurs into the subcapsular renal area or into the perirenal space within Gerota's fascia (Fig. 26). In one small series, the subcapsular space was found to be the most common location for spontaneous hemorrhage.[89] Polkey and Vynalek[93] (in 1933) reported that in 178 cases of spontaneous renal hemorrhage, the subcapsular space was involved in 18.5% of cases, while perirenal, pararenal, or a combination thereof accounted for the remainder.

B. Common Etiologies

In approximately two-thirds of all cases of spontaneous renal hemorrhage, the etiologic factor can be determined preoperatively, using imaging modalities.[94] The reported lesions, diseases, and factors responsible for spontaneous hemorrhage are legion; but renal cell carcinoma is usually the most common reported cause.[90,94–96]

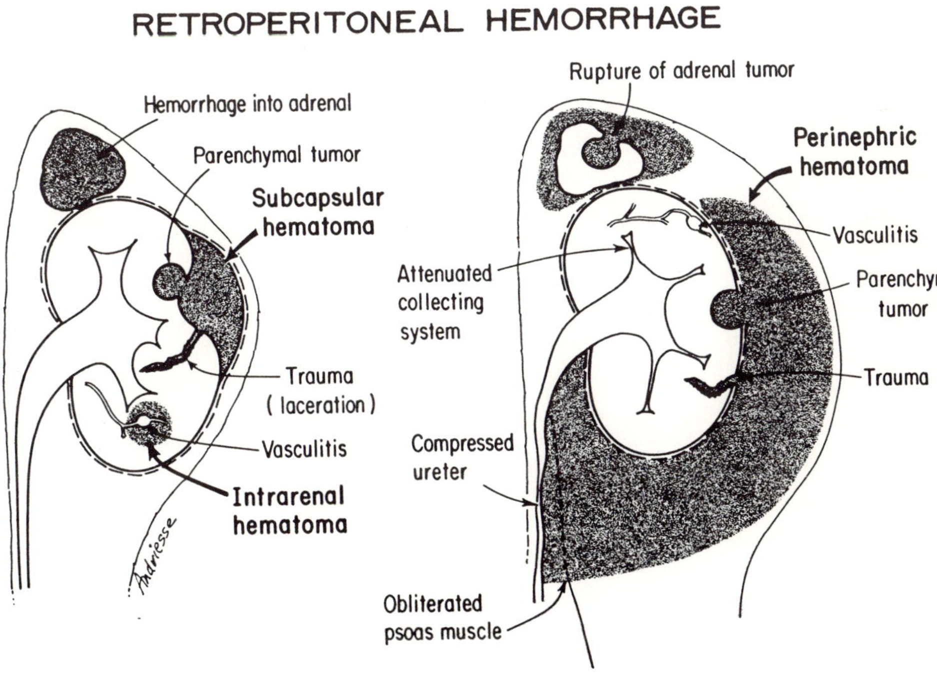

Figure 26: *Diagramatic representation of etiologies and areas of localization of intra- and extrarenal hemorrhage.*

1. Renal Neoplasms

McDougal et al.[90] reported renal neoplasms as the etiologic agent in 57.7% of 78 cases of spontaneous renal hemorrhage. Novicki et al.,[94] in a review of 194 cases, however, found the incidence of renal neoplasm to be 16%, though it was still the most common cause of spontaneous hemorrhage. In both series, renal cell carcinoma was the predominant tumor. Other neoplasms reported include angiomyolipoma (the next most common cause of bleeding), transitional cell carcinoma, Wilms' tumor, adenoma, paraganglioma, angiosarcoma, fibrosarcoma, liposarcoma, lipoma, and reninoma.[89,90,97–99]

Fifty percent of spontaneous renal hemorrhage cases not diagnosed preoperatively will be due to small tumors near the periphery of the kidney.[94] These neoplasms often are not visualized by angiograhy due to their small size or hypovascularity. Pollack and Popky[89] angiographically visualized only one renal cell carcinoma responsible for a subcapsular hematoma in a series of five bleeding neoplasms. The remaining tumors ranged from 5–10 mm in diameter. Morettin and Kumar[96] reported two cases of small papillary renal cell carcinomas with necrosis and bleeding that were not imaged by CT, ultrasound, or angiography. Needle biopsy was also nondiagnostic in these cases, presumably due to the inadequate size of the target lesion.

2. Vascular Lesions

McDougal et al.[90] reported a vascular etiology for spontaneous renal hemorrhage in 23% of cases. These included polyarteritis nodosa and anticoagulation therapy, as well as bleeding diatheses such as hemophilia and polycythemia. Polyarteritis nodosa affects primarily young to middle-aged males. It is a generalized vasculitis with the kidneys involved in 80% of cases.[100] Hemorrhage occurs from rupture of the small intrarenal aneurysms or from leakage through foci of local vessel necrosis. Perirenal hemorrhage is more common than intrarenal hemorrhage.[100]

3. Coagulation Defects

Hemorrhagic complications occur in 7–36% of patients on anticoagulant therapy, even while maintained within a therapeutic range.[101] Of those patients with a hemorrhagic complication, genitourinary bleeding occurs in 40%.[102] While hematuria is the most common presenting symptom, spontaneous retroperitoneal hemorrhage may also occur. As previously mentioned, isolated intrarenal and pararenal hematomas may be the result of anticoagulation.

4. Inflammation

The incidence of inflammatory lesions as the cause of spontaneous renal hemorrhage ranges from 16 to 27%.[90,94] Diseases reported include pyelonephritis, tuberculosis, renal abscess, and chronic nephritis.

5. *Mechanical*

Mechanical etiologies of renal hemorrhage are rare, and include hydronephrosis of whatever cause and calculus disease. Hemorrhage has been reported both with and without associated infection. The incidence due to mechanical cause is approximately 4%.[90,94]

6. *Cystic Disease*

Bosniak and Ambos[103] reported a case of massive retroperitoneal hemorrhage due to rupture of one of the cysts in polycystic kidney disease. Brown[104] described a simple renal cyst with massive hemorrhage into the retroperitoneum, which at surgery was found to be due to a ruptured artery in the cyst wall.

7. *Trauma*

In a comprehensive review of renal injuries, Hessel and Smith[105] found that perirenal hematomas resulted from blunt trauma in 86% of cases, and from penetrating trauma in 14%. Ganji et al.[106] reported five cases of traumatic rupture of renal cell carcinomas, and concluded that traumatic rupture is more likely to occur in kidneys with pre-existing disease. In addition to renal cell carcinoma, predisposing lesions include congenital anomalies, hydronephrosis, tuberculosis, calculus disease, other neoplasms, hemangioma, nephritis, and coagulopathies.

Certainly, iatrogenic trauma must also be included in this discussion of renal hematomas. Diagnostic large needle core biopsy of the kidney (nephrology type biopsy) is associated with a high incidence of perirenal hematoma, some of which are clinically important. Ginsburg et al.[107] studied 25 patients by computerized tomography following closed needle biopsies and found renal hematomas in 60% of the patients. In 33%, the hematomas were moderate to large in size. Rosenbaum et al.[108] noted the incidence of post-biopsy perirenal hematoma to be as high as 85%.

8. *Idiopathic*

The reported incidence of spontaneous idiopathic renal hemorrhage ranges from 4 to 15%.[90,94,105]

C. Imaging Modalities

1. *Plain Film of the Abdomen*

Radiographic visualization of structures in the abdomen is dependent upon the contrast between bone, water (solid viscera, blood, urine), fat, and air. Differential absorption of photons in the x-ray beam produces the contrast between these structures. Collections of blood in the extraperitoneal spaces related to the kidney (subcapsular, perirenal, pararenal) often result in localizing radiologic signs. The bowel gas pattern may suggest the presence, location, and size of a retroperitoneal hematoma. A nonspecific sign is ileus.[109] A more specific sign is displacement of both large and small bowel gas-filled loops. Moderate sized collections yield discrete findings, while massive retroperitoneal hematomas may result in bowel gas being totally displaced to the contralateral side of the abdomen. In rare instances of intraperitoneal rupture of the hematoma, gas-filled loops of bowel can be seen floating centrally, producing a radiographic picture similar to that seen with ascites. A large soft tissue mass, representing the hematoma, may be evident, its axis vertically oriented. With an acute bleed, calcifications are not to be expected, unless present in a preexisting renal lesion such as a renal cell carcinoma or tuberculous kidney, or in calculus disease of the kidney.

The transverse mesocolon curves cephalad from right to left. A larger portion of the right kidney lies above the mesocolon, and a larger portion of the left kidney lies below. McCort[110] has found right perirenal hematomas to be supramesocolic in location in 82% of cases, while on the left, the hematoma is inframesocolic in 81% of cases. In the majority of cases, therefore, a right perirenal hematoma compresses the second portion of the duodenum, displaces the right transverse colon caudad, and pushes the ascending colon and small bowel medially. On the left, the hematoma most frequently elevates the left transverse colon, pushes the small bowel medially, and compresses the descending colon against the left abdominal wall (Fig. 27a).

Aside from alterations in the bowel gas pattern, soft tissue changes are usually evident. The ipsilateral diaphragm may be elevated, the renal outline obliterated, and the psoas muscle margin obscured. The diagnostic value of the absent psoas margin must be viewed with a certain amount of skepticism, however, as approximately only 25% of normal individuals exhibit unequal definition of the psoas borders.[111] Also, slight rotation of the patient or mild spinal scoliosis can cause radiographic loss of the psoas margin.

2. Intravenous Urography

The intravenous urogram with nephrotomography remains the initial step in evaluating a patient with suspected renal hemorrhage. This procedure can demonstrate opacification of the displaced renal capsule and fascia, presumably visualized because of their hypervascularity.[112] The subcapsular hematoma itself may be seen as a nonopacifying mass between the nephrogram and the renal capsule when visualized. The renal capsule is often sharply deflected over the margin of the subcapsular mass and the adjacent renal margin is flat or concave. The kidney may show delayed or decreased visualization, or nonfunction. The latter is more likely with subcapsular bleeds than perirenal hematoma. The collecting system may be distorted due to pressure effects of the hematoma, may be attenuated due to increased intrarenal pressure (Fig. 27b), or may exhibit mass effect from an associated intrarenal component of the hematoma or preexisting renal lesion responsible for the hematoma.

Should hemorrhage occur into the perirenal space, there may also be delayed or decreased function of the kidney with attenuation of the collecting system due to pressure from the surrounding hematoma. Retrograde pyelography in this instance, as with subcapsular hematoma, will usually demonstrate normally distensible collecting systems (Fig. 27c).

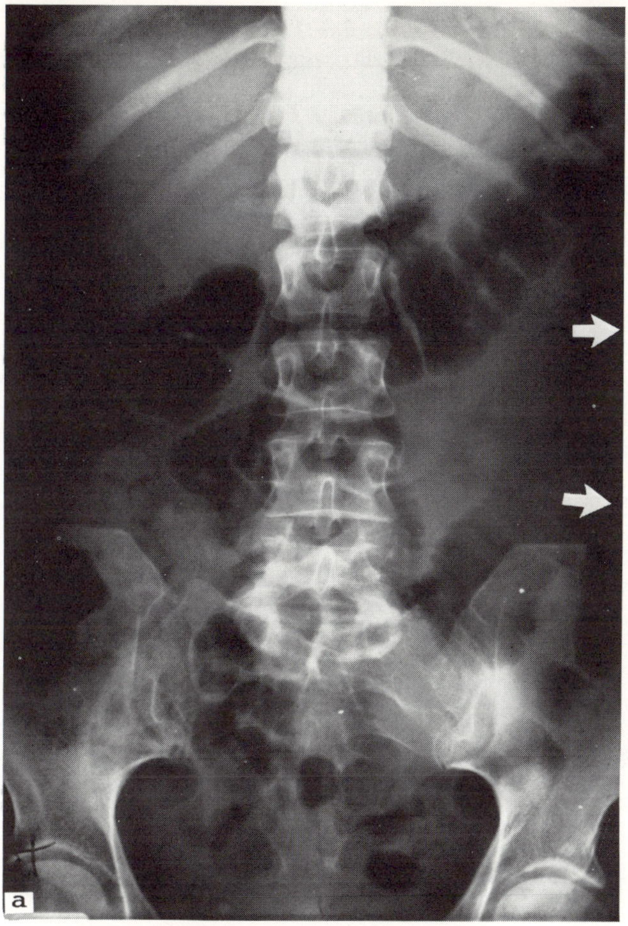

Figure 27: *Large left retroperitoneal hemorrhage in patient with metastatic melanoma and sudden onset of hypotension.*

a. *Plain film reveals loss of left psoas margin and compression of descending colon laterally against abdominal wall (arrows). (Continued.)*

Since perirenal fat and fascia are more yielding than is the renal capsule, there is less likely to be distortion of the renal margin by a perirenal hematoma. Perirenal bleeds often coalesce and localize posterolaterally to the lower renal pole due to the predominance of perirenal fat in this area (path of least resistance).[112] This inferior extension may result in medial displacement of the proximal ureter.

It is important to note whether significant compression of the kidney by surrounding hematoma exists. Resultant perirenal fibrosis may eventually culminate in hypertensive problems,[113] especially following subcapsular bleeds. Page's classic experiments have proven that circumferential compression of the kidney on a chronic basis will produce renin-dependent hypertension.[114]

The subcapsular hematoma may evolve if it is not rapidly resorbed or surgically evacuated. Clot within the hematoma may disintegrate and liquefy after several months. The lesion may then become expansile by drawing in fluid from the capillary beds of the renal capsule.[115] This results in the radiographic picture of a subcapsular, avascular, cystic mass with a thick capsule that may opacify by nephrotomography. The capsule may calcify with age.

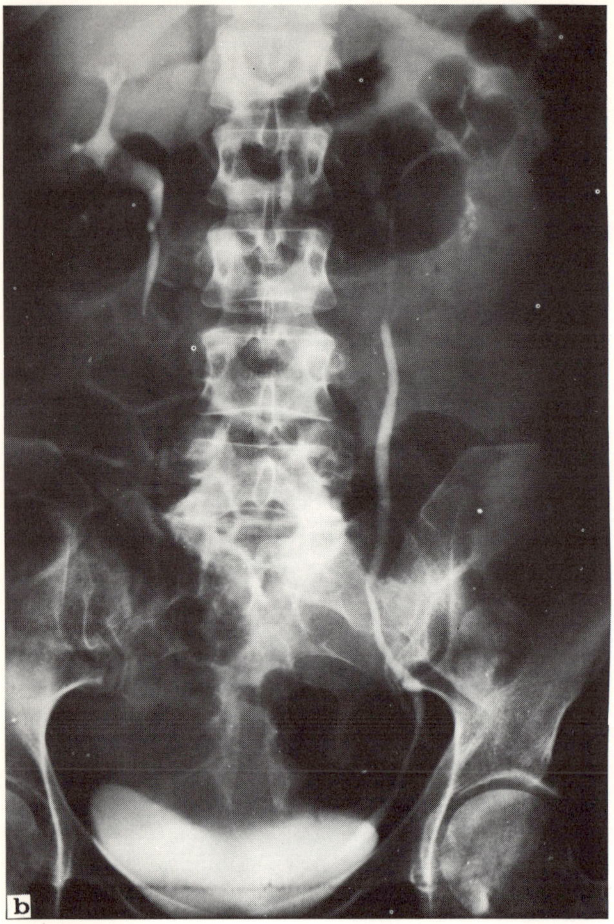

Figure 27: **b.** *Urogram film shows attenuated intrarenal collecting system secondary to circumferential compression of kidney by hematoma. (Continued.)*

Figure 27: **d.** *CT section demonstrates the large hematoma surrounding the contrasted kidney with lucent areas within hematoma (arrows) representing perirenal fat. (Bleeding presumed secondary to small metastatic focus in retroperitoneum.)*

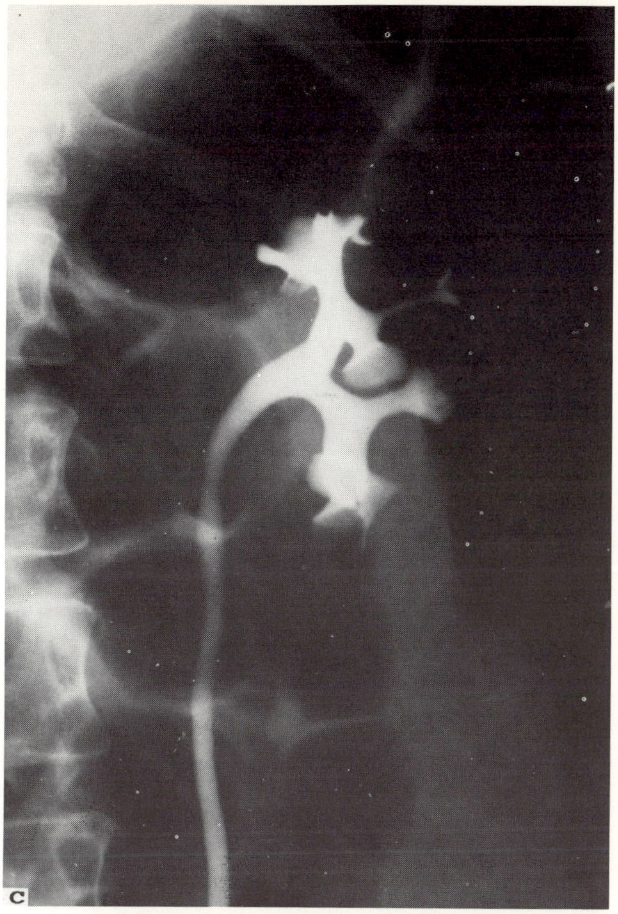

Figure 27: **c.** *Retrograde pyelogram causes normal distention of collecting system. (Continued.)*

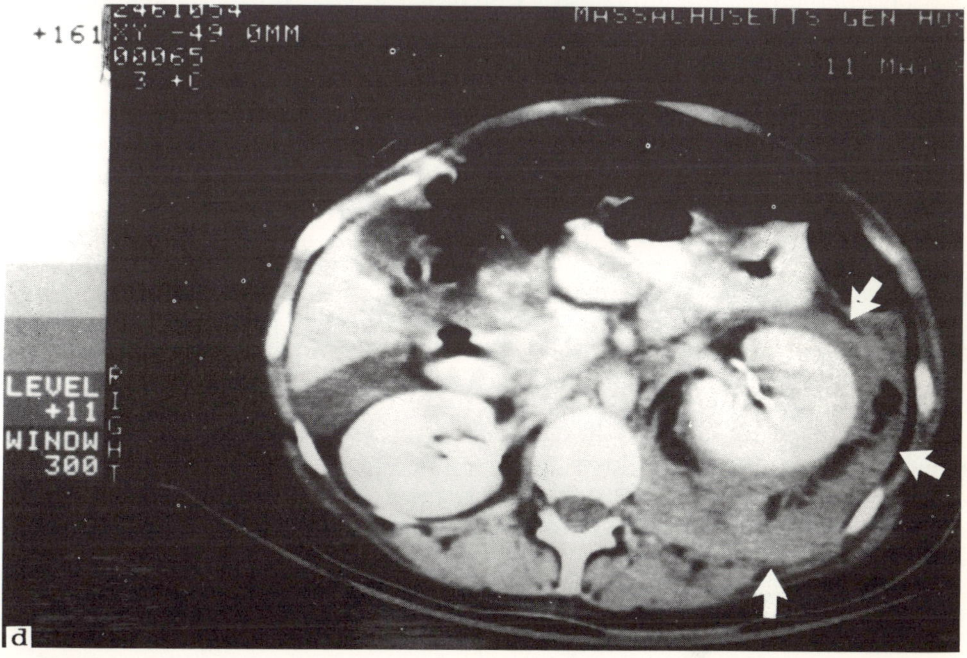

3. *Ultrasonography*

The perinephric space is relatively avascular, obviating the usefulness of angiography and radionuclide studies. Ultrasound evaluation based on anatomic changes is thus more helpful in the evaluation of retroperitoneal hematoma.[116] Acute hematomas may exhibit no or very weak internal echoes,[117] or may appear homogenously solid.[69] The walls may be ill-defined, though the extent of the hematoma is often demonstrable. As liquefaction and clot retraction progress, hyperechoic areas may develop within the hematoma.[118] The evolving hematoma may contain septations, solid debris, or fluid-solid interfaces that are gravity dependent. The wall may remain irregular, or may become elliptical or circular and well defined.[117] Perirenal fibrosis can lead to the Page kidney, which by ultrasound demonstrates a complex mass (fluid, fibrosis) surrounding essentially normal renal parenchyma.[113]

It is difficult, if not impossible, to differentiate one type of fluid from another with ultrasonography. The diagnosis of hemorrhage can usually be strongly suggested on the basis of the history and clinical course of the patient.[119] However, organizing hematomas can be indistinguishable from abscesses.[120] Thus, the value of ultrasound lies in detecting a fluid collection and defining its location and, to a lesser degree, its extent.

4. *Computed Tomography*

The more conventional roentgenologic modalities employed to evaluate retroperitoneal hemorrhage are heavily reliant on inferential findings, and thus lack both sensitivity and specificity. However, on CT sections, retroperitoneal hemorrhage is seen as an abnormal soft tissue density (Fig. 27d), which may obscure, compress, or displace adjacent retroperitoneal structures. The acute hematoma may be well localized or diffusely spread throughout the ipsilateral retroperitoneum. The attenuation values associated with the hematoma vary from 20 to 60 HU, depending upon its age.[121] As the hematoma ages, there may be nonuniform clot resolution with resultant areas of lower and higher CT density. These changes in attentuation values have been shown to correlate well with reduction in hemoglobin content and increase in water content.[122] Within 5 days after an acute bleed, the attenuation value may drop to one-half of its original value due to liquefaction.[123] As with ultrasonography, an abscess may exhibit similar CT findings, and again the clinical background is necessary to determine the final diagnosis. Other entities that may be confused with a hematoma include retroperitoneal tumors, cysts, and urinomas. The attendant attenuation values should be helpful in differentiating these lesions. Thus, when urography suggests the possibility of retroperitoneal or perirenal abnormality, CT becomes the method of choice for further evaluation,[124] especially for follow-up of perirenal hematomas of whatever etiology.

Engelstad et al.[125] found that in 91% of CT examinations, contrast enhancement did not obscure the findings. However, in patients with calcifications, hemorrhage, or contrast extravasation, nonenhanced images were required in conjunction with contrasted sections for accurate diagnosis. It is recommended, therefore, that pre- and post-contrast images be obtained in patients with suspected retroperitoneal hemorrhage. This is especially true in cases of subcapsular hematoma, where the attenuation values of the hematoma and enhanced compromised parenchyma may be somewhat similar and the hematoma could conceivably be missed. On the nonenhanced images, the renal parenchyma has an attenuation value of about 30 HU, which contrasts with the fresh subcapsular hematoma attenuation of 40–60 HU. If attenuation values are not obtained, the resultant film may simulate the appearance of a compressed rim of renal parenchyma (the hematoma) surrounding a less dense collecting system (the renal parenchyma) and can be mistaken for hydronephrosis.[126] Following contrast enhancement, there is an increased attenuation of the renal parenchyma while the hematoma remains virtually unchanged, causing an "inversion" of the differential densities[127] (Fig. 28 a,b).

As with urography, angiography, and ultrasonography, CT may be useful in detecting renal lesions that have precipitated an acute bleed. As with the other modalities, small peripheral neoplasms may be missed. However, should a lesion be seen, CT has the added advantage of being able to determine tissue types in some cases—for example, the fluid density of a cyst or presence of fat in an angiomyolipoma, liposarcoma, or lipoma[128] (Fig. 29 a,b).

Studies have shown that the true extent of renal injuries associated with hemorrhage cannot be accurately determined from intravenous urography with

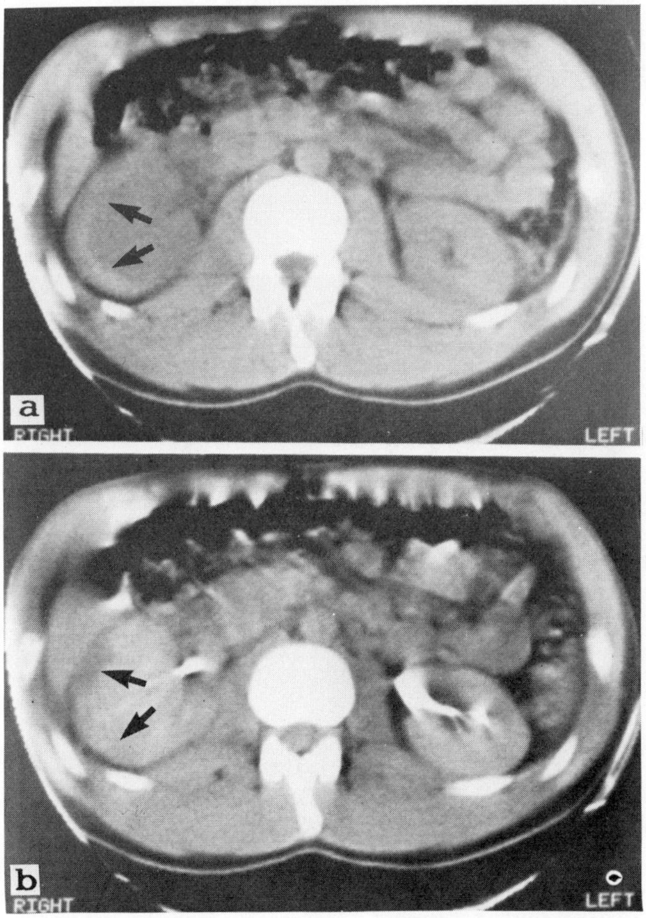

Figure 28: *Subcapsular hematoma in patient suffering blunt abdominal trauma.* **a.** *Precontrast CT scan shows subcapsular hematoma (arrows) as rim of high attenuation surrounding renal parenchyma.* **b.** *Post-contrast section shows enhancement of parenchyma, but not of hematoma ("inversion of densities"). (From: Amis ES Jr, Cronan JJ, Pfister RC. Pseudohydronephrosis on noncontrast computed tomography.* **J Comput Assist Tomogr.** *6:511–513, 1982.) (Continued.)*

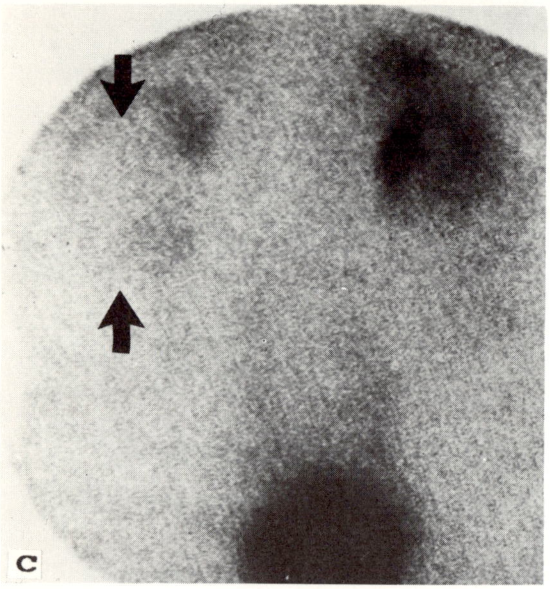

Figure 28: **c.** *Anterior radionuclide renal scan shows minimal function in lower two-thirds right kidney indicative of fracture and contusion (arrows).*

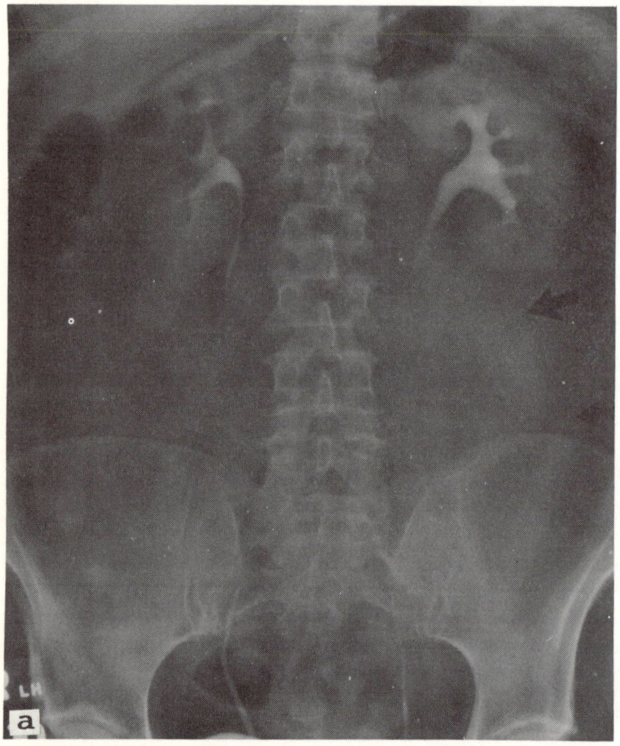

Figure 29: *Angiomyolipoma presenting with acute perirenal hemorrhage.*
a. *Urogram shows mass below left kidney obliterating psoas margin (arrows). (Continued.)*

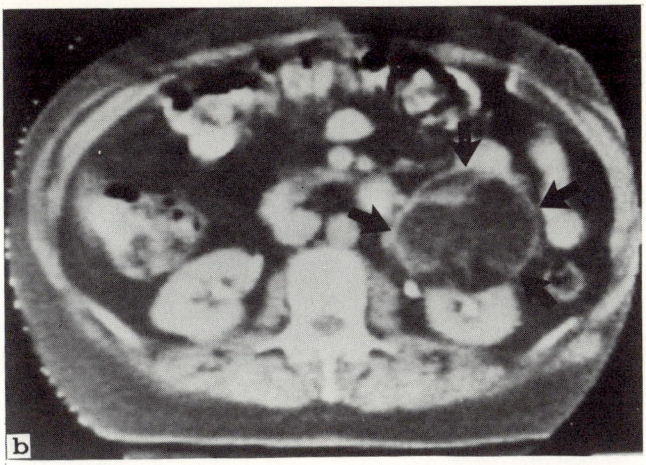

Figure 29: b. *CT section through lower pole of left kidney demonstrates a large anterior mass (arrows) with predominant fat density.*

nephrotomography alone, with the full extent of renal injury depicted in only 70–85% of cases.[129] CT, on the other hand, has been more accurate in determining the type and extent of parenchymal injuries, the presence of perirenal hematomas, and any extravasation or urine.[130] Federle et al.[129] classified renal trauma into three categories. Type I is a contusion or minor cortical laceration without disruption of the pyelocalyceal system (75–85% of renal injuries); type II is a complete laceration or renal fracture that communicates with the collecting system (10%); and type III is a shattered kidney or disruption of the renal pedicle (5%). In type I injuries, small areas of nonfunction may be seen on the nephrographic phase of the CT examination, with persistent accumulations of contrast in these areas on delayed sections.[131] In type II and III lesions, the fracture or kidney fragments may be easily seen by CT. Following pedicle damage, the nonfunctioning kidney can still be seen on CT, allowing determination of its integrity. These determinations require scans before and after contrast media administration.

A useful adjunct of CT is its ability to study the entire peritoneal cavity and retroperitoneum for associated injuries, which are present in 10–20% of cases of blunt trauma, and in greater than 50% of cases of penetrating trauma.[129]

5. Radionuclide Renal Scintigraphy

Radionuclide studies also may be useful in evaluating patients with renal trauma. The currently available agent of choice is Tc-99m-glucoheptonate, which labels the cortex by tubular concentration, and also provides images of the collecting system by glomerular filtration. Chopp et al.[132] reported that nephrotomography detected only 11 of 17 angiographically proven renal injuries, while the glucoheptonate scan was positive in 16 of the 17 cases. Following renal contusion, there is mild to moderate decrease in radioactivity on the involved side in a generalized or segmental pattern. Discrete areas of low activity indicate segmental contusions, intrarenal hematomas, infarcts, or lacerations[133] (Fig. 28c). Renal fracture will present as a distinct band of absent activity through the full width of the kidney. If there is extravasation, a collection of activity may be noted outside the confines of the kidney. A perirenal hematoma is suggested by a halo of decreased activity surrounding the kidney. Koenigsberg et al.[134] found that when a radionuclide study is normal in suspected renal trauma, subsequent angiography revealed no significant injury. Finally, radionuclide studies provide a noninvasive method for follow-up of renal trauma patients.

D. Specific Considerations

1. Adrenal Hemorrhage

Normal adrenals are well protected, and thus rarely affected by trauma,[135] except in the neonatal period when the adrenal size is roughly one-half that of the kidney.[136] Moderate or repeated small bleeding episodes may occur within the adrenal, resulting in enlargement or rupture of the gland with bleeding extending into the retroperitoneum. This retroperitoneal hematoma may occasionally perforate into the peritoneal cavity.[137]

Neonatal adrenal hemorrhage is a well-recognized entity with several postulated etiologies, including birth trauma, sepsis, burns, blood dyscrasias, mismatched transfusions, hypoxia, shock, thrombocytopenia, and disseminated intravascular coagulation.[37,138] A palpable abdominal mass is often the presenting sign. Prolonged jaundice is a frequent accompaniment.[139] The incidence has been established by autopsy series at 1.7 cases in 1,000 births.[140] The bleeding is unilateral in greater than 80% of cases.[140] The right side is more commonly affected than the left, possibly due to direct transmission of caval venous pressures through the shorter right adrenal vein.[138] Based on clinical suspicion, rapid radiologic evaluation is imperative. On plain films, if bleeding is confined to the gland, there may be a paucity of upper abdominal gas due to the mass effect. Retroperitoneal rupture may result in the intestinal gas being displaced to the contralateral side. With intraperitoneal rupture, hemoperitoneum results in bulging flanks and centrally floating bowel loops.

The most important phase of excretory urography is the total body opacification. This may reveal a homogenous lucency in the suprarenal region, which is sharply defined by the opacified adjacent structures.[139] The circumference of the adrenal gland may be opacified, and the ipsilateral kidney is usually displaced inferiorly with its upper pole flattened by the mass.[140] Ultrasonographic examination will demonstrate an echolucent mass, felt to represent the central hematoma of the adrenal.[137] A complex mass may be seen if there is a combination of hemorrhage and necrosis.

Differential diagnosis includes complete duplication of the collecting system with obstructed upper pole moiety, neuroblastoma, Wilms' tumor, and Wolman's familial xanthomatosis.[139,140] Neuroblastoma is rare in the neonatal period, presents a mottled appearance on total body opacification, and by ultrasonography exhibits a predominance of solid over cystic elements. Calcifications, if present, are usually fine and granular, not rim-like. Wilms' tumor is also rare in the neonatal period, and infrequently calcifies. Wolman's familial xanthomatosis is a rare entity occurring during the first 3 months of life, in which the adrenals are large bilaterally and remain roughly neonatal size. Dense calcifications are usually present.[139]

Complete duplication with an obstructed upper pole may be the most easily confused differential. Lucency above the displaced renal collecting system both by total body opacification and sonography is the expected finding, though the clinical setting should suggest neonatal adrenal hemorrhage as the correct diagnosis. Both could exist simultaneously.

Should the child survive, a rim of calcification may be seen as early as 12 days of age[139] (Fig.30). By 2 months, a coalescence of the calcification accompanies a general reduction in the size of the mass, with progression to a local, small suprarenal calcification such as those occasionally encountered in the adult.[141]

Adrenal hemorrhage after the neonatal period suggests the probability of bleeding into or rupture of an adrenal tumor. As mentioned previously, traumatic adrenal hemorrhage is rare, though it has been reported on an iatrogenic basis following adrenal vein catheterization.[142] Other reported nontumoral causes of intra-adrenal hemorrhage include pregnancy, burns, bleeding diathesis (including anticoagulation), cardiovascular disease, severe stress, sepsis, and the Waterhouse-Friderichsen syndrome.[143,144] In the latter syndrome, adrenal hemorrhage occurs most commonly as a response to meningococcal infection.[138] There is usually associated necrosis and infarction, and the adrenals are often enlarged due to the hemorrhage.[138,145]

Adrenal tumors reported in association with hemorrhage include adrenal carcinoma,[146] neuroblastoma,[147] and pheochromocytoma.[143,147] The latter appears to be the more common cause, and the hemorrhage may often be massive and rupture into the retroperitoneal space,[143] though bleeding may be confined intratumorally, even in small tumors.[147]

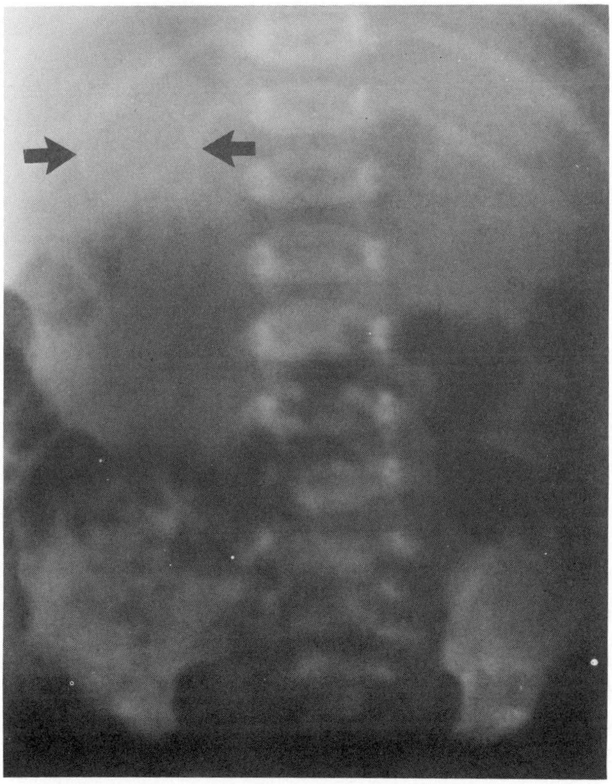

Figure 30: *Rim calcification seen in suprarenal region of newborn approximately 1 month after neonatal adrenal hemorrhage (arrows).*

Adrenal pseudocysts may be the end result of liquefaction of encapsulated intra-adrenal blood of whatever etiology with wall calcifications occurring in 15%.[138] Further bleeding can occur into adrenal cysts.[121]

In the radiological evaluation of the adrenals, the plain film of the abdomen is useful only if calcifications are present. Intravenous urography with nephrotomography may demonstrate lesions larger than 2.5 cm,[148] or glands large enough to displace the kidney with a resultant reversal of its axis.

Ultrasonographic evaluation of the adrenals may be technically difficult to perform and accurately interpret, especially on the left, due to overlying bowel gas and rib structures. Resolution is in the range of 2–3 cm.[149] If the adrenal is significantly enlarged, or if the patient is very thin, sonography becomes more accurate. Isolated hemorrhage within the gland may appear as a sonolucent lesion, or fine internal echoes may be seen. Hemorrhage into a pheochromocytoma will have a similar appearance,[138] while bleeding into a larger necrotic tumor such as a neuroblastoma may exhibit a mixed cystic-solid pattern.

Computed tomography is currently the modality of choice for imaging the adrenals. Even normal adrenal glands can be seen on CT in 85–90% of patients studied.[142,150] On CT sections, the normal right adrenal is most commonly seen as a vertical linear streak dorsal to the inferior vena cava, with its posterior portion extending between the right lobe of the liver and the spine. It is cephalad to the medial border of the kidney. The normal left adrenal is triradiate in configuration and lies anterior to the upper pole of the left kidney.[151] The thickness of the limbs of either gland should not exceed 1 cm. This is probably the most useful measurement in determining pathological involvement.[150] Another sensitive indicator of an abnormal adrenal is a change in the margin from concave or straight to convex. A spherical gland is never normal.[142]

Clinically significant hemorrhage within the adrenal should be easily detectable with CT. However, the etiology of the bleeding may not be apparent, as hemorrhage into a pre-existing lesion may have resulted in significant effacement of the lesion. Retroperitoneal bleeding will almost certainly obscure small adrenal lesions, while larger lesions may still be recognizable. The CT appearance of an intra-adrenal hemorrhage is that of a cyst-like lesion within the gland. This is secondary to blood contained within a narrow capsule of tumor tissue.[147] Indeed, the entire gland may be so effaced that only a cystic suprarenal lesion remains. Attenuation values of these lesions, however, will be consistent with blood. If acute, the values will be 40–60 HU, decreasing with time as the solid elements are resorbed. Percutaneous needle aspiration may be helpful in determining the diagnosis.[138] In the absence of other predisposing causes, adrenal tumor must be excluded as the source of hemorrhage.

REFERENCES

1. Marx WJ, Patel SK. Renal fascia: Its radiographic importance. *Urology*. 13:1–7, 1979.
2. Amin M, Blandford AT, Polk HC. Renal fascia of Gerota. *Urology*. 7:1–3, 1976.
3. Thornbury JR, McCormick TL, Silver TM. Anatomic/radiologic classification of renal cortical nodules. *AJR*. 134:1–7, 1980.
4. Felson B, Moskowitz M. Renal pseudo-tumors: The regenerated nodule and other lumps, bumps and dromedary humps. *Am J Roentgenol Radium Ther Nucl Med*. 107:720–729, 1969.

5. Pollack HM, Edell S, Morales JO. Radionuclide imaging in renal pseudotumors. *Radiology*. 111:639–644, 1974.
6. Older RA, Korobkin M, Workman J, Cleeve DM, Cleeve LK, Sullivan D, Webster GD. Accuracy of radionuclide imaging in distinguishing renal masses from normal variants. *Radiology*. 136:443–448, 1980.
7. Wolfson JJ, Stowell DW. Aberrant renal papilla simulating intrarenal mass: Report of two cases. *Radiology*. 93:812–814, 1969.
8. Binder R, Korobkin M, Clark RE, Palubinskas AJ. Aberrant papillae and other filling defects of the renal pelvis. *Am J Roentgenol Radium Ther Nucl Med*. 114:746–752, 1972.
9. Koehler PR, Kyaw MM. Hematuria. *Med Clin North Am*. 59:201–232, 1975.
10. Lee LW, Davis E, Jr. Gross urinary hemorrhage: Symptom, not a disease. *JAMA*. 153:782–784, 1953.
11. Jonsson K, Owman T. Roentgenologic aspects of haematuria. *Scand J Urol Nephrol*. 10:229–234, 1976.
12. Prien EL Sr. The analysis of urinary calculi. *Urol Clin North Am*. 1:229–240, 1974.
13. Margolin EG, Cohen LH. Genitourinary calcification: An overview. *Semin Roentgenol*. 17:95–100, 1982.
14. Lalli AF. Renal Parenchymal calcifications. *Semin Roentgenol*. 17:101–112, 1982.
15. Daniel WW Jr, Hartman GW, Witten DM, Farrow GM, Kelalis PP. Calcified renal masses: A review of ten years experience at the Mayo Clinic. *Radiology*. 103:503–508, 1972.
16. Kikkawa K, Lasser EC. "Ring-like" or "rim-like" calcification in renal cell carcinoma. *Am J Roentgenol*. 107:737–742, 1969.
17. Mencini RA. Calcification in a renal mass. *Semin Roentgenol*. 17:90–91, 1982.
18. Pollack HM, Banner MP, Martinez LO, Hodson CJ. Diagnostic considerations in urinary bladder wall calcification. *AJR*. 136:791–797, 1981.
19. Miller SW, Pfister RC. Calcification in uroepithelial tumors of the bladder: Report of 5 cases and survey of the literature. *Am J Roentgenol*. 121:827–831, 1974.
20. Witten DM. High-dose urography and nuclear medicine techniques. Presented at 3rd Annual Postgraduate Course, The Society of Uroradiology, San Diego, CA. Jan. 12, 1981.
21. Newhouse JH, Pfister RC. The Nephrogram. *Radiol Clin North Am*. 17:213–226, 1979.
22. Evans JA, Dubilier W, Monteith JC. Nephrotomography: A preliminary report. *AJR*. 71:213–223, 1954.
23. Pfister RC, Shea TE. Nephrotomography: Performance and interpretation. *Radiol Clin North Am*. 9:41–62, 1971.
24. Moreau J-F. Renal failure after urographic contrast media. Presented at 3rd Annual Postgraduate Course, The Society of Uroradiology, San Diego, CA, Jan. 12, 1981.
25. Shehadi WH. Contrast media adverse reactions: Occurrence, recurrence and distribution patterns. *Radiology*. 143:11–17, 1982.
26. Van Sonnenberg E, Pfister RC, Neff CC. An eight-year review of the treatment of intravenous contrast induced hypotensive reactions. Presentation at The Radiological Society of North America, Dallas TX, Nov. 16–20, 1980.
27. Barbaric Z. Renal fascia in urinary tract disease. *Radiology*. 118:561–565, 1976.
28. Hann L, Pfister RC. Renal subcapsular rim sign: New etiologies and pathogenesis. *AJR*. 138:51–54, 1982.
29. McLaughlin AP III, Pfister RC. Spontaneous rupture of renal cysts into the pyelocalyceal system. *J Urol*. 113:2–7, 1975.
30. Hidvegi RS. Bilateral intrarenal hematomas from anticoagulants. *J Can Assoc Radiol*. 27:250–254, 1976.
31. Kaiser JA, Jacobs RP, Korobkin M. Submucosal hemorrhage of the renal collecting system. *Am J Roentgenol*. 125:311–313, 1975.
32. Thompson JS, McAlister WH. Subepithelial hemorrhage in the renal pelvis and ureter simulating pyeloureteritis cystica. *Pediatr Radiol*. 3:156–157, 1975.

33. Komolafe F. The "spaghetti sign": An uncommon radiologic sign of upper urinary tract hemorrhage. *AJR*. 137:1062, 1981.
34. Hillman BJ, Silvert M, Cook G, Stanisic T, Bjelland J, Claypool HR, Haber K, Mellins HZ. Recognition of bladder tumors by excretory urography. *Radiology*. 138:319–323, 1981.
35. Elkin M. Tumors of the urinary tract. In: *Radiology of the Urinary System*. Elkin M. Boston, Little, Brown and Co., 1980, pp. 405–419.
36. Scully RE, Galdabini JJ, McNeely BU. Case records of the Massachusetts General Hospital. Case 8-1981. *New Engl J Med*. 304:469–474, 1981.
37. Amis ES Jr, Cronan JJ, Yoder IC, Pfister RC. Impressions on floor of female bladder: "The female prostrate." *Urology*. 19:441–446, 1982.
38. Navani S, Bosniak MA, Shapiro JH, Kaufman S. Varied radiographic manifestations of urinary tract bleeding. *J Urol*. 100:339–343, 1968.
39. Lytton B, Brooks, M, Spencer RP. Absorption of contrast material from the urinary tract during retrograde pyelography. *J Urol*. 100:779–782, 1968.
40. Pfister RC, Newhouse JH. Interventional percutaneous pyeloureteral techniques. I. Antegrade pyelography and ureteral perfusion. *Radiol Clin North Am*. 17:344–350, 1979.
41. Mellins HZ. Radiology of the urinary tract. Urography and cystourethrography. In: *Urology*, 4th d. Harrison JH, Gittes RF, Perlmutters AD, et al., Eds. Philadelphia, WB Saunders Co., 1978, pp. 222–270.
42. McAninch LN, Mostafa HM. Pyelocancerous backflow: A diagnostic radiologic sign for renal cell carcinoma. *J Urol*. 105;491, 1971.
43. Rankin RS, Wegenke JD, Madsen PO. Pseudotumor of kidney. *Urology*. 10:68–70, 1977.
44. Copeland JS, Schellhammer PF, Devine CJ Jr. Pyelocancerous backflow: A radiologic finding in renal malignancy. *J Urol*. 115:214–215, 1976.
45. Rosenfield AT, Taylor KJ. Gray scale nephrosonography: Current status. *J Urol*. 117:2–6, 1977.
46. Rosenfield AT, Taylor KJ, Crade M, DeGraaf CS. Anatomy and pathology of the kidney by gray scale ultrasound. *Radiology*. 128:737–744, 1978.
47. Pollack HM, Arger PH, Goldberg BB, Mulholland SG. Ultrasonic detection of nonopaque renal calculi. *Radiology*. 127:233–237, 1978.
48. Brennan RE, Curtis JA, Kurtz AB, Dalton JR. Use of tomography and ultrasound in the diagnosis of nonopaque renal calculi. *JAMA*. 244:594–596, 1980.
49. Green WM, King DL, Casarella WJ. A reappraisal of sonolucent renal masses. *Radiology*. 121:163–171, 1976.
50. Goldstein HM, Green B, Weaver RM Jr. Ultrasonic detection of renal tumor extension into the inferior vena cava. *AJR*. 130:1083–1085, 1978.
51. Lee TG, Henderson SC, Freeny PC, Raskin MM, Benson EP, Pearse HD. Ultrasound findings of renal angiomyolipoma. *J Clin Ultrasound*. 6:150–155, 1978.
52. Hartman DS, Goldman SM, Friedman AC, Davis CJ Jr, Madewell JE, Sherman JL. Angiomyolipoma: Ultrasonic-pathologic correlation. *Radiology*. 139:451–458, 1981.
53. Cronan JJ, Simeone JF, Pfister RC, Newhouse JH, Ferrucci JT, Jr. Cystosonography in the detection of bladder tumors: A prospective and retrospective study. *J Ultrasound Med*. 1:237–241, 1982.
54. Parienty RA, Pradel J, Picard JD, Ducellier R, Lubrano JM, Smolarski N. Visibility and thickening of the renal fascia on computed tomograms. *Radiology*. 139:119–124, 1981.
55. Curtis JA, Brennan RE, Rubin C, Kurtz A, Goldberg BB. Computed tomography of the kidneys. *Comput Tomogr*. 4:17–37, 1980.
56. Federle MP, McAninch JW, Kaiser JA, Goodman PC, Roberts J, Mall JC. Computed tomography of urinary calculi. *AJR*. 136:255–258, 1981.
57. Segal AJ, Spataro RF, Linke CA, Frank IN, Rabinowitz R. Diagnosis of nonopaque calculi by computed tomography. *Radiology*. 129:447–450, 1978.

58. Alter AJ, Peterson DJ, Plautz AC Jr. Non-opaque calculus demonstrated by computerized tomography. *J Urol.* 122:699–700, 1979.
59. Pollack HM, Arger PH, Banner MPL, Mulhern CB Jr, Coleman BG. Computed tomography of renal pelvic filling defects. *Radiology.* 138:645–651, 1981.
60. McClennan BL, Stanley RJ, Melson GL, Levitt RG, Sagel SS. CT of the renal cyst: Is cyst aspiration necessary? *AJR.* 133:671–675, 1979.
61. Hattery RR, Williamson B Jr, Stephens DH, Sheedy PF II, Hartman GW. Computed tomography of renal abnormalities. *Radiol Clin North Am.* 15:401–418, 1977.
62. Sagel SS, Stanley RJ, Levitt RG, Geisse G. Computed tomography of the kidney. *Radiology.* 124:359–370, 1977.
63. Weyman PJ, McClennan BL, Stanley RJ, Levitt RG, Sagel SS. Comparison of computed tomography and angiography in the evaluation of renal cell carcinoma. *Radiology.* 137:417–424, 1980.
64. Becker JA, Kinkhabwala M, Pollack H, Bosniak M. Angiomyolipoma (hamartoma) of the kidney: An angiographic review. *Acta Radiol (Diag).* 14:561–568, 1973.
65. Hansen GC, Hoffman RB, Sample WF, Becker R. Computed tomography diagnosis of renal angiomyolipoma. *Radiology.* 128:789–791, 1978.
66. Bosniak MA. Angiomyolipoma (hamartoma) of the kidney: A preoperative diagnosis is possible in virtually every case. *Urol Radiol.* 3:135–142, 1981.
67. Sherman JL, Hartman DS, Friedman AC, Madewell JE, Davis CJ, Goldman SM. Angiomyolipoma: Computed tomographic-pathologic correlation of 17 cases. *Am J Roentgenol.* 137;1221–1226, 1981.
68. Baert AL, Wilms G, Marchal G, DeMayer P, DeSomer F. Contrast enhancement by bolus technique in the CT examination of the kidney. *Radiologe.* 20:279–287, 1980.
69. Seidelmann FE, Cohen WN, Bryan PJ. Computed tomographic staging of bladder neoplasms. *Radiol Clin North Am.* 15:419–440, 1977.
70. Kwok-Liu JP, Zikman JM,. Cockshott WP. Carcinoma of the urachus: The role of computed tomography. *Radiology.* 137:731–734, 1980.
71. Lisbona R, Derbekyan V, Rosenthall L. Observations on renal scanning and intravenous urology in acute segmental renal infarction. *Clin Nucl Med.* 6:253–257, 1981.
72. Mettler FA, Christie JH. The scintigraphic pattern of acute renal vein thrombosis. *Clin Nucl Med.* 5:468–470, 1980.
73. Quigley JM, Druy EM, Rich JI. Acute renal vein thrombosis with a diagnostic renal scintigram. *AJR.* 137:1066–1068, 1981.
74. Amis ES Jr. Cronan JJ, Pfister RC. Filling defects in small bowel urinary conduits. *AJR.* 137:787–792, 1981.
75. Yoder IC, Pfister RC. Radiology of colon loop diversion: Anatomic and urodynamic studies of the conduit and ureters in children and adults. *Radiology.* 127:85–92, 1978.
76. McCallum RW. The adult male urethra. Normal anatomy, pathology and method of urethrography. *Radiol Clin North Am.* 17:227–244, 1979.
77. Richter MW, Lytton B, Myerson D, Grnja V. Radiology of genitourinary trauma. *Radiol Clin North Am.* 11:593–631, 1973.
78. McLaughlin AP III, Pfister RC. Double catheter technique for evaluation of urethral injury and differentiating urethral from bladder rupture. *Radiology.* 110:716–719, 1974.
79. Newhouse JH, Pfister RC. Antegrade pyelography. In: *Interventional Radiology.* Athanasoulis CA, Pfister RC, Greene RE, et al., Eds. Philadelphia, WB Saunders Co., 1982, pp. 437–454.
80. Pfister RC, Newhouse JH. Percutaneous nephrostomy: Types of catheters for drainage, occlusion, dilation and fiber optics for endoscopy. In: *Interventional Radiology.* Athanasoulis CA, Pfister RC, Greene RE, et al., Eds. Philadelphia, WB Saunders Co., 1982, pp. 467–496.
81. Gill WB, Lu CT, Thomsen S. Retrograde brushing: A new technique for obtaining histologic and cytologic material from ureteral, renal pelvic and renal caliceal lesions. *J Urol.* 109:573–578, 1973.

82. Pfister RC, Newhouse JH. Interventional percutaneous pyeloureteral techniques. II. Percutaneous nephrostomy and other procedures. *Radiol Clin North Am.* 17: 351–363, 1979.
83. Jackman RJ, Stevens GM. Benign hemorrhagic renal cyst. Nephrotomography, renal arteriography and cyst puncture. *Radiology.* 110:7–13, 1974.
84. Amis ES Jr., Cronan JJ, Yoder IC, Pfister RC, Newhouse JH. Renal cysts: Curios and caveats. *Urol Radiol.* 4:199–209, 1982.
85. Harris RD, Goergen TG, Talner LB. The bloody renal cyst aspirate: A diagnostic dilemma. *J Urol.* 114:832–835, 1975.
86. Pfister RC, Newhouse JH. Percutaneous biopsy of the urinary tract. In: *Interventional Radiology.* Athanasoulis CA, Pfister RC, Greene RE, et al., Eds. Philadelphia, WB Saunders Co., 1982, pp 426–436.
87. Wunderlich CRA. *Handbuch der pathologie und therapie.* 2nd ed. Stuttgart. Ebner & Seubert, 1856.
88. Beh WP, Barnhouse DH, Johnson SH, Marshall M Jr, Price SE Jr. A renal cause for massive retroperitoneal hemorrhage-renal angiomyolipoma. *J Urol.* 116:372–374, 1976.
89. Pollack HM, Popky GL. Roentgenographic manifestations of spontaneous renal hemorrhage. *Radiology.* 110:1–6, 1974.
90. McDougal WS, Kursh ED, Persky L. Spontaneous rupture of the kidney with perirenal hematoma. *J Urol.* 114:181–184, 1975.
91. McCallum RW, Munro TG. Spontaneous retroperitoneal hemorrhage due to renal cell carcinoma. *J Can Assoc Radiol.* 25:110–112, 1974.
92. Thornbury JR. Perirenal anatomy: Normal and abnormal. *Radiol Clin North Am.* 17:321–331, 1979.
93. Polkey HJ, Vynalek WJ. Spontaneous nontraumatic perirenal and renal hematomas: Experimental and clinical study. *Arch Surg.* 26:196–218, 1933.
94. Novicki DE, Turlington JT, Ball TP Jr. The evaluation and management of spontaneous perirenal hemorrhage. *J Urol.* 123:764–765, 1980.
95. Degusseau B, Chousterman P, Bourquelot P, Druet P. Spontaneous pure subcapsular renal hematoma. Two cases. *Nouv Presse Med.* 8:3149–3151, 1979.
96. Morettin LB, Kumar R. Small renal carcinoma with large retroperitoneal hemorrhage: Diagnostic considerations. *Urol Radiol.* 3:143–148, 1981.
97. Gilbert JT. Spontaneous rupture of hypernephroma simulating the acute surgical abdomen. *Am Surg.* 26:136–140, 1960.
98. Barret F, Sellier N, Affre J, Leclerc J, Helenon C, Bigot JM. Subcapsular renal hematoma: Report of two cases revealing benign cortical tumors. *Ann Radiol.* (Paris) 23:671–674, 1980.
99. Dunnick NR, Hartman DS, Ford KK, Davis CJ Jr, Amis ES Jr. The Radiology of juxtaglomerular tumors. *Radiology.* 147:321–326, 1983.
100. Peterson C, Willerson JT, Doppman JL, Decker JL. Polyarteritis nodosa with bilateral renal artery aneurysm and perirenal hematomas: Angiographic and nephrotomographic features. *Br J Radiol 43:62–66, 1970.*
101. Hodin E, Dass T. Spontaneous retroperitoneal hemorrhage complicating anticoagulant therapy. *Ann Surg.* 170:848–851, 1969.
102. Zweifler AJ, Coon WW, Willis PW. Bleeding during oral anticoagulant therapy. *Am Heart J.* 71:118–123, 1966.
103. Bosniak MA, Ambos MA. Polycystic kidney disease. *Semin Roentgenol.* 10: 133–143, 1975.
104. Brown CD. Massive spontaneous renal cyst hemorrhage. *JAMA.* 239:1418–1419, 1978.
105. Hessel SJ, Smith EH. Renal trauma: A comprehensive review and radiologic assessment. *CRC Crit Rev Clin Radiol Nucl Med.* 5:251–293, 1974.
106. Ganji H, Bryan R, Cohn I Jr. Traumatic rupture of hypernephroma. *Am J Surg.* 116:120–122, 1968.

107. Ginsburg JC, Fransman SL, Singer MA Cohanim M, Morrin PA. Use of computerized tomography to evaluate bleeding after renal biopsy. *Nephron.* 26:240–243, 1980.
108. Rosenbaum R, Hoffstein PE, Stanley RJ, Klahr S. Use of computerized tomography to diagnose complications of percutaneous renal biopsy. *Kidney Int.* 14:87–92, 1978.
109. Drew JH. Ileus in retroperitoneal haematoma. *Med J Aust.* 1:246–248, 1973.
110. McCort JJ. Plain film diagnosis of perirenal hemorrhage. *Radiol Clin.* (Basel) 47: 280–294, 1978.
111. Elkin M, Cohen G. Diagnostic value of the psoas shadow. *Clin Radiol.* 13:210–217, 1962.
112. Myers MA, Whalen JP, Evans JA. Diagnosis of perirenal and subcapsular masses: Anatomic-radiologic correlation. *Am J Roentgenol.* 121:523–538, 1974.
113. Chamorro HA, Forbes TW, Padkowsky GO, Wholey MH. Multi-imaging approach in the diagnosis of Page kidney. *AJR.* 136:620–621, 1981.
114. Page IH. The production of persistent arterial hypertension by cellophane perinephritis. *JAMA.* 113:2046–2048, 1939.
115. Downs RA. Liquified subcapsular hematomas of kidney. *Urology.* 4:519–523, 1974.
116. Conrad MR, Freedman M, Weiner C, Freeman C, Sanders RC. Sonography of the Page kidney. *J Urol.* 116:293–296, 1976.
117. Doust BD, Quiroz F, Stewart JM. Ultrasonic distinction of abscesses from other intra-abdominal fluid collections. *Radiology.* 125:213–218, 1977.
118. McCullough DL, Leopold GR. Diagnosis of retroperitoneal fluid collections by ultrasonography: A series of surgically proved cases. *J Urol.* 115:656–659, 1976.
119. Sample WF. Renal, adrenal, retroperitoneal and scrotal ultrasonography. In: *Diagnostic Ultrasound.* (Text and cases.) Sarti DA, Sample WF, Eds. Boston, GK Hall Medical Publishers,1980, pp. 268–279.
120. Scheible W, Talner LB. Gray scale ultrasound and the genitourinary tract: A review of clinical applications. *Radiol Clin North Am.* 17:281–300, 1979.
121. Sagel SS, Siegel MJ, Stanley RJ, Jost RG. Detection of retroperitoneal hemorrhage by computed tomography. *AJR.* 129:403–407, 1977.
122. Korobkin M, Callen PW, Fisch AE. Computed tomography of the pelvis and retroperitoneum. *Radiol Clin North Am.* 17:301–319, 1979.
123. Schaner EG, Balow JE, Doppman JL. Computed tomography in the diagnosis of subcapsular and perirenal hematoma. *AJR.* 129:83–88, 1977.
124. Williamson B Jr, Hattery RR, Stephens DH, Sheedy PF II. Computed tomography of the kidneys. *Roentgenol.* 13:249–255, 1978.
125. Engelstad BL, McClennan BL, Levitt RG, Stanley RJ, Sagel SS. The role of precontrast images in computed tomography of the kidney. *Radiology.* 136:153–155, 1980.
126. Amis ES Jr, Cronan JJ, Pfister RC. Pseudohydronephrosis on noncontrast computed tomography. *J Comput Assist Tomogr.* 6:511–513, 1982.
127. Baert AL, Wilms G. Marchal G, DeMayer P, De Somer F. Contrast enhancement by bolus technique in CT examination of the kidney. *Radiologe.* 20:279–287, 1980.
128. Stephens DH, Sheedy PF, Hattery RR, Williamson B Jr. Diagnosis and evaluation of retroperitoneal tumors by computed tomography. *AJR.* 129:395–402, 1977.
129. Federle MP, Kaiser JA, MC Aninch JW, Jeffrey RB, Mall JC. The role of computed tomography in renal trauma. *Radiology.* 141:455–460, 1981.
130. Federle MP, Goldberg HI, Kaiser JA, Moss AA, Jeffrey RB Jr, Mall JC. Evaluation of abdominal trauma by computed tomography. *Radiology.* 138:637–644, 1981.
131. Kuhn JP, Berger PE. Computed tomography in the evaluation of blunt abdominal trauma in children. *Radiol Clin North Am.* 19:503–513, 1981.
132. Chopp RT, Hekmat-Ravan H, Mendez R. Technetium-99m glucoheptonate renal scan in diagnosis of acute renal injury. *Urology.* 15:201–206, 1980.
133. McConnell BJ, McConnell RW, Guiberteau MJ. Radionuclide imaging in blunt trauma. *Radiol Clin North Am.* 19:37–51, 1981.
134. Koenigsberg M, Blaufox MD, Freeman LM. Traumatic injuries of the renal vasculature and parenchyma. *Semin Nucl Med.* 4:117–132, 1974.

135. McCort JJ. Intraperitoneal and retroperitoneal hemorrhage. *Radiol Clin North Am.* 14:391–405, 1976.
136. Lawson EE, Teele RL. Diagnosis of adrenal hemorrhage by ultrasound. *J Pediatr.* 92:423–26, 1978.
137. Eklof, O. Large asymptomatic adrenal haematomas in the neonate. *Acta Radiol.* (Diagn) (Stockh)11:481–488, 1971.
138. Mitty HA, Yeh H-C. Non-neoplastic lesions (of adrenal). In: *Radiology of the Adrenals with Sonography and CT.* Mitty HA, Yeh H-C, Eds. Philadelphia, WB Saunders Co., 1982, pp. 210–223.
139. Rose J, Berdon WE, Sullivan T, Baker DH. Prolonged jaundice as presenting sign of massive adrenal hemorrhage in newborns. Radiographic diagnosis by IVP with total-body opacification. *Radiology.* 98:263–272, 1971.
140. Eklof O, Grotte G, Jorulf H, Lohr G, Ringertz H. Perinatal hemorrhagic necrosis of the adrenal gland: A clinical and radiological evaluation of 24 consecutive cases. *Pediatr Radiol.* 4:31–36, 1975.
141. Brill PW, Krasna IH, Aaron H. An early rim sign in neonatal adrenal hemorrhage. *AJR.* 127:289–291, 1976.
142. Karstaedt N, Sagel SS, Stanley RJ, Melson GL, Levitt RG. Computed tomography of the adrenal gland. *Radiology.* 129:723–730, 1978.
143. Lawson DW, Corry RJ, Paton AS, Daggett WM, Austen WG. Massive retroperitoneal adrenal hemorrhage. *Surg Gynecol Obst* 129:989–994, 1969.
144. Korobkin M, White EA, Kressel HY, Moss AA, Montagne JP. Computed tomography in the diagnosis of adrenal disease. *AJR.* 132:231–238, 1979.
145. Alexander ES, Clark RA. Computed tomography in the diagnosis of abdominal hemorrhage. JAMA. 248:1104–1107, 1982.
146. Stephens DH, Williamson B, Jr. Sheedy PF II, Hattery RR, Miller WE. Computed tomography of the retroperitoneal space. *Radiol Clin North Am.* 15:377–390, 1977.
147. Yeh HC, Mitty HA, Rose J, Wolf BS, Gabrilove JL. Ultrasonography of adrenal masses: Unusual manifestations. *Radiology.* 127:475–483, 1978.
148. Sample WF, Sarti DA. Computed tomography and gray scale ultrasonography of the adrenal gland: A comparative study. *Radiology.* 128:377–383, 1978.
149. Curtis JA, Brennan RE, Kurtz AB. Evaluation of adrenal disease by computed tomography. *Comput Tomogr.* 4:165–168, 1980.
150. Montagne JP, Kressel HY, Korobkin M, Moss, AA. Computed tomography of the normal adrenal glands. *AJR.* 130:963–966, 1978.
151. Brownlie K, Kreel L. Computer assisted tomography of normal suprarenal glands. *J Comput Assist Tomogr.* 2:1–10, 1978.

Chapter 8

Angiography in the Diagnosis and Control of Genitourinary Hemorrhage

Laura Feldman, M.D., and Christos A. Athanasoulis, M.D.

I. Diagnostic Angiography and Venography

A. Introduction

Angiography can be a powerful tool for both the diagnosis and therapy of urologic hemorrhage. Pathologic lesions can be diagnosed, bleeding sites can be localized, and hemorrhage can be stopped or slowed using selective embolization techniques.

Initial diagnostic measures depend on the etiology and rapidity of bleeding. Blunt and penetrating trauma are the most frequent causes of hemorrhage that we study angiographically. After initial evaluation and the stabilization of the patient, a plain film of the abdomen, intravenous urography, computed tomography and/or retrograde cystogram may be performed (see Chapter 7). If there is nonvisualization of one kidney or there is evidence of significant renal trauma, or if pelvic hemorrhage is present, an angiogram is performed. Arteriography has a high degree of accuracy in detecting injury to the renal pedicle, renal parenchymal disruption, subcapsular or perinephric hematoma, arteriovenous fistula formation, as well as arterial extravasation both in the kidney and in the pelvis. Moreover, the angiographic catheter can then be used to embolize arterial bleeding sites selectively, thus reducing or eliminating hemorrhage with a minimum of tissue loss.

The development of angiographic techniques for localizing and controlling hemorrhage in the genitourinary tract followed its successful use in gastrointestinal hemorrhage. If bleeding is rapid enough, i.e. greater than 0.5 cc/min in experimental models,[1] the bleeding site can be demonstrated by the extravasation of radiopaque contrast. Unlike the gastrointestinal tract, the genitourinary tract is not amenable to the vasoconstrictive effects of vasopressin. Therefore,

From Bern MM (ed.): *Urinary Tract Bleeding: Diagnosis and Control by Medical, Radiologic, and Surgical Techniques*. Mount Kisco, NY, Futura Publishing Co., Inc., 1985.

arterial occlusion is required to obtain hemostasis. This is accomplished either by injecting fragments of embolic material through the catheter or by occluding the artery with an inflatable balloon. This latter approach is used for cases of major vessel transection and provides an opportunity to stabilize the patient in preparation for surgical repair of the transected vessel.

Patients with subacute or chronic hematuria may come to angiography following routine work-up, including urography, nephrotomography, cytoscopy, and ultrasound or CT if no apparent cause for bleeding has been detected. This group represents only 5% to 8% of patients with hematuria.[23] Although the diagnostic yield is low (angiographic diagnosis is made in 12% to 15% of such cases), vascular lesions such as hemangioma, aneurysm, arteriovenous malformation, renal vein varices, renal artery embolus, vasculitis, or tumor occur with enough frequency to warrant angiography.[45]

B. Services to be Provided

To provide optimal angiographic services, a commitment must be made by a skilled angiographic team on a 24-hour basis. In addition, a nurse and a clinical physician should be available to manage an unstable patient while the angiographer and radiology technician devote their attention to the procedure. Patient monitoring equipment including ECG and pressure monitoring devices, wall-mounted oxygen and suctioning capacity as well as resuscitation equipment are mandatory if critically ill patients are to be examined and treated in an angiographic suite. Acutely bleeding patients should be brought to angiography after being stabilized as completely as possible with large caliber intravenous lines, ongoing blood and fluid replacement, and central venous and intra-arterial lines if appropriate.

C. Technique

The procedure is performed using mild sedation and local anesthesia. If the patient is bleeding from the upper genitourinary tract, an initial abdominal aortogram is performed. A radiopaque pigtail, ring, or straight catheter with multiple sideholes and tip occluder is introduced into the femoral artery and advanced under fluoroscopic control to a level just above the origin of the renal arteries. An arteriogram is obtained providing an overall anatomic "road map." It demonstrates the number of renal arteries on each side and may reveal extravasation of contrast from a renal artery, from lumbar arteries, or from an unexpected mesenteric source. It may also demonstrate additional retroperitoneal pathology that may be missed if selective renal arteriogrpahy is performed initially. It also helps to avoid the misdiagnosis of renal infarct or avascular mass that may result from selective injection into only one of multiple renal arteries (Fig. 1).

A percutaneous transfemoral approach is most commonly used. However, if the femoral artery is unavailable, either because of massive pelvic trauma or atherosclerotic disease, a transaxillary approach may be used.

After the abdominal aortogram, the catheter is exchanged for a preshaped endhole catheter and the appropriate renal and/or lumbar arteries are selectively catheterized and injected, using magnification, pharmacoangiography, and multiple projections if appropriate.

In patients with suspected lower genitourinary bleeding, such as patients with pelvic trauma, a pelvic arteriogram is initially performed. The catheter then is exchanged and selective hypogastric artery injections are filmed.

Venous angiography is occasionally efficacious. It can be useful in patients with renal hemorrhage that remains unexplained after arteriography by demonstrating pathology such as renal vein varices. In addition, transitional cell carcinomas may become evident during renal venography with simultaneous administration of approximately 8 mg of epinephrine into the corresponding renal artery. In patients with pelvic hemorrhage secondary to trauma, venous studies have not been helpful. Either no site of extravasation is seen or, as in patients with transection of an iliac vein, extensive hemorrhage necessitates immediate surgical exploration, bypassing angiography entirely.

When a site of contrast extravasation is seen, either in the kidney or elsewhere in the retroperitoneum or pelvis, the catheter may be advanced as selectively as possible and the bleeding site embolized. A variety of embolic materials may be used depending upon the clinical circumstances. When further injection of contrast demonstrates no additional extravasation, embolization is complete and the catheter is withdrawn. Manual compression at the groin for approximately 15 minutes should result in hemostasis.

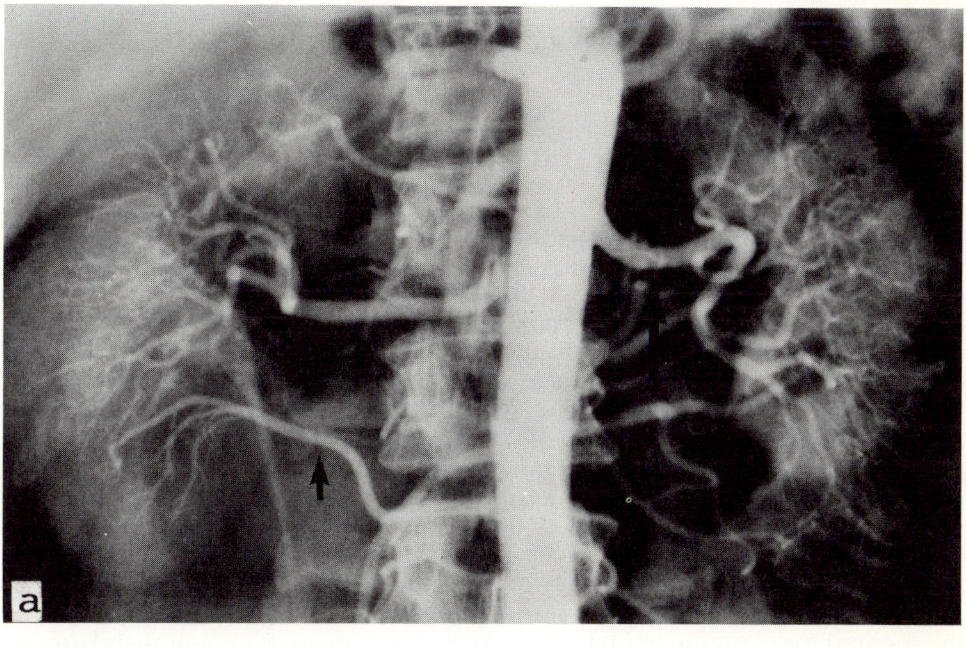

Figure 1: *Multiple renal arteries.* **a.** *Normal aortogram with three right renal arteries (small arrows) and one left renal artery (large arrow).(Continued.)*

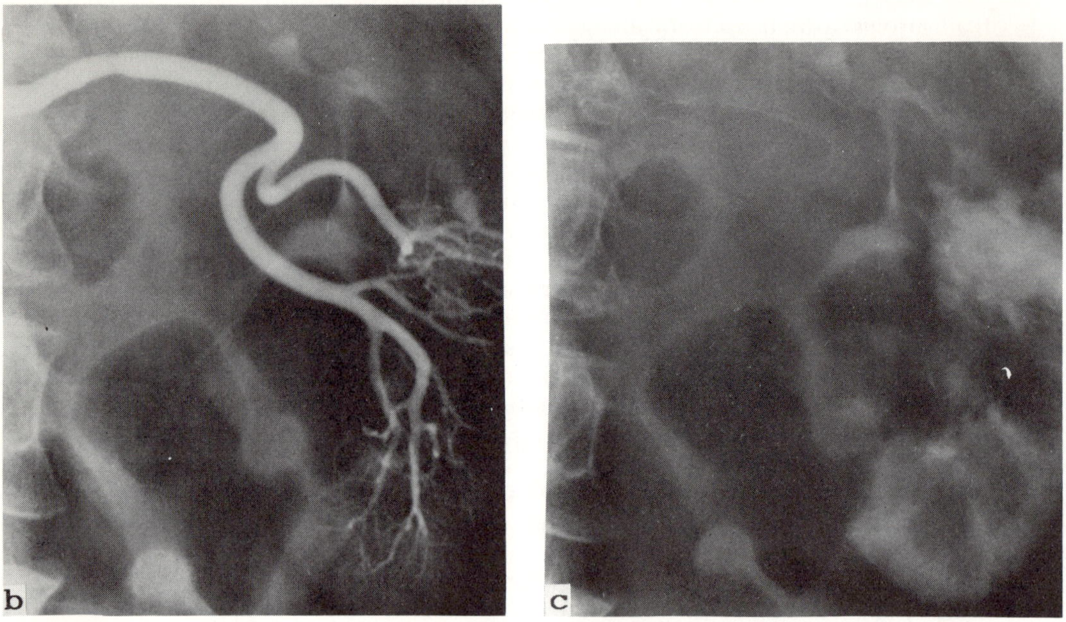

Figure 1: **b, c.** *Different patient than* **a.** *Selective arteriogram of one of two left renal arteries, early and late phase. The segmental nephrogram could be confused with a traumatized kidney.*

II. Angiographic Anatomy

A. Normal Renal Arteriography and Venography

In 75% of patients there is a single renal artery supplying each kidney, usually originating at the L1-L2 level. Accessory renal arteries can be identified anywhere from the lower thoracic aorta to the iliac arteries. The right renal artery is usually higher and longer with its origin slightly more anterior than that of the left. The main renal artery often gives rise to other retroperitoneal branches: renal capsular branches and pelvoutaric branches, the inferior adrenal artery, the gonadal branches and, occasionally, the inferior phrenic artery. The main renal artery classically bifurcates into a smaller more superior dorsal branch and a larger ventral branch. These then divide into segmental branches and subdivide further into interlobar branches that course to the corticomedullary junction. The arcuate arteries arise at this juncture and run parallel to the cortex, giving rise to small intralobar branches that penetrate the cortex. Small intrarenal communications (for example between intralobar branches and arcuate branches), and extrarenal communications (for example between perforating branches) arising from arcuate arteries and capsular branches are present and may provide collateral flow.

The arterial phase lasts for approximately 4 seconds after the beginning of a 2-second injection of contrast material into the renal artery. The nephrogram phase normally lasts up to 10 seconds. Its duration depends on renal blood flow. Renal size and the outline and thickness of the cortex (normally 7–10 mm) can be determined during this phase. The renal veins are often poorly seen unless a high dose injection is performed (i.e. using 30 cc of contrast as opposed to the usual 10-12 cc). The veins normally appear 10-12 seconds after arterial injection. Direct renal venography, however, is often necessary to demonstrate renal venous anatomy satisfactorily. Intrarenal venous branches can be optimally visualized when venography is performed immediately after the injection of epinephrine into the corresponding renal artery (Fig. 2). Multiple right renal veins are quite common, occurring with a frequency of 15–20%.[6] There is no correlation between the number of renal veins and the number of corresponding renal arteries. Unlike the arterial circulation, there is free anastomosis of multiple veins and of the intrarenal venous branches.

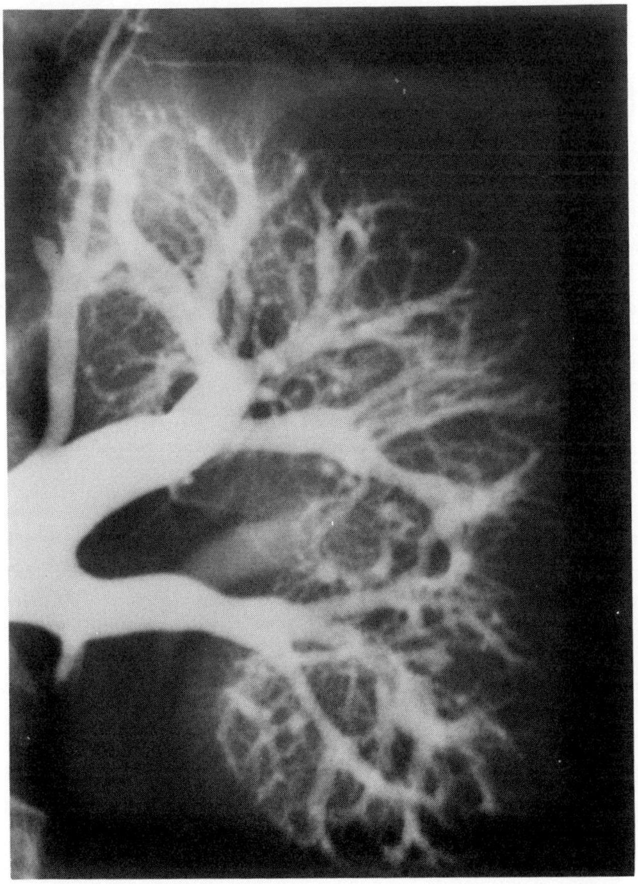

Figure 2: *Epinephrine assisted renal venogram. Renal venogram obtained with simultaneous injection of 8 micrograms epinephrine into renal artery.*

B. Normal Pelvic Arterial Anatomy

The common iliac artery occasionally gives origin to a major branch, such as an accessory renal artery or the iliolumbar artery, but usually gives origin to only small branches to the peritoneum, psoas major, and ureter. It then bifurcates into the external iliac artery, which terminates as the common femoral artery after giving off the inferior epigastric and deep circumflex iliac arteries, and the internal iliac (hypogastric) artery. The hypogastric artery has the most variable branching pattern of any artery in the body[7] but classically bifurcates into anterior and posterior divisions. Commonly, the posterior division gives rise to the iliolumbar artery, the lateral sacral artery, and the superior gluteal artery. The anterior division supplies the superior and inferior vesicular arteries, the inferior gluteal artery, the internal pudendal artery, the obturator artery, the middle hemorrhoidal artery, and the uterine artery. There are many variations of this branching pattern, however.

III. Upper Genitourinary Tract Hemorrhage

A. Trauma

The most common indication for patients to undergo angiography for upper genitourinary hemorrhage is blunt abdominal trauma, usually the result of a motor vehicle accident. Other etiologies include penetrating trauma, athletic injuries, and iatrogenic trauma, such as that caused by renal biopsy or following surgery. In cases of blunt trauma, if intravenous urography fails to demonstrate one kidney or reveals evidence of major injury, such as extravasation of contrast or marked distortion of the pelvocalyceal system, arteriography should be performed. Angiography is the only modality capable of definitely diagnosing arterial thrombus or laceration, aneurysm or arteriovenous fistulae formation, or renal vein thrombosis. It will also demonstrate parenchymal disruption as well as intrarenal, subcapsular, and perirenal hematomas. It may aid in assessing the degree of tissue loss and the eventual prognosis. Angiography may reveal underlying renal abnormalities, the incidence of which is unusually high in renal trauma patients. This is true especially in children, in whom from 15% to 22% have underlying pathology,[89] most commonly hydronephrosis. Solitary kidneys and renal tumors are also seen more frequently in renal trauma patients than in the population as a whole.[8]

Arteriography may also diagnose unanticipated extrarenal pathology such as splenic rupture, hepatic laceration, mesenteric thrombosis, or lumbar artery hemorrhage. An aggressive radiologic approach is suggested if there is any clinical suspicion of renal trauma since 15% of trauma patients do not manifest even microscopic hematuria[9] and the degree of hematuria does not necessarily correlate with degree of damage.

The advent of computed tomography is altering the role of angiography in the emergency evaluation of renal hemorrhage in the stable patient. With a normal or equivocal intravenous urogram in the presence of persistent symptoms, computed tomography may exclude the need for angiography altogether.[10,11] It can accurately diagnose intrarenal and perirenal hematomas, renal lacerations and infarcts, as well as extravasation of contrast into the collecting system. Computed tomography can also detect additional intra-abdominal or pelvic injuries without further expenditure of time or contrast.[12] However, if a trauma patient is not hemodynamically stable or if the intravenous urogram suggests renal pedicle injury, angiography should be expeditiously performed.

With major vascular disruption, there is a time constraint for successful reconstructive surgery after which renal viability is no longer present. Successful surgical repairs have been reported as long as 19 hours after injury.[13] Finally, even a normal arteriogram may be of value in managing patients with suspected renal trauma by allowing a conservative approach with early discharge from the hospital rather than prolonged and costly inpatient observation.

B. The Angiographic Findings in Trauma

1. *Arterial Extravasation*

Extravasation of contrast material during the arteriographic phase is the sine qua non of renal hemorrhage (Fig. 3). If extravasation is massive, surgery may be indicated, perhaps facilitated by the placement of a temporary balloon occlusion catheter in the renal artery for preoperative hemostasis. If the bleeding is less

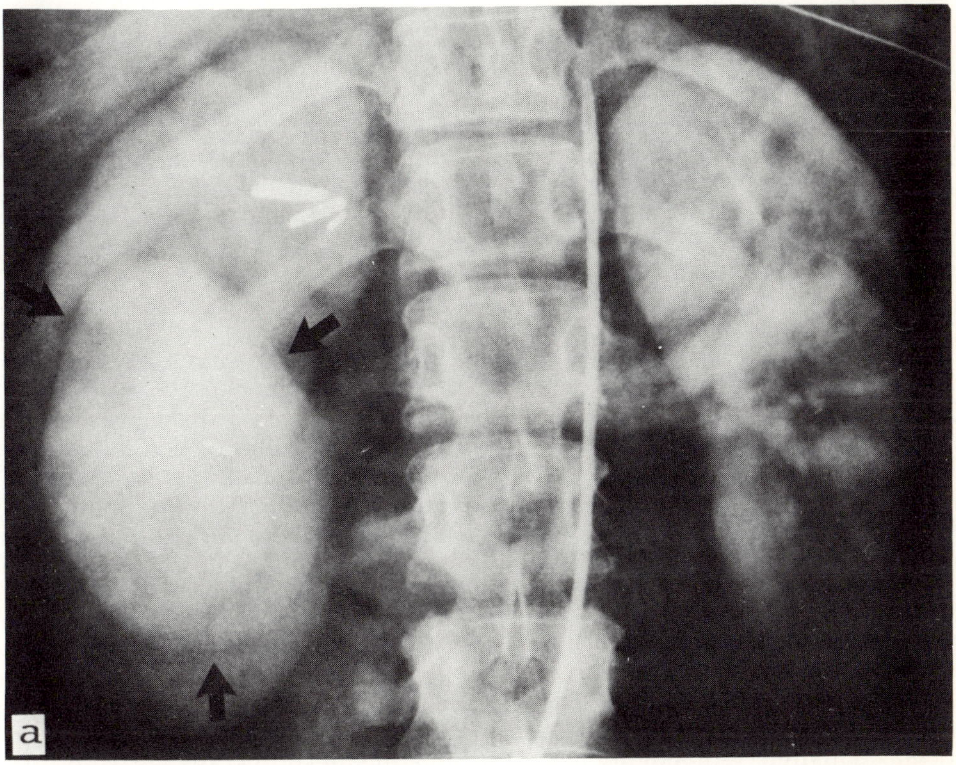

Figure 3: *Extravasation of contrast material in a patient with renal trauma.* **a.** *Late phase of aortogram shows contrast extravasation in right kidney (arrows). (Continued.)*

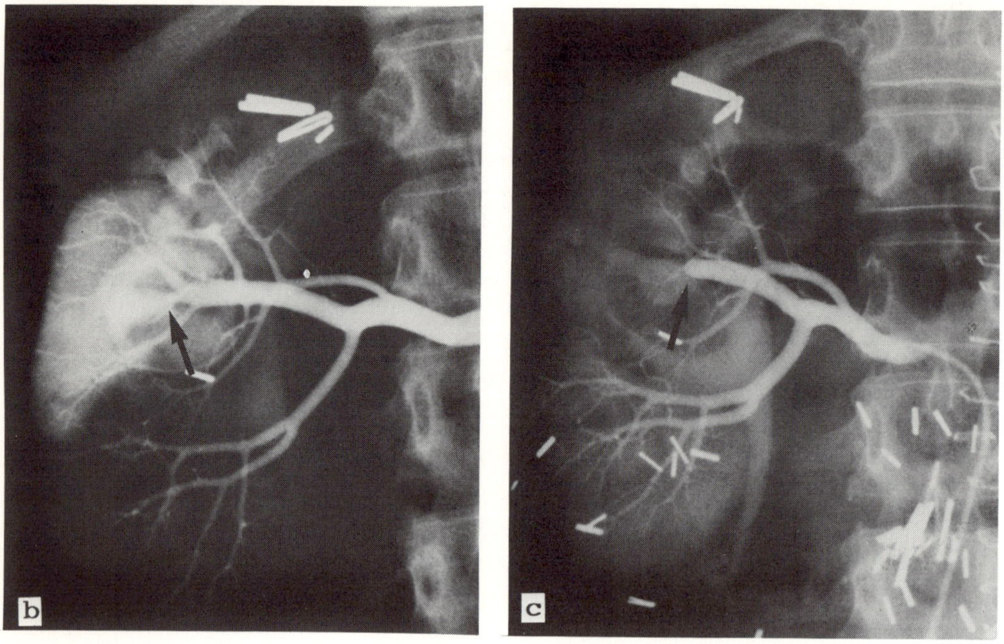

Figure 3: **b.** *Renal arteriogram shows the site of extravasation (arrow).* **c.** *Surgical repair was unsuccessful. Arrow points to detachable balloon occluding the bleeding branch.*

catastrophic, angiographic embolization therapy, sacrificing a minimum of renal tissue, may be the treatment of choice. This will be discussed in detail later.

2. *Intrarenal Hematoma*

An intrarenal hematoma is indicated by displacement and stretching of intrarenal vessels around an avascular mass. Surrounding edema may result in poor visualization of the corticomedullary junction and a mottled nephrogram. Diminished staining of the renal parenchyma adjacent to the hematoma in comparison with the remainder of the kidney indicates diminished vascularity in this region.[14] If such an area of poor viability is large, needle aspiration of the hematoma or surgical decompression is suggested to prevent loss of functioning renal tissue. However, an uncomplicated intrarenal hematoma often resorbs spontaneously.

3. *Subcapsular Hematoma*

If the renal capsule remains intact, a superficial renal bleed may produce a subcapsular hematoma characterized angiographically by flattening of the renal outline, usually at the lateral border (Fig. 4), and elevation of the renal capsule, which may be visualized as a paper-thin curved structure of increased density parallel to the cortex. A subcapsular hematoma is self-limited because of tampo-

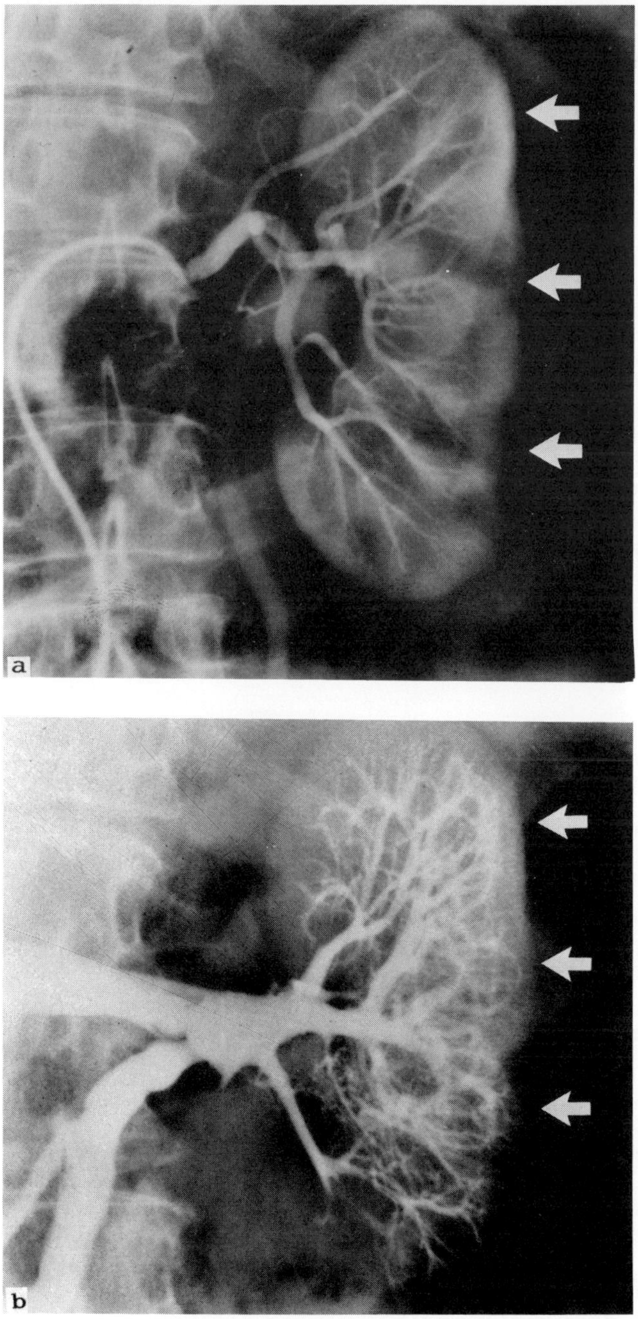

Figure 4: *Subcapsular hematoma. Arterial* **(a)** *and venous* **(b)** *phase. Observe flattening of the lateral margin of the kidney (arrow).*

nade, but the consequent renal compression may result in hypertension. Capsular branches will be displaced away from the capsule if there is an additional perirenal component to the hematoma.

4. *Perirenal Hematoma*

Hematomas in the perirenal space may become quite large. A soft tissue flank mass is observed characteristically, obscuring the renal outline and psoas margin and possibly displacing the kidney, ureter, or bladder, depending upon its size. Angiography reveals the renal contour to be relatively unaffected and the capsular arteries to be displaced from the capsule.

5. *Renal Vascular Pedicle Injuries*

Traumatic avulsion of the renal artery is uncommon (Fig. 5). When present, it causes massive retroperitoneal bleeding in patients who are usually too unstable to undergo angiography. Renal artery thrombosis secondary to blunt trauma may result from acute stretching of the vascular pedicle with subsequent intimal tear which produces a thrombus (Figs. 6,7). Early diagnosis of this lesion is mandatory since revascularization will be successful in restoring renal function only if performed soon after the injury. An acute arterial cutoff with dilatation of the segment of renal artery proximal to the occlusion is the classic angiographic picture. Renal venous injuries such as thrombosis or avulsion are rare. Renal vein thrombosis is suggested on the arteriogram by slow flow of contrast and prolonged nephrogram phase. It should be confirmed by renal venography.

6. *Infarct*

Thrombosis of a peripheral branch artery is indicated angiographically by an abrupt arterial cutoff. This lesion is frequently seen following blunt trauma to the kidney and may result in a localized area of infarction. Lang states that if the devascularized area is greater than 4 cm in diameter, healing is unlikely.[14] The presence of collateral vessels in the affected area producing a noticeable, if delayed, parenchymal stain is a good prognostic sign. A cortical infarct pattern, seen during the nephrogram as multiple small peripheral infarcts resulting from occlusion of tertiary branches, is occasionally seen.

7. *Post-traumatic Aneurysm*

False aneurysms can be diagnosed best by arteriography (Fig. 8). Their walls lack at least one of the three normal arterial layers and frequently consist of periadventitial tissue only. They probably result from the breakdown of the vascular wall between a small intrarenal hematoma and its adjacent arterial source and are often associated with intrarenal and perirenal hematomas. Extraparenchymal aneurysms are best treated surgically. However, surgical therapy for small intrarenal aneurysms often results in nephrectomy because of technical difficulties approaching the lesion. Selective transcatheter embolization has been successfully used under these circumstances.[15,16]

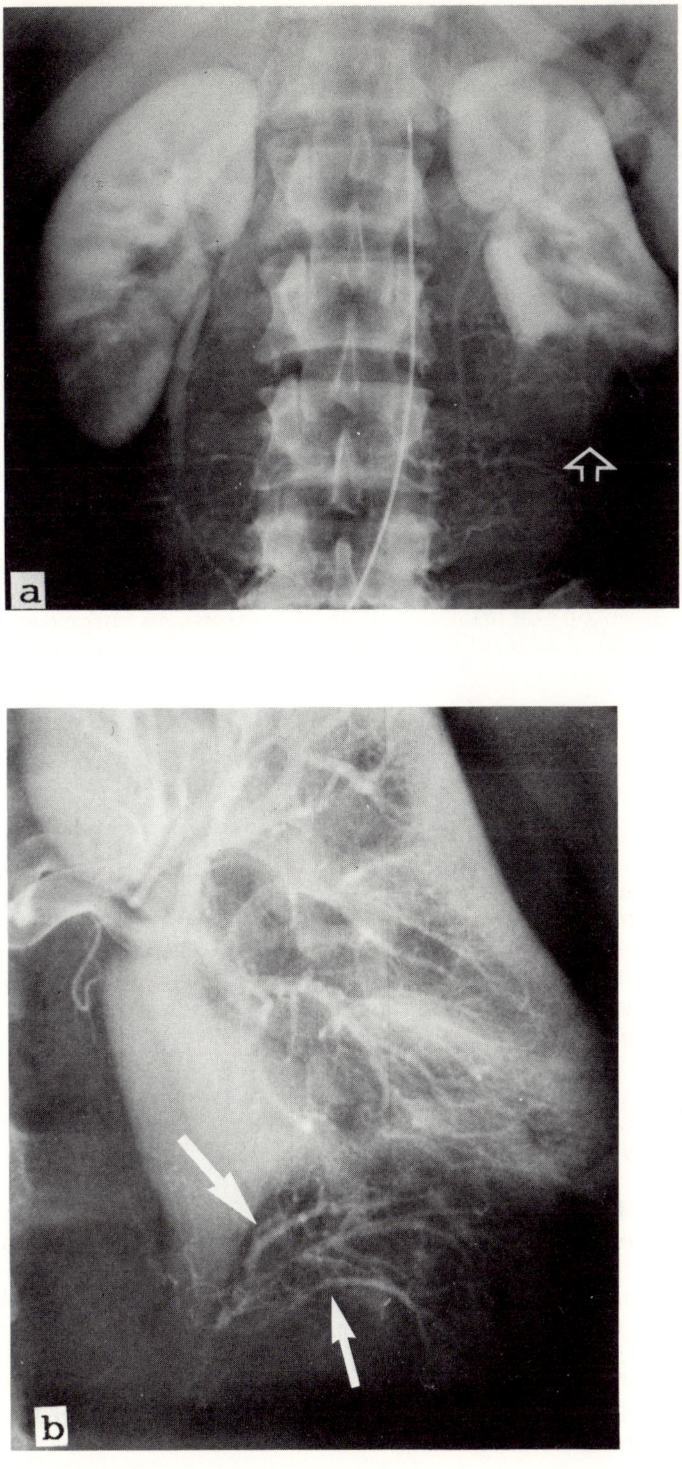

Figure 5: *Avulsion of accessory renal artery in a patient with hypertension after trauma.*
a. *Aortogram shows absent nephrogram in the lower pole of the left kidney (arrow).*
b. *Selective arteriogram demonstrates intrarenal collateral opacification of avulsed accessory renal artery (arrows).*

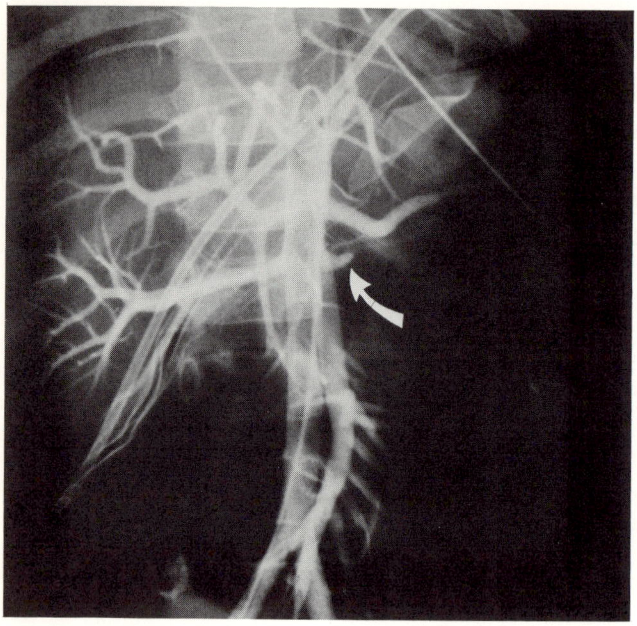

Figure 6: *Thrombosis of renal artery secondary to trauma. Arrow points to thrombosed left renal artery.*

8. Arteriovenous Fistula

Although post-traumatic arteriovenous fistula formation can result from blunt trauma, or after surgical procedures such as cyst puncture, partial nephrectomy, or nephrolithotomy, by far the most common etiology is percutaneous renal biopsy (Figs. 9, 10). It is estimated that approximately 15% of patients undergoing biopsy will develop arteriovenous fistulae.[17] Pre-existing hypertension is present in 75% of these cases.[18] Most post-biopsy fistulae will remain asymptomatic and approximately 70% will heal spontaneously. However, complications from the fistulae including massive renal hemorrhage, hypertension, or high output heart failure may necessitate intervention. Arteriovenous fistulae can appear immediately after trauma or may become manifest years later. (The fistula site may be quite small.) The diagnosis is made by angiography, which demonstrates early filling of a draining vein.

The viability of the parenchyma distal to the fistula can be estimated angiographically. If the siphoning effect of the fistula is such that the distal parenchymal stain is mottled or significantly diminished, ischemic necrosis with probable hypertension may be anticipated and early intervention is suggested.[14] A small arteriovenous fistula with a homogenous distal parenchymal stain, on the other hand, will most likely close spontaneously without clinical sequelae. Interventional options include surgical ligation of the feeding artery, partial nephrectomy, or angiographic embolization.

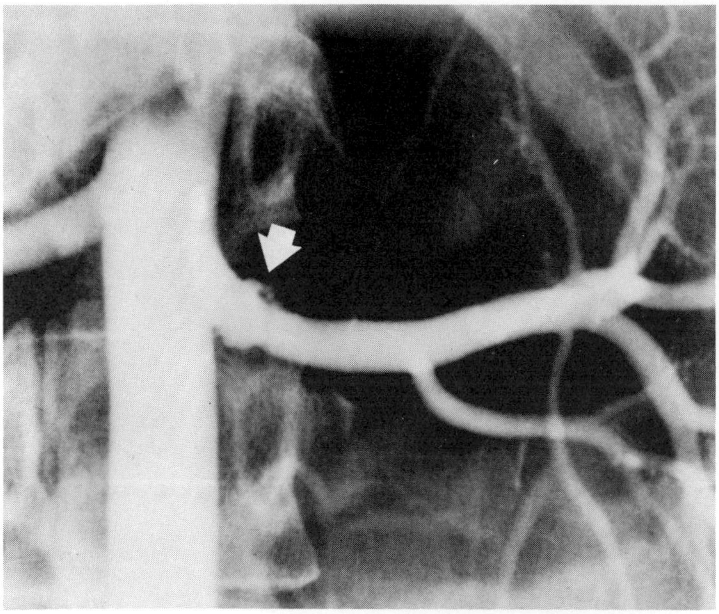

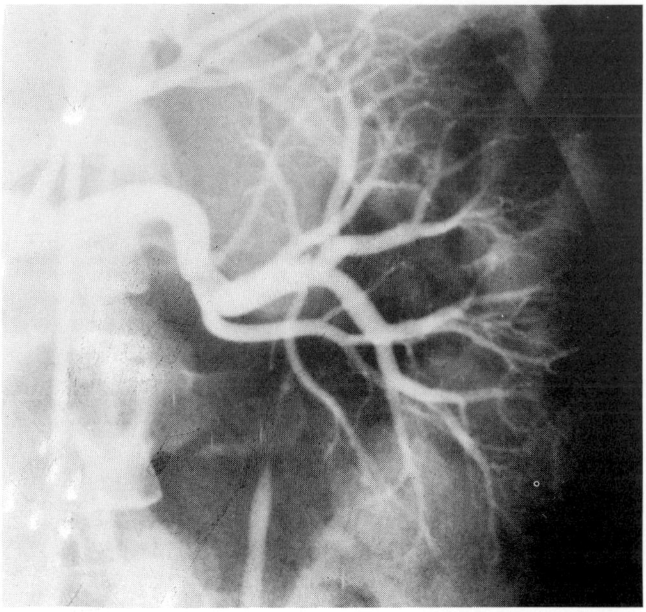

Figure 7: *Post-traumatic intimal tear of renal artery.*

a. *Arrow points to disruption of left renal artery.*

b. *Celiac arteriogram following splenorenal bypass.*

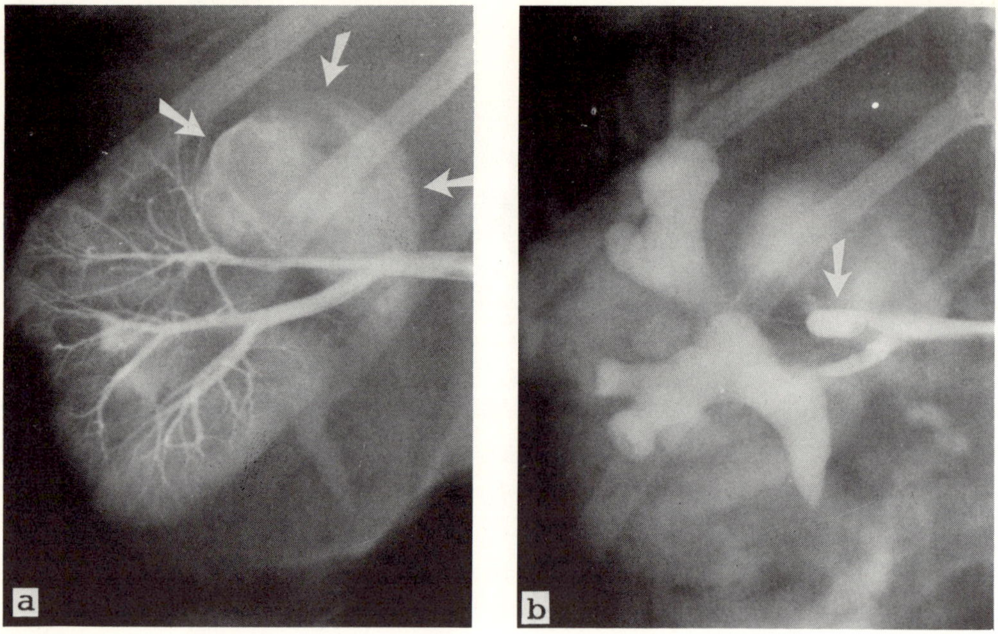

Figure 8: *Post-traumatic false aneurysm.* **a.** *Arrows point to contrast accumulation in false aneurysm after transection of upper pole renal artery branch in a patient with hematuria.* **b.** *Temporary occlusion of renal artery with a Fogarty balloon catheter (arrow) allowing for preoperative hemodynamic stabilization.*

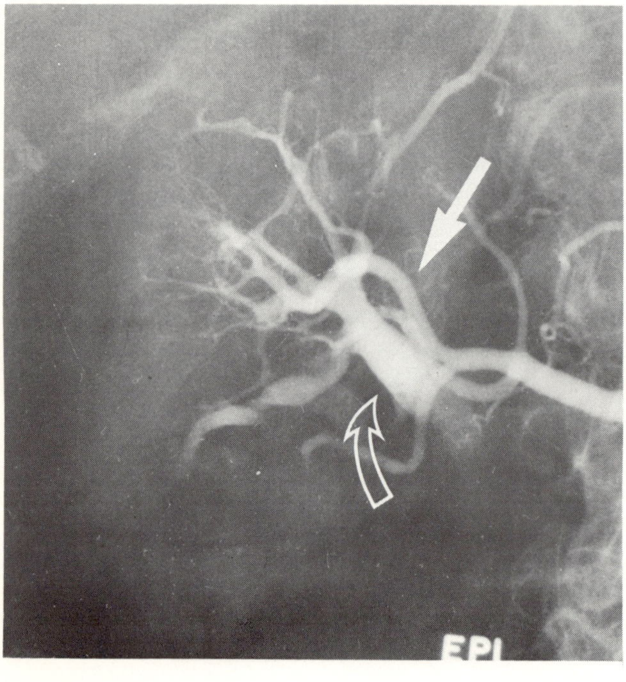

Figure 9: *Arteriovenous fistula after cyst puncture. There is simultaneous arterial (closed arrow) and venous (open arrow) opacification.*

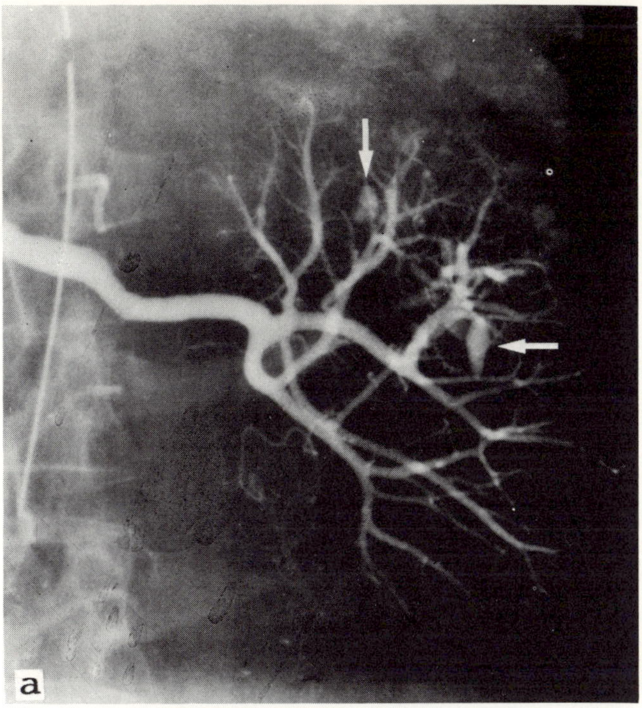

Figure 10: *Post-biopsy arteriovenous fistulae with hemorrhage.* **a.** *Arteriogram show extravasation (arrows) (Continued.)*

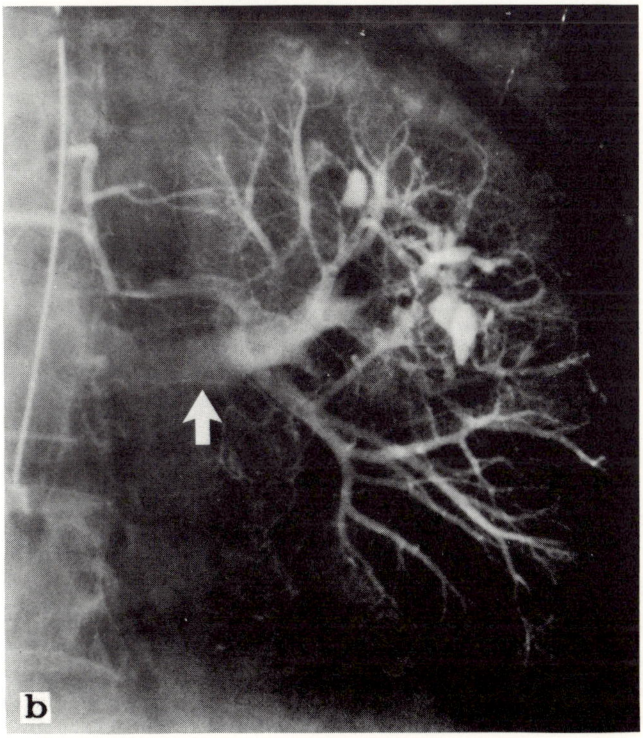

Figure 10: **b.** *There is early opacification of the renal vein (arrow).*

9. *Parenchymal Tears (Fig. 11)*

Parenchymal tears range from a single laceration manifested on the arteriogram as disruption of the cortical margin to a shattered kidney divided into multiple fragments. Tears are associated with perirenal hematomas and occasionally with extravasation of contrast outside the capsule. The arteriogram can again be used to determine the degree of viability of the renal tissue; mottled parenchymal opacification suggests vascular embarrassment and poor viability. If the radius of such an area of vascular compromise exceeds 2 cm, Lang reports a high incidence of subsequent late hemorrhage, vascular thrombosis, and urinoma formation.[14] Shattered kidneys are treated aggressively, usually with nephrectomy. Renal lacerations are often treated more conservatively in an attempt to avoid significant tissue loss.[8]

10. *Trauma to Renal Pelvis and Ureter*

The role of angiography in the diagnosis and management of trauma to the renal pelvis and ureter is limited. These structures are infrequently injured in

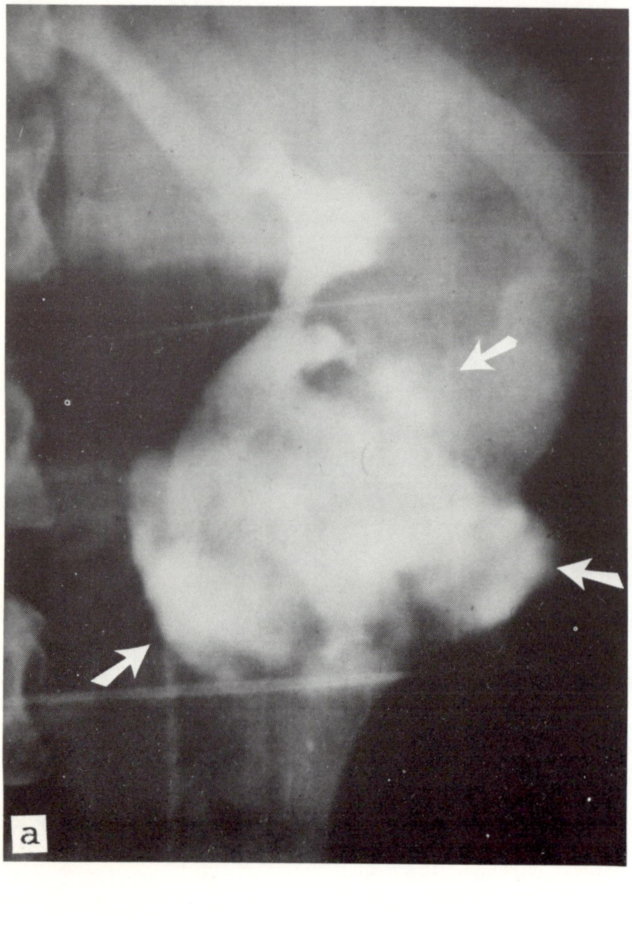

Figure 11: *Intrarenal hematoma.*
a. *Intravenous urogram shows disruption of collecting system (arrows). (Continued.)*

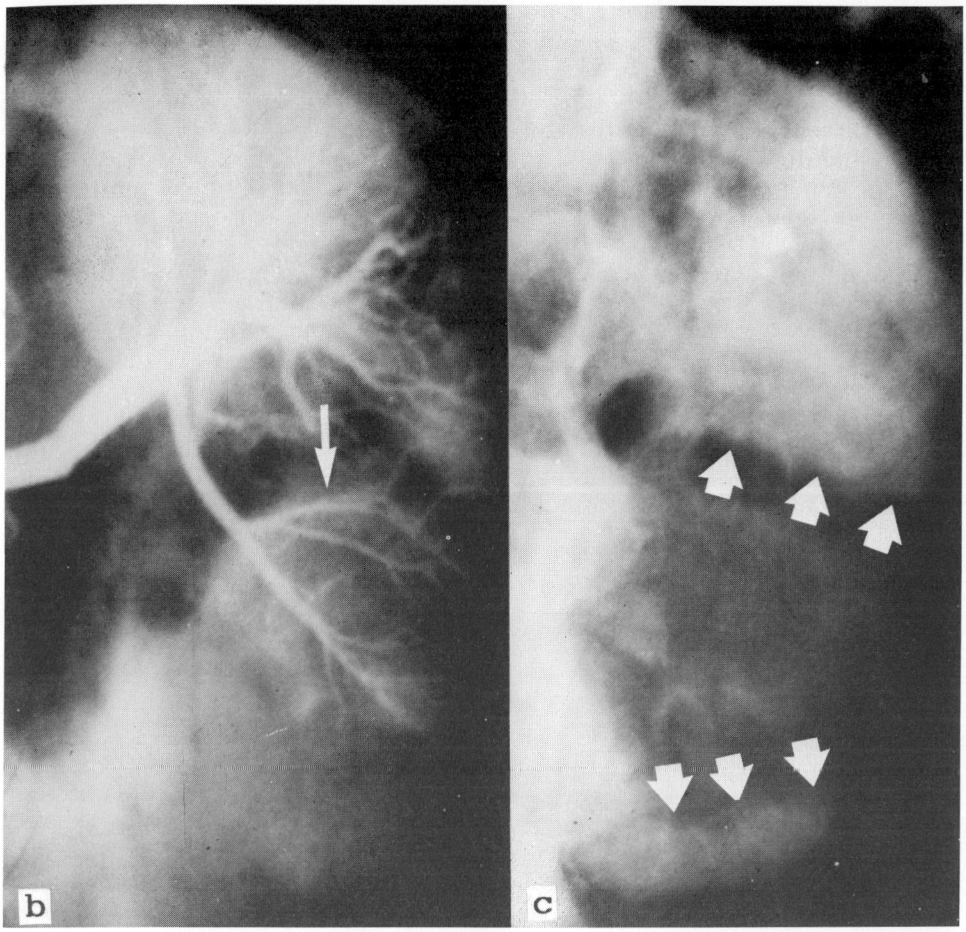

Figure 11: **b.** *Arteriogram shows stretching of intrarenal branches (arrow) but no extravasation.* **c.** *Nephrogram phase shows defect due to intrarenal hematoma (arrows).*

blunt trauma. Iatrogenic damage following surgical accident or other instrumentation are most common. While they may occasionally present with genitourinary hemorrhage in the form of a retroperitoneal hematoma, angiographic visualization of the site of extravasation or other major vascular abnormality is quite rare. More often, these patients present with urinoma rather than with bleeding.

C. Vascular Lesions

Angiography is the only diagnostic modality for many of the vascular lesions that cause upper genitourinary hemorrhage. Arteriography or venography will, in addition, provide an anatomical "road map" for surgical therapy or may provide alternative angiographic treatment.

1. *Arteriovenous Fistulae* (Fig. 12)

Arteriovenous fistulae can be classified into two major categories: congenital or acquired. The angiographic diagnosis is made in both forms by early visualization of a draining vein or veins. In addition, a region of hypoperfusion or infarction distal to the fistula may be seen. The congenital form of arteriovenous malformations accounts for approximately 25% of abnormal arteriovenous communications. They are usually cirsoid in appearance with multiple communications between artery and vein. Acquired arteriovenous fistulae have solitary communications and may occur secondary to a ruptured aneurysm, from blunt trauma or renal biopsy, or from inflammatory diseases such as bacterial infection or granulomatous disease. Acquired fistulae may also develop from tumors eroding into adjacent vessels in patients with hypernephroma or after nephrectomy as a stump fistula.

The presenting symptoms of arteriovenous fistulae include genitourinary hemorrhage, hypertension, and high output heart failure. Patients may become symptomatic years after the etiologic event. Angiographic therapy may be employed[19] as described later in the text.

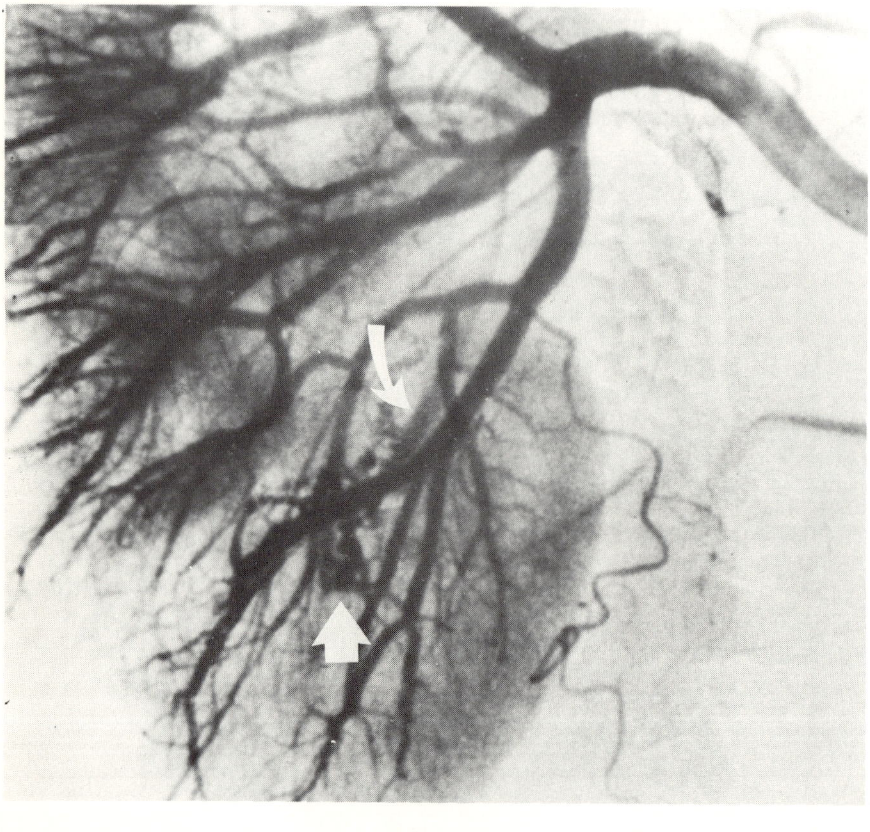

Figure 12: *Congenital arteriovenous malformation. Cirsoid appearance (arrow) with early filling of draining vein (curved arrow).*

2. *Hemangioma*

Renal hemangiomas are similar in appearance to the cirsoid congenital arteriovenous fistulae. Both may be characterized by multiple small tortuous clusters of vessels. However, early venous drainage is absent in hemangiomas. Sometimes its differentiation from a hypervascular renal tumor may be difficult, but the absence of arterial encasement, of any mass effect, and of staining or pooling during the nephrogram phase are characteristic of hemangioma. Gross hematuria is the most common clinical presentation.

3. *Renal Aneurysm*

Renal artery aneurysms are most often due to atherosclerosis. Other causes include trauma, tumor (e.g. angiomyolipoma), vasculitis (e.g. periarteritis nodosa) fibromuscular hyperplasia, and infection. They are commonly located near the hilum with calcification in 25% to 50% of cases[20] (Fig. 13). Angiography demonstrates a localized arterial dilation that may be saccular or fusiform (Fig. 14). There is no opacification of an early draining vein(s) unless erosion and fistula formation has occurred. In fact, if the aneurysm is large enough, there may be delayed flow through the artery resulting in distal ischemia manifested angiographically by collateral formation and clinically by hypertension. Under these circumstances, selective renal vein renin samples should be obtained. Angiography cannot distinguish reliably between true and false aneurysms. Approximately 10% of aneurysms are bilateral; therefore, careful investigation of the contralateral kidney is imperative. Approximately 6% go on to rupture.[21] Extraparenchymal aneurysms are best treated surgically. Intrarenal aneurysms,

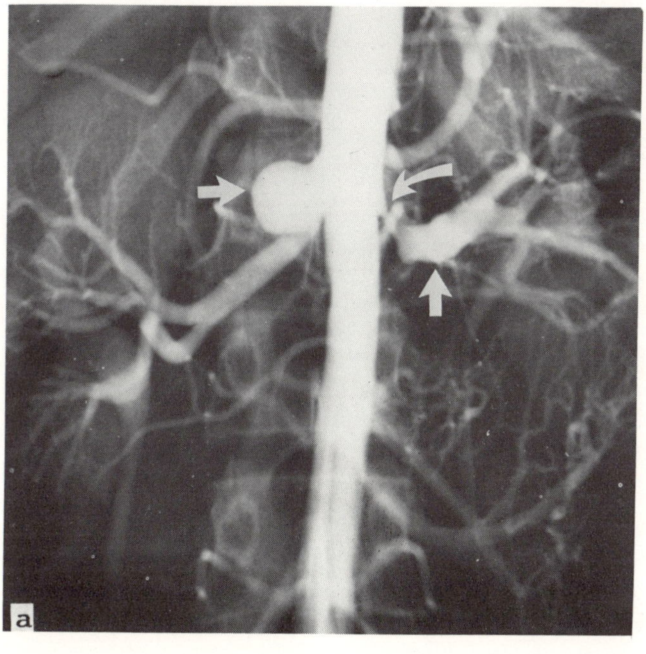

Figure 13: *Renal artery aneurysm in a patient with neurofibromatosis.* **a.** *Aortogram shows aneurysms of both left and right renal arteries (arrows). Stenosis of proximal left renal artery (curved arrow). (Continued.)*

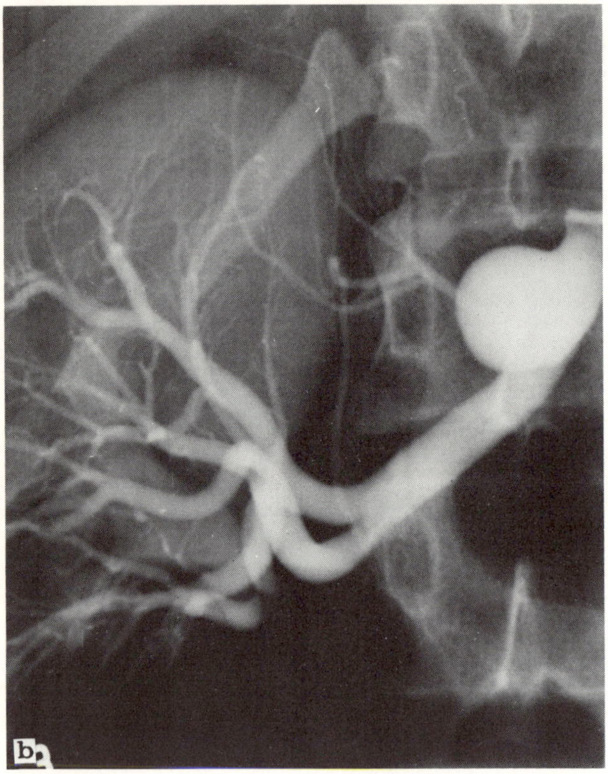

Figure 13: **b.** *Selective arteriogram demonstrates relationship of aneurysm to origin of renal artery.*

however, present technical difficulties, and surgical therapy frequently results in nephrectomy. Therefore, interest in angiographic embolization of such lesions has flourished.

4. *Polyarteritis Nodosa*

This is a vascular disease of unknown etiology that occasionally presents with retroperitoneal hemorrhage.[22] Fibrinoid necrosis of small and medium sized arteries results in an angiographic picture of peripheral aneurysms at the level of the interlobar and arcuate arteries along with irregular narrowing of arterial walls with stenosis and occlusion of small intraparenchymal vessels (Fig. 15). Renal involvement occurs in at least 80% of patients. While these findings may be seen with other forms of necrotizing angitis, angiography can be a useful diagnostic tool in patients in whom the diagnosis is suspected but muscle biopsy has been unrevealing. Similar angiographic changes are frequently seen in the liver, the spleen, and the mesenteric vessels.

5. *Hemorrhagic Infarct*

Hemorrhagic infarct is an occasional cause of renal hemorrhage, particularly in patients with valvular cardiac disease or left ventricular aneurysm and

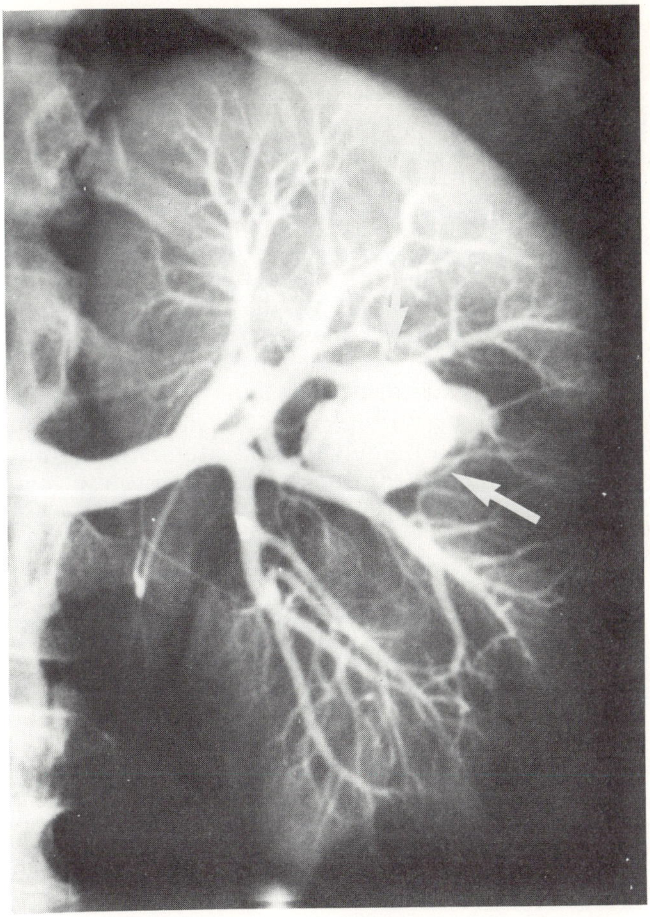

Figure 14: *Intrarenal aneurysm (arrows).*

thrombus formation. It may result in an intrarenal, subcapsular, or perirenal hematoma, as well as gross or microscopic hematuria. An abrupt arterial cutoff is seen angiographically.

6. *Renal Vein Lesions*

Renal varices are controversial as a cause of genitourinary hemorrhage. Patients with otherwise unexplained renal bleeding have occasionally been demonstrated to have renal vein varices. However, a recent series of 132 consecutive renal venograms reported by Beckman[23] revealed eight patients (6%) with varices, only one of whom had hematuria that was not attributable to another lesion. Therefore, renal vein varices may merely represent an incidental finding rather than a true pathologic lesion.

Venography may reveal a solitary varix or a network of veins. Varices are almost always central: that is, at the hilum or at the entrance site of the left gonadal vein. Left-sided varices are much more common. Since the left renal vein courses between the aorta and the superior mesenteric artery, it is thought that compression may result in variceal formation. The "nutcracker phenomenon,"[24] a related diagnosis, has been postulated as a cause of hematuria as well. In this, venography reveals an abrupt cutoff of the left renal vein with collateral formation and a pressure gradient across the vein.

Hematuria can occur with acute renal vein thrombosis. The arteriographic findings include renal enlargement, slow washout of contrast during the arterial phase, with branch arteries stretched around an edematous kidney, delayed nephrogram, no opacification of the renal vein, and possibly opacification of venous collaterals. An inferior vena cavagram will fail to show the normal washout of unopacified blood in the region of the inflow from the renal vein. It may show propagation of thrombus into the inferior vena cava. Selective renal venography, performed carefully so as not to dislodge the clot, will demonstrate intraluminal thrombus or occlusion of the main renal vein or its branches. However, a false positive selective examination due to the inflow of unopacified blood from a kidney with good antegrade flow is a potential diagnostic error. For the detection of small thrombi, therefore, simultaneous intra-arterial epinephrine should be administered during the intravenous injection of contrast.

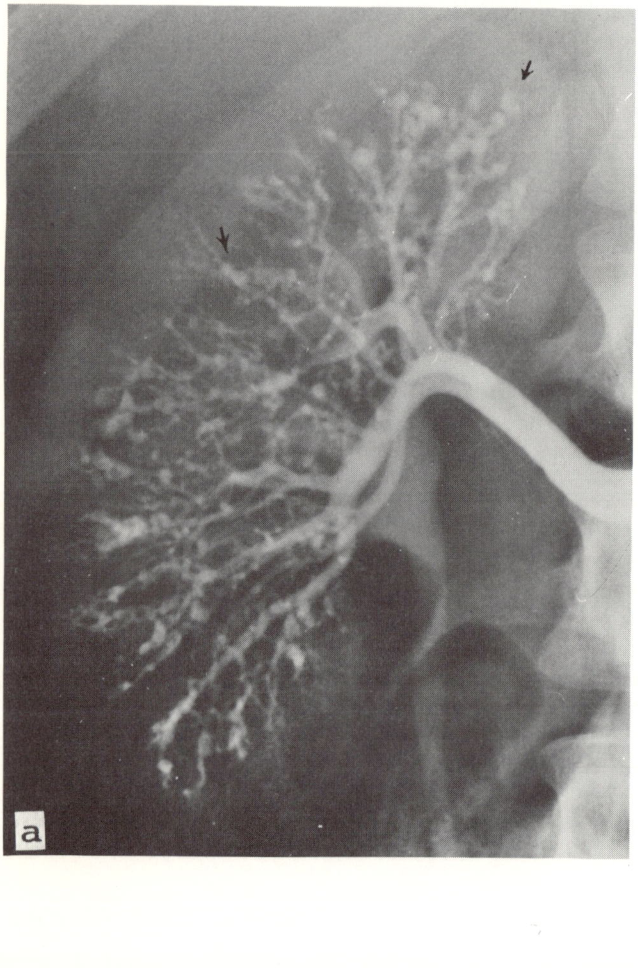

Figure 15: *Periarteritis nodosa.* **a.** *Arterial and* **b.** *nephrogram phase show characteristic multiple small intrarenal aneurysms. (Continued.)*

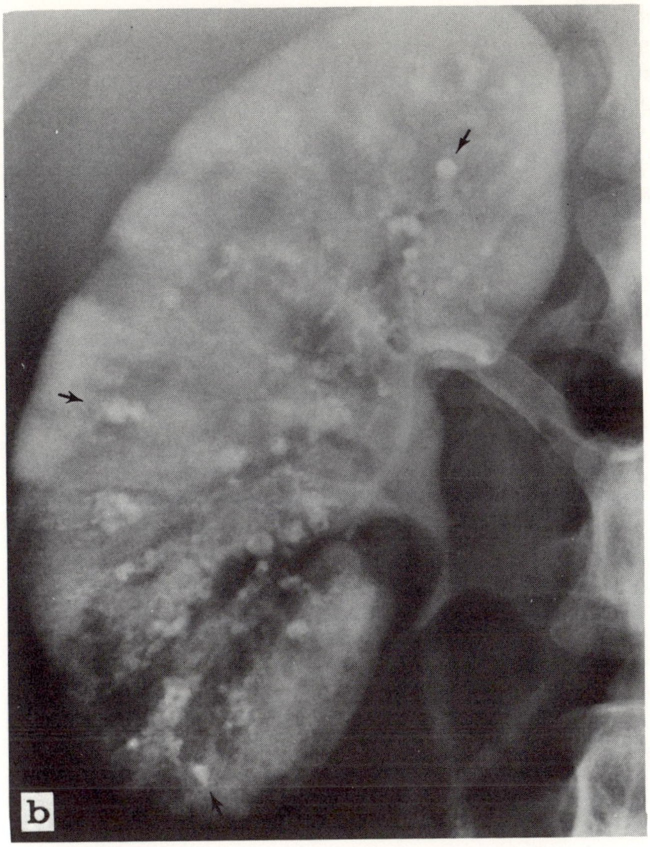

Figure 15: b.

D. Renal Mass Lesions

Any of the renal tumors, either primary or metastatic, may present with genitourinary hemorrhage. While the diagnosis is usually made prior to angiography, angiography can occasionally demonstrate a small tumor missed by other techniques (Figs. 16, 17) and can be used to evaluate the extent of involvement, renal vein or inferior vena cava extension of tumor, or metastatic spread to the contralateral kidney or other abdominal structures. Preoperative embolization of large hypervascular tumors can reduce intra-operative blood loss (Fig. 18). Moreover, if the patient is not a surgical candidate, selective angiographic embolization may provide hemostasis with a minimum of tissue loss.

The typical hypernephroma is a hypervascular mass lesion with arteriovenous shunting, pooling of contrast, neovascularity, encasement, and stretching of the arteries. The renal vein or inferior vena cava can be involved by tumor or thrombus, which may be visualized after high dose (30 cc) selective arterial injection of contrast (Fig. 18). Venous collaterals may opacify if the renal vein is occluded. Since hypernephromas are avascular in up to 10% of cases and hypovascular in another 15–30%, the characteristic tumor blush with pooling of contrast and arteriovenous shunting will then be absent. Pharmacoangiography using intra-arterial epinephrine during the renal arteriogram can be of value in

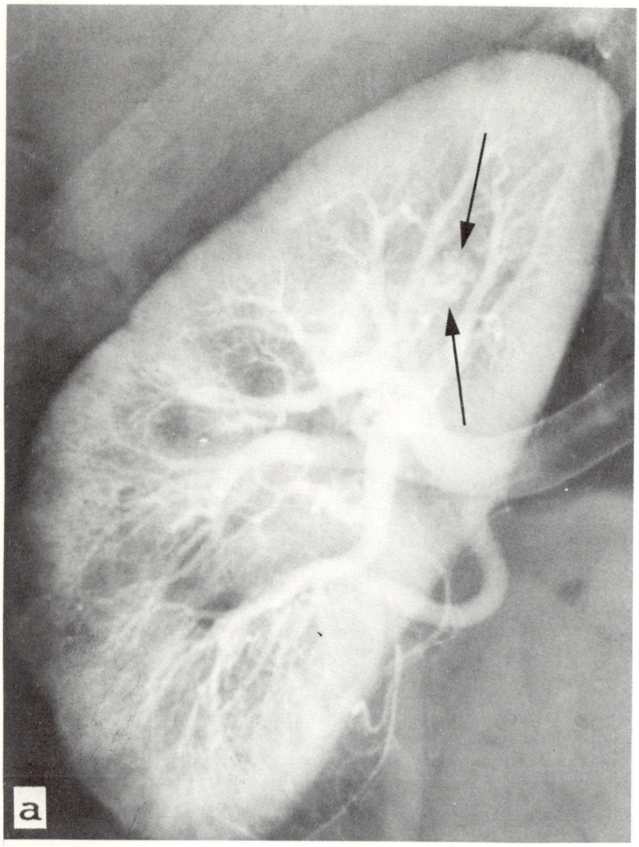

Figure 16: *Small renal cell carcinoma in a patient with Von Hippel Lindau syndrome. Selective arteriogram* **(a)** *and magnification view* **(b)**. *Arrows point to small vascular lesion. (Continued.)*

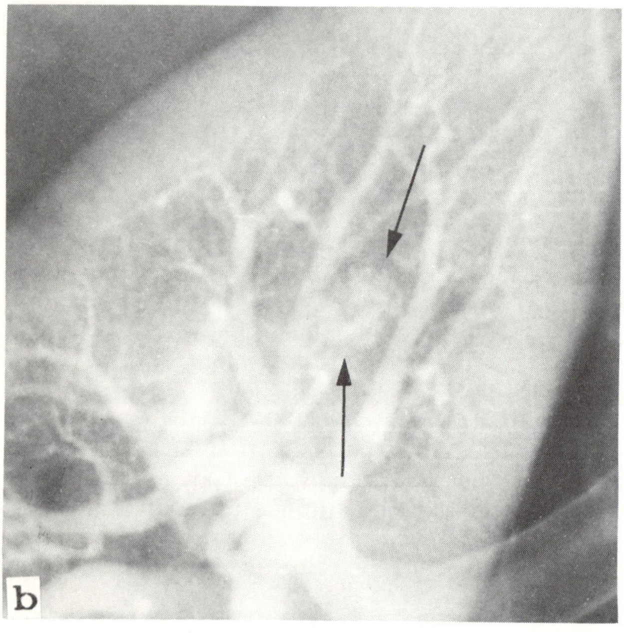

Figure 16: b.

these cases to enhance the demonstration of tumor vessels, encasement, or occlusion of veins during venography.

Angiomyolipomas, or hamartomas, are frequently difficult to differentiate from hypernephromas. An increase in fat observed on plain film or computed tomography will be the diagnostic key. The arteriogram may demonstrate multiple arterial aneurysms, particularly when the tumor is part of the syndrome of tuberous sclerosis, in which case the tumors are often small, multiple, and bilateral.

The vascularity of metastatic tumors characteristically reflects the vascularity of the primary lesion. Therefore, the diagnosis is often made by demonstration of encasement and mass effect, since most metastatic tumors are hypovascular. Squamous cell and transitional cell carcinomas are also hypovascular as well and thus are poorly visualized on angiography. However, vascular encasement, prominent pelvoureteric arteries, and neovascularity may be seen (Fig. 19).

Benign cysts may present with bleeding. Although ultrasound or computed tomography are ideal diagnostic modalities for cysts, they may remain unsuspected prior to angiography. Angiography will characteristically reveal a sharply demarcated mass lesion with pencil-thin rim, smooth margins, and a "beak" formed by compressed normal parenchyma adjacent to the cyst. No neovascularity or other hallmark of tumor is seen.

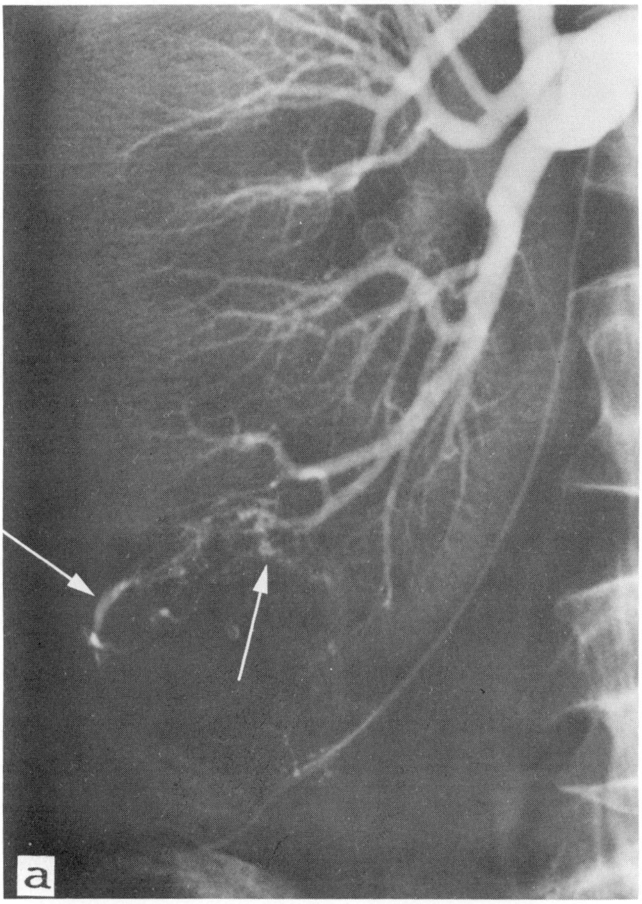

Figure 17: *Small occult renal cell carcinoma seen only by angiography.* **a.** *Arrows point to tumor vascularity in lower pole of kidney. (Continued.)*

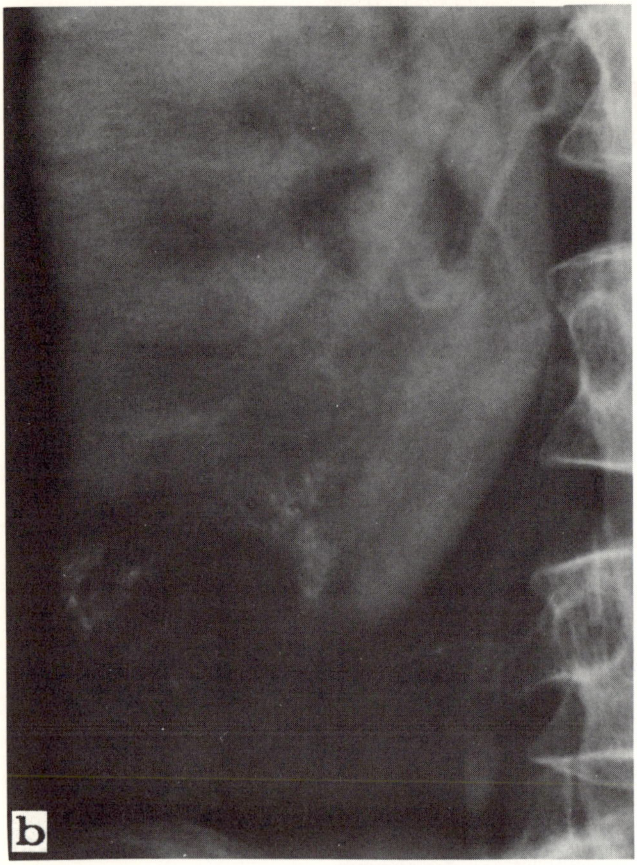

Figure 17: **b.** *Nephrogram phase with retained vascular stain.*

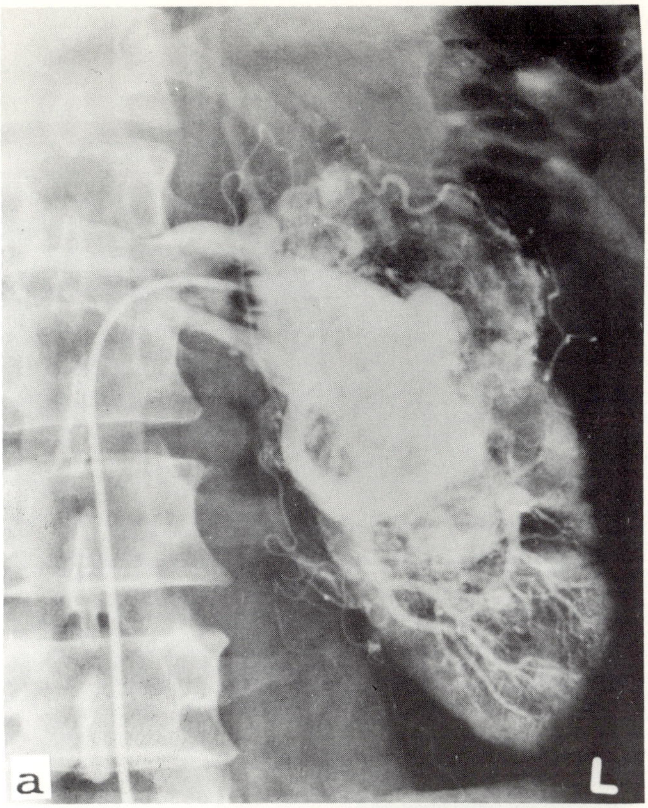

Figure 18: *Hypernephroma with preoperative embolization.* **a.** *High dose selective arteriogram showing large hypernephroma with arteriovenous shunting, neovascularity, and tumor stain (arrows). (Continued.)*

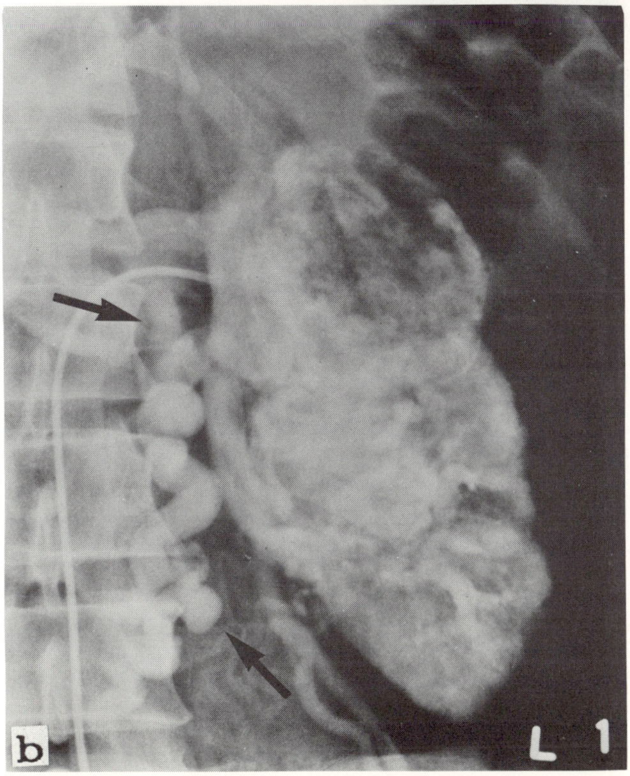

Figure 18: **b.** *Later phase shows occlusion of renal vein with large venous collaterals (arrows). (Continued.)*

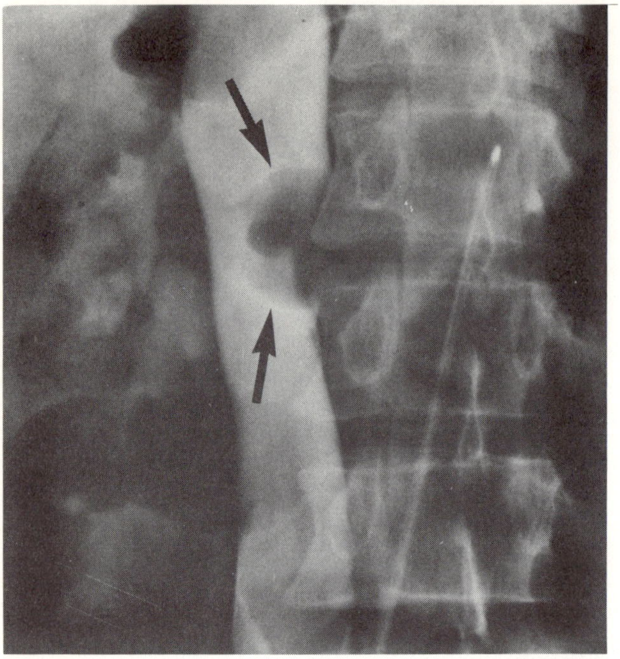

Figure 18: **c.** *Inferior vena cavagram shows extension of tumor into inferior vena cava (arrows). (Continued.)*

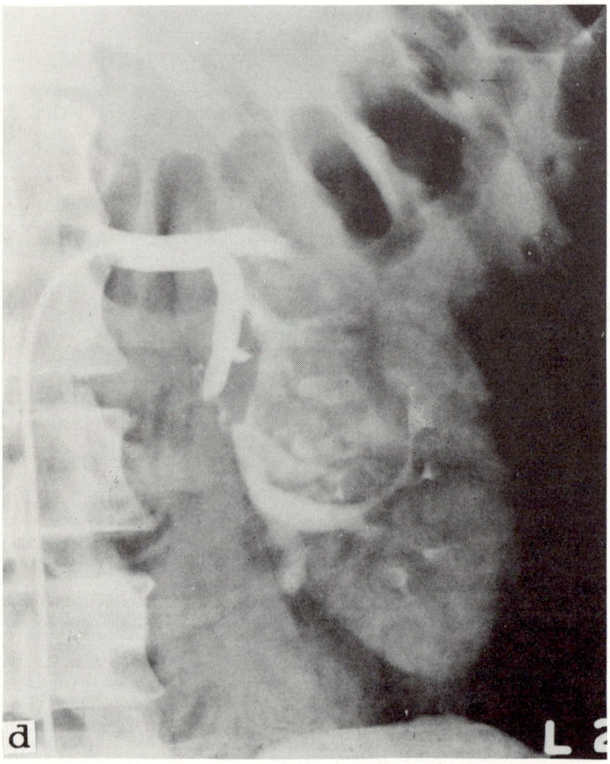

Figure 18: **d.** *After embolization, there is complete occlusion of the renal artery.*

Figure 19: *Transitional cell carcinoma.* **a.** *Minor irregularities of arteries in region of renal pelvis (arrows). (Continued.)*

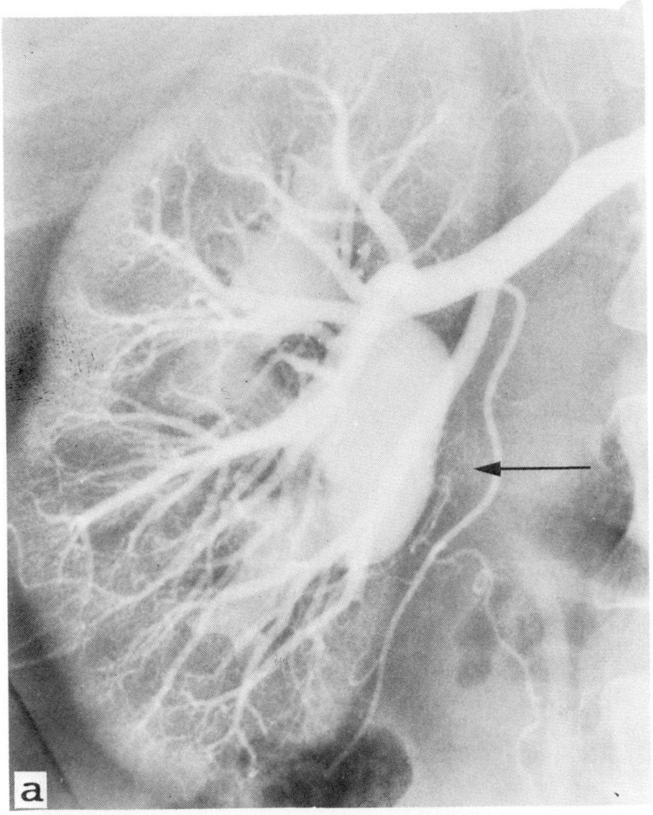

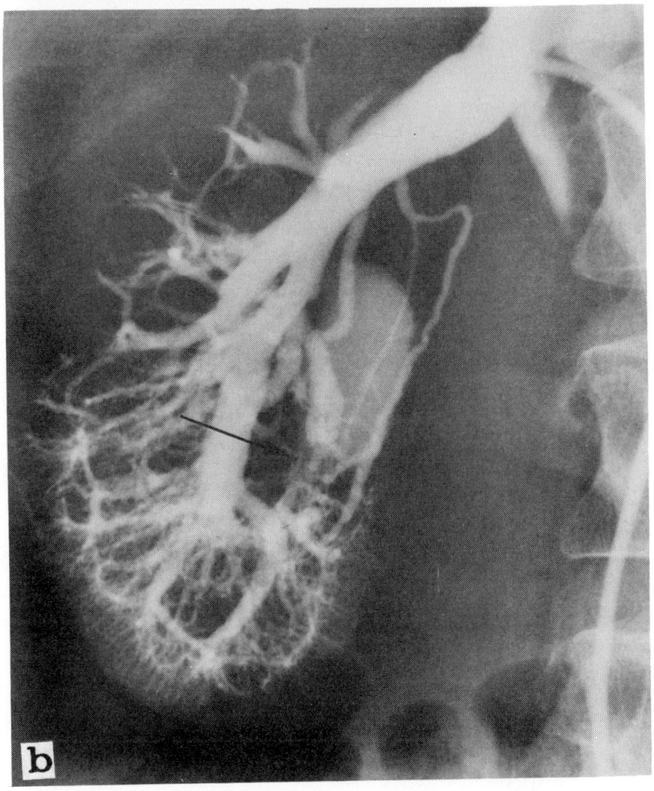

Figure 19: **b.** *Epinephrine assisted renal venogram shows encasement by tumor of a major vein (arrow).*

E. Chronic Parenchymal Disease, Hydronephrosis, Polycystic Disease, and Systemic Disease

Other renal diseases may present with gross or microscopic hematuria. The presence of nephritis or hydronephrosis is usually previously known. Angiography is certainly not the optimal diagnostic modality; however, angiographic changes are occasionally the first clue to the underlying pathology. Both chronic glomerulonephritis and pyelonephritis demonstrate thinning of the cortex with poor definition of the corticomedullary junction. Glomerulonephritis is usually bilateral with uniform distribution of changes throughout each kidney and smooth renal contours. Chronic pyelonephritis, on the other hand, tends to be asymmetrical with one kidney more severely affected than the other. It is nonuniform within the kidney, particularly affecting the upper and lower poles, causing cortical scarring.

Hydronephrosis classically shows a rapidly tapering main renal artery, the result of diminished renal blood flow. The artery is displaced superiorly and gently curves around a dilated renal pelvis. There is marked reduction in cortex with a relatively smooth renal outline during the nephrogram phase.

The adult form of polycystic disease may present with hematuria. A routine radiologic workup including intravenous urography and ultrasound should be sufficient for the diagnosis. The angiographic findings include large kidneys with arterial stretching and displacement around the cysts and irregular renal outlines with multiple avascular lesions, the "Swiss cheese appearance," in the nephrogram phase.

Anticoagulants are a common cause of urologic bleeding, and hematuria is the most common hemorrhagic complication of anticoagulant therapy.[25] Intrarenal hematomas, subcapsular hematomas, or perirenal hematomas may occur. Angiographic demonstration of a site of extravasation is extremely uncommon. The symptoms and findings should disappear after the discontinuation of anticoagulation.

Constitutional bleeding diatheses, such as hemophilia and von Willebrand's disease, may result in urologic hemorrhage as well. Angiography may demonstrate a hematoma but is otherwise nondiagnostic.

Hematuria may be seen with acute or chronic systemic diseases such as sickle cell disease or sickle trait. The few angiograms that have been performed on sickle cell patients have shown a mottled nephrogram and focal cortical ischemia consistent with occlusion of small vessels. Polyarteritis nodosa has been discussed earlier. Other vasculidites may demonstrate angiographic changes similar to those seen in polyarteritis nodosa with irregular narrowing and arterial occlusion but almost always without the peripheral small aneurysms characteristic of the latter disease.

IV. Lower Genitourinary Tract Hemorrhage

A. Trauma

The contribution of angiography to the diagnosis and treatment of lower genitourinary hemorrhage has been most significant in cases of blunt trauma to the pelvis. Patients with pelvic fractures, in particular with fractures of the anterior pelvic rim, may manifest hematuria from bladder contusion or laceration. They often suffer from massive retroperitoneal blood loss as well. Up to 60% of such patients die from the complications of hemorrhage.[26] Arteriography is critically important to localize a bleeding site(s) but also to diagnose traumatic vascular occlusion when present. When a site of extravasation is seen, selective angiographic embolization of the involved hypogastric artery branch is the optimal therapeutic choice (Fig. 20). Embolization can control massive arterial hemorrhage, occluding the vessel at a more distal and, hence, at a more effective site than surgical hypogastric artery ligation. Embolization also avoids the loss of the tamponade effect, which surgical intervention inevitably destroys and which aids in controlling simultaneous venous bleeding.[27]

Depending upon the site of the fracture, several branches of the hypogastric artery may show extravasation. Because of the abundant collateral network in the pelvis, both hypogastric arteries must be studied angiographically. Embolization of only one side is often insufficient for successful control of hemorrhage.

The axillary approach may be necessary in patients with severe trauma because of multiple pelvic fractures and concomitant edema. Both the diagnostic and therapeutic portions of the study can be performed via this route. After embolization and stabilization of the patient, surgical repair of a ruptured bladder or other injury may then be undertaken.

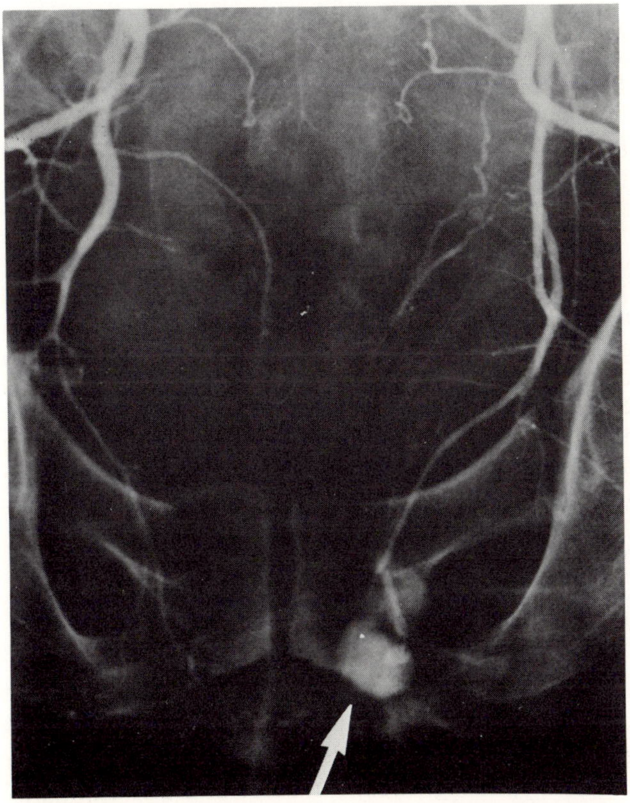

Figure 20: *Bleeding in a patient with pelvic trauma controlled by embolization.* **a.** *Contrast extravasation from obturator branch of hypogastric artery (arrow). (Continued.)*

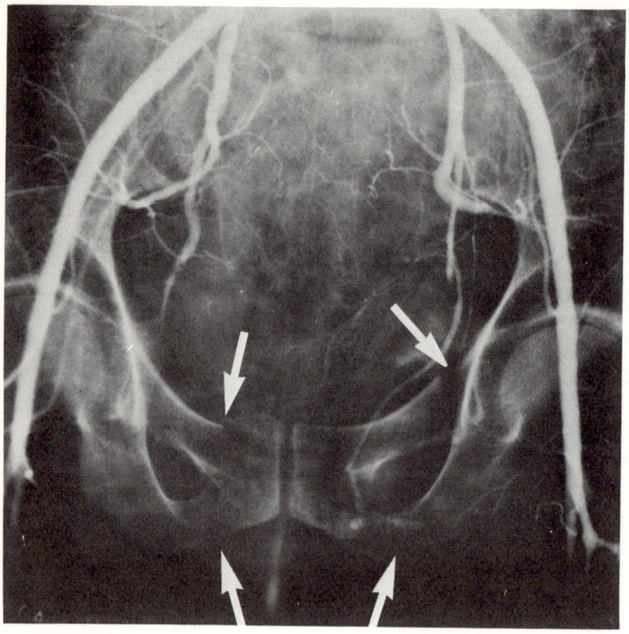

Figure 20: **b.** *No further extravasation after occlusion of branches of both hypogastric arteries with Gelfoam. Arrows point to multiple pelvic fractures.*

Iatrogenic trauma to the lower genitourinary tract, from ileal loop diversion, transurethral prostatectomy, or prostatic needle biopsy, for example, has been successfully diagnosed and treated by angiographic techniques.[28,29] One patient with brisk bleeding from a nephrostomy tube 20 days after an ileal loop diversion was treated with Pitressin infusion into the superior mesenteric artery after arteriography demonstrated extravasation from an ileal branch.[28] Several patients with bleeding from the prostatic bed after instrumentation have been embolized successfully (Fig. 21). Fortunately, the frequency of significant hemorrhage after such procedures is low, and lesser amounts of bleeding may respond to irrigation and clot removal. In the event that these maneuvers fail, angiography can identify and control hemorrhage with minimal risk without subjecting the patient to an additional surgical procedure. The usual site of arterial extravasation in patients with prostatic hemorrhage is one or both internal pudendal arteries. It is important to remember that the rich collateral network of the pelvis mandates bilateral hypogastric artery investigation when angiography is performed. Usually, embolization of branches of both hypogastric arteries is required to insure hemostasis.

B. Lower Genitourinary Neoplasm and Radiation Cystitis

Angiographic diagnosis and therapy of patients with bladder or vaginal hemorrhage from tumor or radiation-induced hemorrhagic cystitis has been quite valuable. Vesicular hemorrhage may be due to bladder wall angioma or arteriovenous malformation, paraganglionoma, carcinoma or lymphoma of the bladder, metastatic implant, or invasion of the bladder by adjacent carcinoma of the cervix, uterus, or colon. Angiographic extravasation of contrast is rarely seen, but some degree of localization is often provided by the neovascularity and

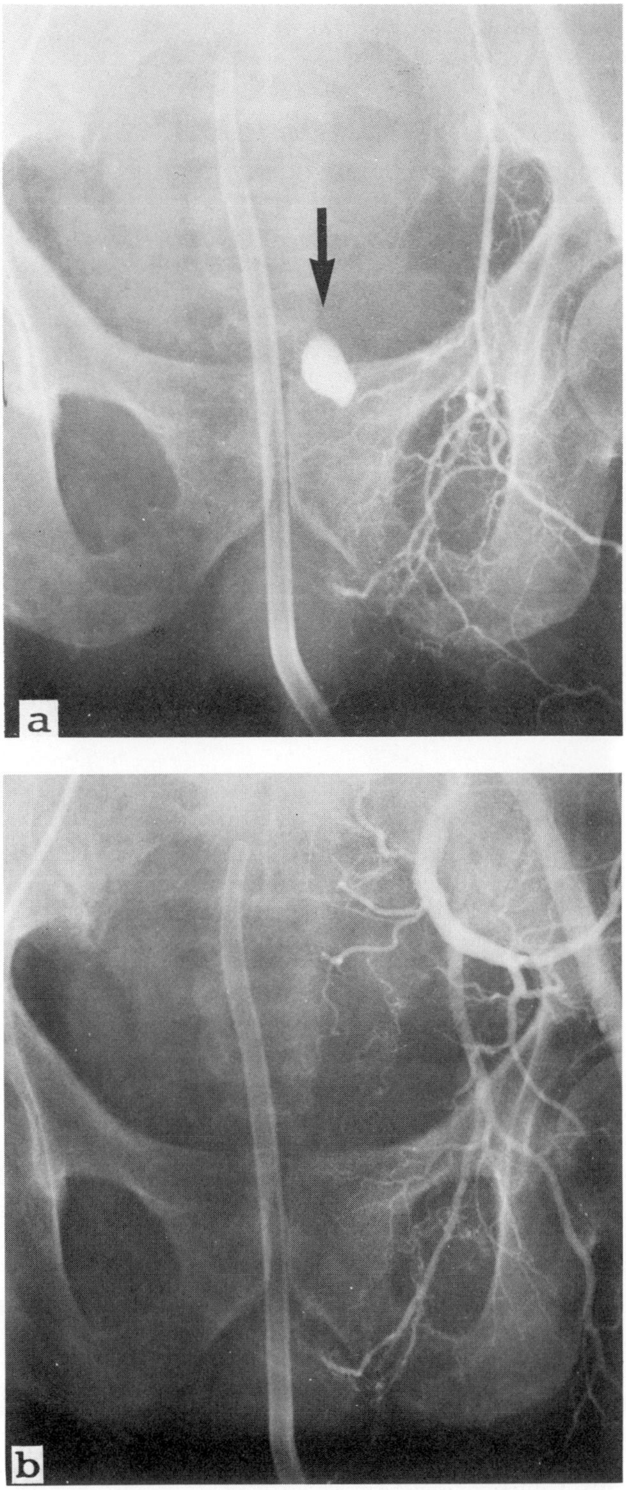

Figure 21: *Prostatic bleeding following needle biopsy controlled by embolization.*
a. *Left hypogastric arteriogram shows extravasation in prostatic bed (arrow).*
b. *No further extravasation after embolization of left hypogastric artery branches with Gelfoam. Extravasation persisted from branches of the right hypogastric artery which was then successfully embolized.*

tumor blush. If the tumor involvement appears to be unilateral, embolization of branches of only one hypogastric artery is performed. If involvement appears diffuse, both hypogastric arteries are angiographically occluded.

Embolization should be as selective as possible, usually occluding branches of the anterior division of the hypogastric artery such as the inferior and superior vesicular arteries. However, particularly in the case of invasion by carcinoma of the cervix with involvement of the vesicovaginal septum and posterior wall of the bladder, branches of the posterior division of the hypogastric artery may supply the tumor as well. In older patients, it is important to determine the patency of the inferior mesenteric artery. If this vessel is occluded secondary to atherosclerosis, the predominant arterial supply to the rectum may be from the hypogastric arteries, and bilateral hypogastric occlusion can then result in rectal necrosis. Moreover, in one reported case[30] of a patient with vaginal bleeding and a rectovaginal fistula secondary to carcinoma of the cervix, extravasation was demonstrated from the superior hemorrhoidal artery, a branch of the inferior mesenteric artery, and not from hypogastric branches at all. The superior hemorrhoidal artery was successfully embolized without ischemic sequelae (Fig. 22). In most patients with vaginal bleeding secondary to carcinoma of the cervix, however, no site of extravasation is demonstrated, and embolization of the

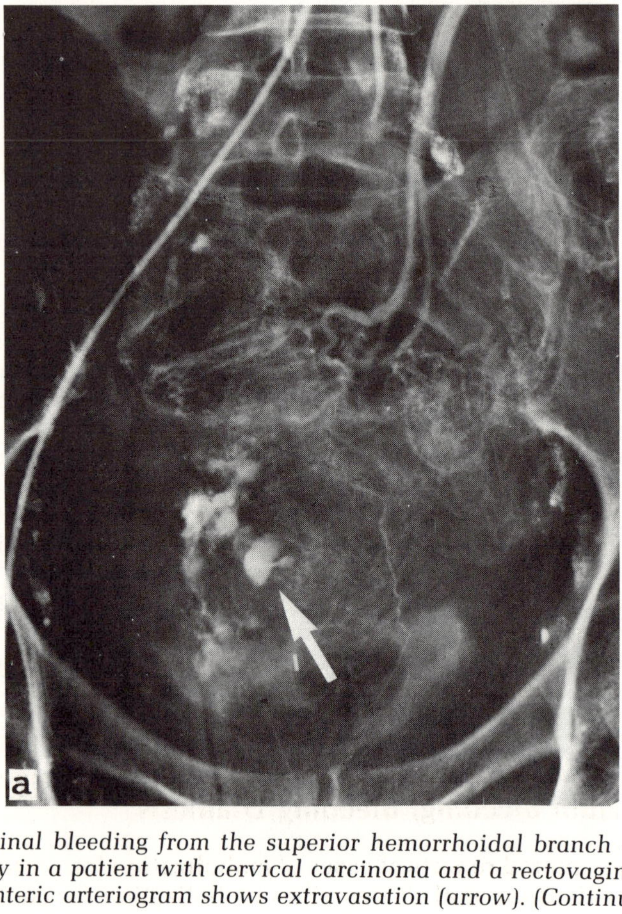

Figure 22: *Vaginal bleeding from the superior hemorrhoidal branch of the inferior mesenteric artery in a patient with cervical carcinoma and a rectovaginal fistula.* **a.** *Inferior mesenteric arteriogram shows extravasation (arrow). (Continued.)*

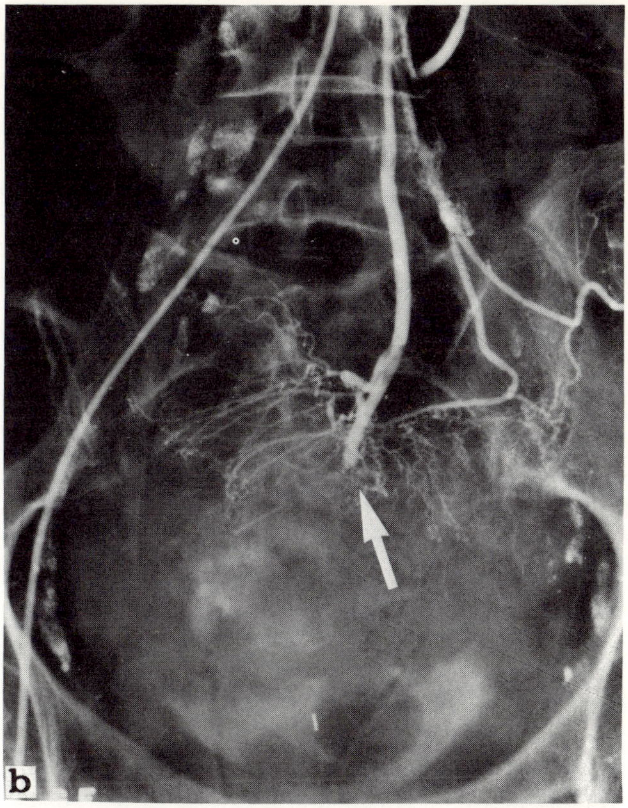

b. *Bleeding controlled after embolization of superior hemorrhoidal branch with Gelfoam (arrow).*

uterine artery or of the anterior division of one or both hypogastric arteries is performed. Pharmacoangiography, using epinephrine or vasopressin, has been employed to help direct the flow of embolic material into abnormal vessels, thereby sparing healthy tissue.[31]

Arteriovenous malformations of the bladder pose different therapeutic problems. Post-embolization recurrence has been frequent despite superselective peripheral embolization because of the multiple small collateral channels that dilate to provide additional feeding arteries after initial embolization. Repeat procedures are frequently necessary.

Patients with hemorrhagic cystitis rarely show a site of contrast extravasation. Angiography may, however, demonstrate a diffuse mucosal bladder blush. The anterior divisions of both hypogastric arteries should be embolized if arteriographic therapy is employed (Fig. 23).

C. Other Causes of Lower Genitourinary Hemorrhage: Post-Partum Bleeding, Bleeding Diathesis

There are scattered reports of cases of embolization for post-partum hemorrhage. One, by Heaston et al.,[32] describes embolization for control of massive

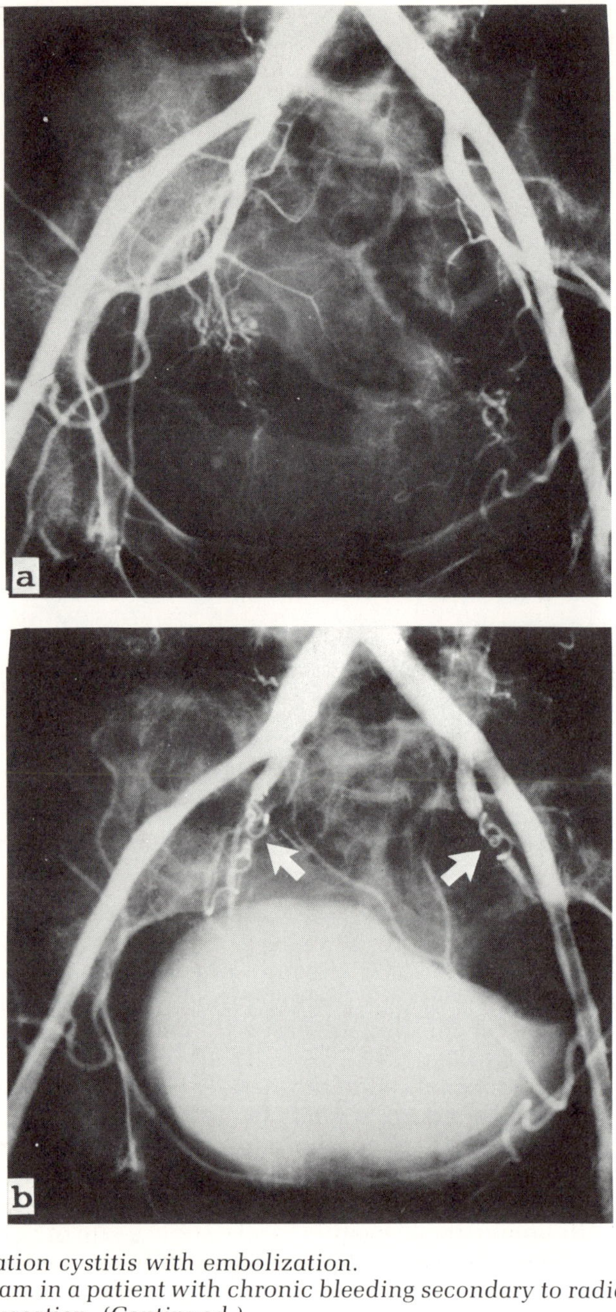

Figure 23. *Radiation cystitis with embolization.*
a. *Pelvic arteriogram in a patient with chronic bleeding secondary to radiation-induced cystitis. No extravasation. (Continued.)*
b. *Embolization of both hypogastric arteries with Gianturco coils (arrows). Bleeding clinically controlled.*

vaginal hemorrhage refractory to packing, hysterectomy, and bilateral hypogastric artery ligation. After ligation of the hypogastric artery, angiographic access to a bleeding site can be quite difficult. In this patient, a collateral route via the profunda femoris artery was negotiated and embolized successfully. A similar case of successful transcatheter occlusion in a patient with cavernous hemangiomas of the pelvis and post-abortion disseminated intravascular coagulopathy has been described.[31]

Bleeding diathesis can, of course, result in lower genitourinary bleeding. In a similar fashion with upper genitourinary hemorrhage, angiography is nondiagnostic but can occasionally be helpful therapeutically.

V. Complications of Angiography

The most common complication is a hematoma at the catheter entry site. This may be the result of faulty arterial compression, multiple catheter exchanges, or bleeding diathesis. Hematomas are unsightly but are usually of no clinical significance. Surgical repair is rarely necessary to control the bleeding. Occasionally, a large hematoma may result in false aneurysm formation. Bleeding from an inadvertently high site of puncture, i.e. above the inguinal ligament, will produce a pelvic retroperitoneal hematoma. It is important to watch for this by carefully monitoring the patient's vital signs after angiography and by initiating blood and fluid replacement if occult blood loss is suspected. Ultrasound or computerized axial tomography may be helpful in establishing the diagnosis. In the axilla, even a 5 cc hematoma within the neurovascular sheath can result in permanent brachial plexus damage. Therefore, at the first sign of neurologic sequelae after a transaxillary study, surgical evacuation of the hematoma should be performed.

Thrombus formation at the puncture site is a potential complication and should be treated surgically if the patient's extremity is cold, painful, and white. Arterial spasm is occasionally encountered, more often in children and teenagers than in adults. Other occasional complications include arteriovenous fistula at the catheter insertion site, dissection secondary to suboptimal passage of a guidewire, and, rarely, infection. There are scattered reports of paralysis after aortography either from embolic material inadvertently entering the arterial supply to the spinal cord or from a direct neurotoxic effect of the contrast.[33]

Minor contrast reactions including urticaria and wheezing are not uncommon. Major contrast reactions including anaphylaxis, angioneurotic edema, shock, and death occur rarely. The mortality for intravascular contrast is one in 40,000 patients.[34] Patients with known allergy to contrast material are pretreated with diphenylhydramine and steroids. The anesthesia department is notified if a severe reaction is anticipated.

Transient renal insufficiency has been reported in from 0% to 12% of patients following angiography. It appears to be somewhat higher for angiography than for intravenous urography.[8] The risk factors predisposing to contrast-induced renal insufficiency include diabetes mellitus, advanced age, hyperuricemia, monoclonal gammopathies, and multiple contrast exposures, dehydration, and underlying renal insufficiency. In a large series of patients, a rise in serum creatinine of at least 2.0 mg/dl within 48 hours of arteriography occurred at a rate of 0.53%.[35] Serum creatinine returned to baseline in three out of four of the cases. To reduce the frequency of this complication, contrast material should always be kept to the minimum that is consistent with adequate diagnostic information and therapy and the patients should be well hydrated before, during, and after the study.

The complications specifically associated with embolization will be discussed at the end of this chapter.

VI. Control of Genitourinary Bleeding with Angiographic Methods

A. Introduction

With the emergence of ultrasound and computed tomography, angiography plays less of a role in the routine diagnosis of genitourinary tract pathology than in the past. However, the emergence of interventional angiographic techniques has extended the available options for control of hemorrhage to include angiography as well as surgery. In cases of bleeding due to pelvic trauma, angiographic embolization is the current treatment of choice.

Transcatheter control of genitourinary hemorrhage developed following successful angiographic therapy for bleeding within the gastrointestinal tract, using both vasoactive infusion, i.e. vasopressin, and embolic occlusion. Outside the gastrointestinal tract, however, vasopressin has little efficacy and it is therefore rarely used in the therapy of genitourinary hemorrhage. The single exception to this is the uncommon case of angiographically demonstrated extravasation from the superior mesenteric artery in a patient with an ileal loop urinary diversion. Here vasopressin infused at a rate of 0.2 to 0.3 U/min for 20 minutes has been successful in permanently controlling hemorrhage.[28,36] Despite this exception, embolic occlusion is the chief angiographic modality for control of genitourinary hemorrhage. Transcatheter intra-arterial chemotherapy infusion has also been utilized for the treatment of hematuria and pain in patients with pelvic tumors.

Angiographic techniques, when feasible, offer several general advantages over the surgical approach. First, cost is reduced, as is the length of the patient's hospital stay. Second, patient discomfort is often much less. Third, in many cases, a single peripheral site of hemorrhage can be identified and selectively occluded, thereby preserving the maximal amount of viable tissue and organ function. This is particularly true for vascular lesions of the kidney and for post-traumatic renal hemorrhage where surgical exploration frequently results in total nephrectomy. Moreover, the inherent tamponade effect provided by the tissue planes around the kidney and in the pelvis remain undisturbed after embolization and can be valuable in controlling concomitant venous oozing. This has been particularly true in the case of pelvic trauma. Finally, in the event that the angiographic procedure is not completely successful in controlling hemorrhage, partial stabilization of the patient may allow surgery to be performed under more optimal conditions rather than as an acute emergency.

B. Embolization

There are many occlusive agents and embolization techniques currently available. The choice depends upon the type of lesion, whether it is benign or malignant, its location, its vascular anatomy, whether occlusion is to be temporary or permanent, and whether proximal, large vessel embolization or peripheral, arteriocapillary obliteration is desired. The site of occlusion should be as selective as possible yet allow adequate treatment of the lesion in order to preserve the maximal amount of normal tissue. This is particularly true when the lesion is benign. When embolizing a malignant lesion, however, extensive embolization is useful for palliation as well as immediate control of hemorrhage. If the hemorrhage is not brisk, it may be advisable to perform the diagnostic and therapeutic portions of the procedure at separate sessions in order to minimize contrast-induced renal toxicity.

1. Agents and Techniques

A variety of catheters and techniques are commonly employed, including coaxial systems, balloon occlusion catheters, and inflatable detachable balloons. Familiarity with multiple techniques is necessary to gain access to sites of hemorrhage and to avoid pitfalls and complications.

Occlusive agents can be categorized by their degree of permanence and by their site of occlusion within the arterial system.[37] Autologous clot and surgical gelatin (Gelfoam) are absorbable agents. Autologous clot, even modified with aminocaproic acid, usually lyses within 48 hours. Gelfoam, the most popular embolic material, is reabsorbed within days to weeks. It is easily available and is ideal for many situations, especially in the management of non-neoplastic sources of bleeding and for the preoperative embolization of large hypernephromas where permanent occlusion is not necessary.

Polyvinyl alcohol sponge (Ivalon) is a permanent occlusion. It can be obtained in either particulate or granular form. The latter form is available in microspheres which lodge at the arteriolar level and which are useful for permanent occlusion of nonresectable tumors.

Isobutyl-cyanoacrylate (Bucrylate) is a frequently used liquid that polymerizes when it comes in contact with blood and can produce total obliteration of the target vascular bed. It is therefore commonly used for arteriovenous malformations where proximal occlusion of the feeding vessel alone will merely result in revascularization of the lesion by collaterals. It is particularly efficacious when there is a large rent in the vessel, as sometimes occurs with trauma-induced bleeding, where particulate matter such as Gelfoam is less effective. However, Bucrylate is currently approved for experimental use only by the Federal Drug Administration, making it of limited general usefulness for now.

Newer liquid agents such as Ethibloc[38] (a corn protein mixed with alcohol and contrast) and 95% ethanol[39] are currently under investigation for permanent occlusion at the capillary level. Ethanol is gaining increasing acceptance for preoperative hypernephroma embolization.

Permanent agents that occlude at a proximal level are Gianturco coils and detachable balloons. With these agents, the site of occlusion is similar to that obtained by surgical ligation. The coils are made of stainless steel and are available in sizes commonly ranging from 2.5 mm to 8 mm in diameter. Coils may be used in conjunction with smaller particulate agents, such as Gelfoam, for a combination of both distal and proximal occlusion. When using coils preoperatively for hypernephroma, it is important to place the coils sufficiently distal within the renal artery so that cross-clamping of the renal pedicle will not transect the coil, thereby sending the proximal fragment back into the aorta to be carried distally into the pelvis or the lower extremity.

Detachable flow-directed mini-balloons are of limited usefulness since they are expensive and cumbersome to use. However, they offer the distinct advantage of easy retrieval prior to detachment if the initial site of placement is not optimal. They are particularly useful in the therapy of arteriovenous fistulae where a large communication must be effectively occluded without the passage of embolic material through the fistula.

Occasionally used agents include silicon spheres, transcatheter electrocoagulation, and tissue staining with contrast media, all rarely used within the genitourinary system.

Double lumen balloon occlusion catheters are valuable for emergency preoperative control of hemorrhage, as well as for the prevention of reflux during embolization with particulate matter. In the case of exsanguinating hemorrhage, a 2 French Fogarty catheter can be introduced through a standard angiographic catheter for emergency stabilization prior to surgery if a double lumen balloon catheter is not available.

2. *Embolization for Trauma*

Embolization for trauma, particularly pelvic trauma, and for preoperative management of hypernephroma are the two situations that have generated large series of patients. The surgical approach to massive hemorrhage from pelvic trauma often proves unsatisfactory. Surgical ligation of the hypogastric arteries provides only proximal occlusion of a vascular bed that has a vast collateral supply. The leading cause of death in patients with pelvic fractures treated surgically is blood loss.[40] Angiography, on the other hand, offers precise localization and distal embolization of bleeding sites, thereby virtually eliminating the problem of collateral supply, and does so without disrupting the retroperitoneum. It can also identify concomitant splenic, renal, or hepatic injury. Matalon[41] reported a series of 18 patients embolized after pelvic trauma in which hemorrhage was clinically controlled in 17 patients, with blood transfusion requirements reduced from an average of 32.1 units prior to the procedure to 5.2 units during the 48 hours after the procedure. The only angiographic complication was reflux of a Gelfoam pledget with distal embolization requiring popliteal embolectomy (Fig. 24). Lang[31] reported an additional series of 15 patients who underwent embolization for pelvic hemorrhage. In all but one patient, bleeding was controlled. The remaining patient was maintained in a positive pressure suit for several hours after the procedure and suffered large areas of skin necrosis and decubitus ulcers, probably as a result of the combined effects of the suit and the embolization. Multiple additional small series verify the efficacy of embolization therapy for pelvic fracture hemorrhage.[42–45]

Embolization within the kidney for post-traumatic hemorrhage has been performed in a few scattered cases[16,46-49] with considerable reported success. The major advantage of subselective renal embolization over a surgical approach is the relative preservation of viable tissue. Chuang[50] reports successful renal embolization in six of seven patients with post-traumatic bleeding. No patient in this series developed hypertension. In fact, this complication has not been a problem with small intrarenal branch embolization, regardless of the underlying etiology of the bleed.[51] Embolization for control of upper and lower post-traumatic hemorrhage, as well as in most cases of non-neoplastic hemorrhage, should include temporary occlusive agents, i.e. Gelfoam, to maximize the possibility of recanalization and restitution of vascular supply.

Intrarenal aneurysms, both congenital and post-traumatic, have been successfully treated using Gelfoam with minimal tissue loss and no clinical sequelae[15,16,52,53] (Fig. 25). Extraparenchymal aneurysms are best managed by the vascular surgeon.

Small post-biopsy arteriovenous fistulae frequently close spontaneously but can be successfully embolized if intervention is required. The largest series of six patients with arteriovenous fistula embolization was reported by Cho[54] with no significant complications, although transient hypertension was noted in two patients. Larger fistulae require use of different agents, since the small particulate matter such as Gelfoam or clot may pass through the fistula and lodge in the lungs. Stainless steel coils and detachable balloons have been used here.[55,56] Transcatheter electrocoagulation has been employed in arteriovenous fistula closures as well.[57] When there are multiple arterial feeders to an abnormal capillary bed, as in congenital arteriovenous malformations, isobutyl-cyanoacrylate has been quite useful. This agent forms a cast of the lesion, obliterating it in its entirety, thereby reducing the chance of collateral supply revascularizing the malformation.[58] Ethanol at 95% may offer the same degree of efficacy in this situation with greater safety, availability, and ease of use. Both of

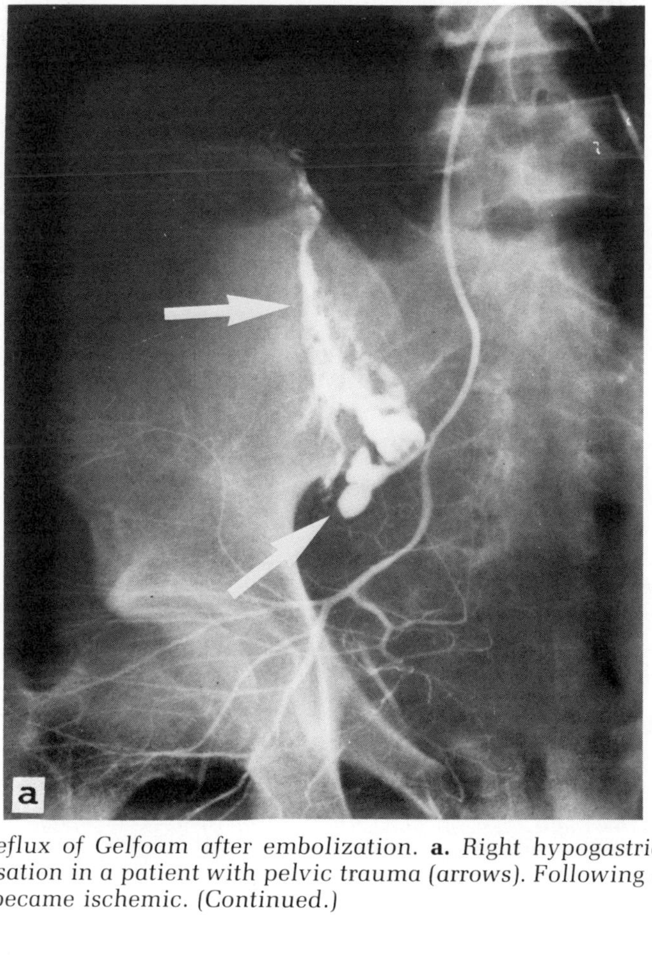

Figure 24: *Reflux of Gelfoam after embolization.* **a.** *Right hypogastric arteriogram shows extravasation in a patient with pelvic trauma (arrows). Following embolization, the right foot became ischemic. (Continued.)*

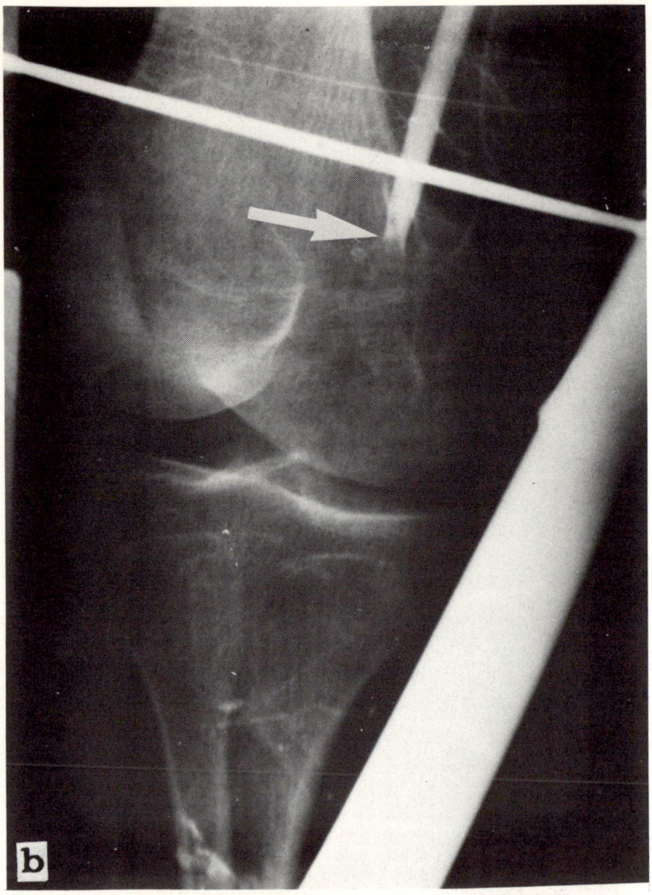

b. *Femoral arteriogram shows embolic occlusion of the popliteal artery by a Gelfoam pledget.*

these substances can be deposited superselectively using very small (3 French) catheters, thereby minimizing tissue loss (Fig. 26).

Hemorrhage from malignant lesions should be treated with permanent agents unless the embolization is performed as a preoperative procedure, in which case permanence is not necessary. Unlike benign lesions, bleeding with malignancy arises from abnormal tissue in which healing is not likely to occur. Moreover, embolization should be as extensive as necessary to control pain and tumor bulk.

Preoperative embolization for large hypernephromas has become a routine procedure in many centers. There are several large series reported: 100 patients in a series by Chuang,[59] 90 patients in a series by Hlava.[60] Transcatheter occlusion decreases operative blood loss, reduces anesthesia time, and facilitates the separation of tissue planes at surgery by creating post-embolization edema. It may also spark an enhanced immunologic response as a result of tumor necrosis. Gelfoam,[60] Ivalon,[61] stainless steel coils,[55] and, more recently, 95% ethanol[39] have been used. Chuang et al.[59] have reported a series of 49 patients

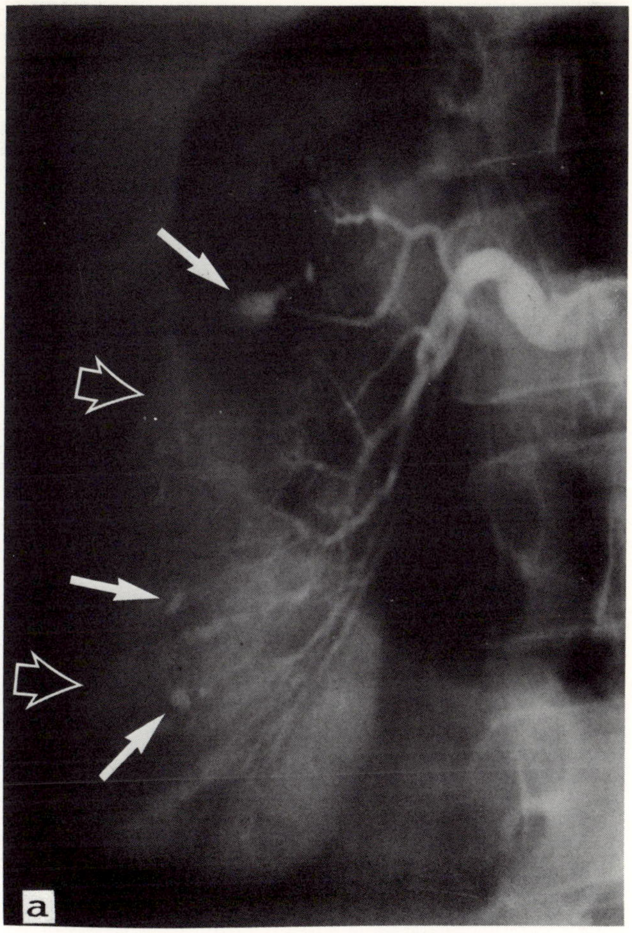

Figure 25: *Ruptured intrarenal aneurysm in a patient with arteritis.* **a.** *Renal arteriogram shows multiple intrarenal aneurysm (arrows). There is extravasation of contrast (superior arrow) and a subcapsular hematoma (open arrows). (Continued.)*

with limited metastases who were embolized with Gelfoam and coils up to 11 days prior to nephrectomy and then treated with progesterone postoperatively. This group of patients showed a marked improvement of the response rate when compared to other patients receiving other modes of therapy. For patients who are not surgical candidates because of widespread metastases, embolization has been performed to control hematuria or pain.[39,59] It has also been useful in the therapy of an inoperable hypernephroma in a solitary kidney. Permanent agents that occlude at a peripheral level, such as Ivalon granules, isobutyl-cyanoacrylate,[62] or ethanol, should be used in these circumstances. In patients in whom both radiation therapy and embolization are anticipated, radiation therapy should proceed embolization because post-occlusion ischemia may render the tumor relatively radio-resistant.

Several small series of patients treated by embolization for hemorrhage secondary to pelvic neoplasm have been reported[62-65] (Fig. 27). Surgery is often

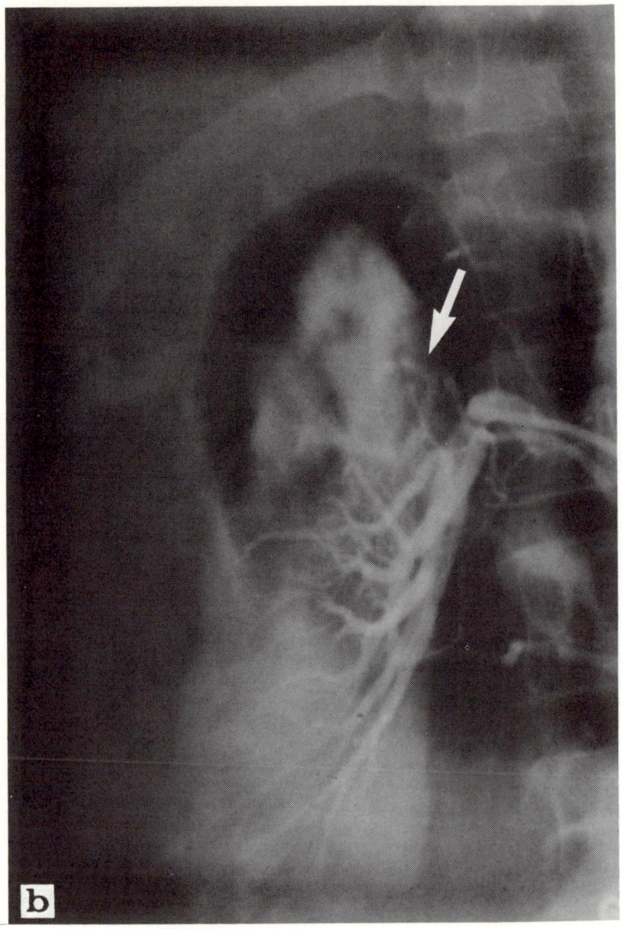

b. *After branch occlusion with Gelfoam (arrow) there is no further extravasation. The patient remained normotensive.*

technically difficult in these patients because of extensive tumor spread or radiation-induced fibrosis. Carmignani[65] performed nine such procedures for massive hematuria secondary to cancer of the bladder, cervix, or prostate using isobutyl-cyanoacrylate and/or Gelfoam. There was immediate cessation of hemorrhage in all nine cases, with rebleeding in one patient who developed collateral blood supply to the neoplasm. These collateral vessels were then embolized and there was no recurrent bleeding. One patient in this series suffered an unusual complication – the development of a Brown-Sequard syndrome which gradually cleared. Embolization has been successfully employed for hemorrhage from radiation-induced cystitis[63,66] and for vaginal bleeding secondary to cervical carcinoma.[30,62,63] As with tumor embolization elsewhere, permanent occlusive agents should be used.

Nonmalignant lower genitourinary tract hemorrhage, such as post-partum hemorrhage or bladder hemorrhage secondary to an angioma or cystitis, can be

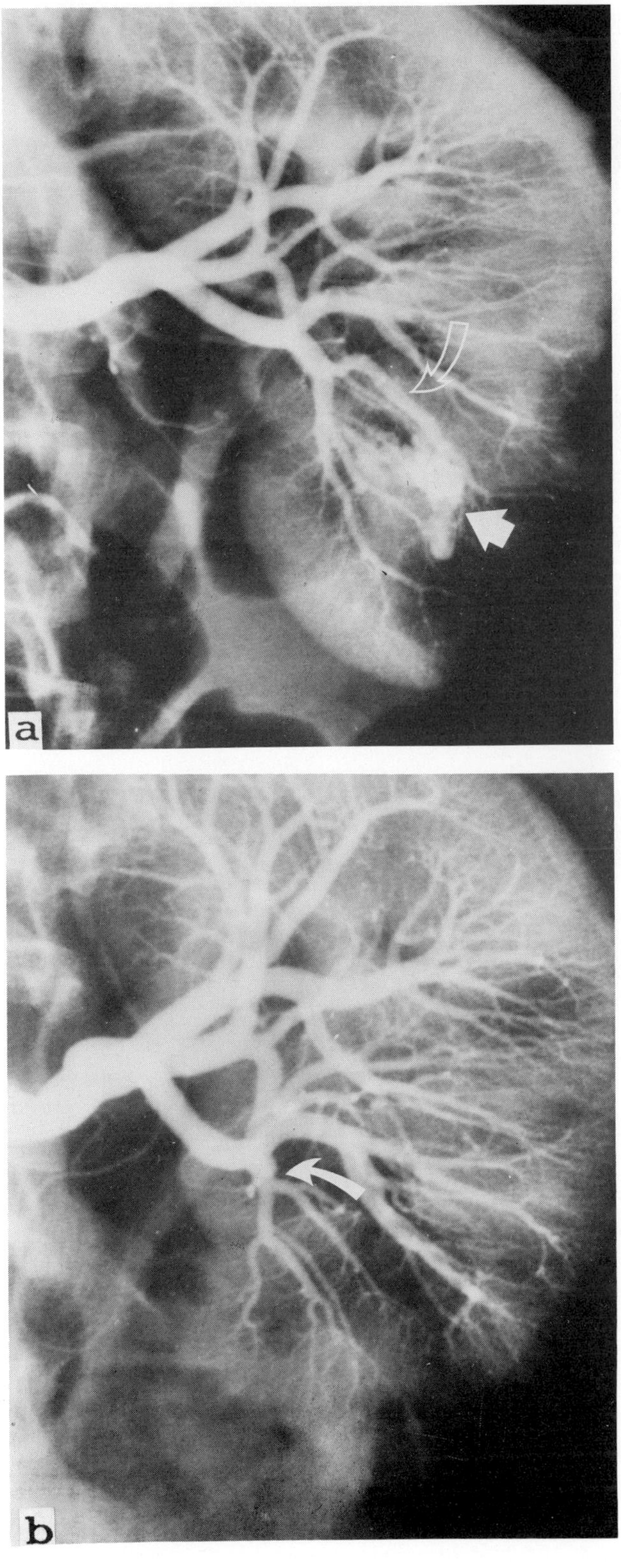

Figure 26: *Congenital arteriovenous malformation with embolization.* **a.** *Arteriovenous malformation (arrow) with dilated feeding artery (open arrow).* **b.** *Embolization of feeding branch (arrow) with clinical control of bleeding. The patient remained normotensive.*

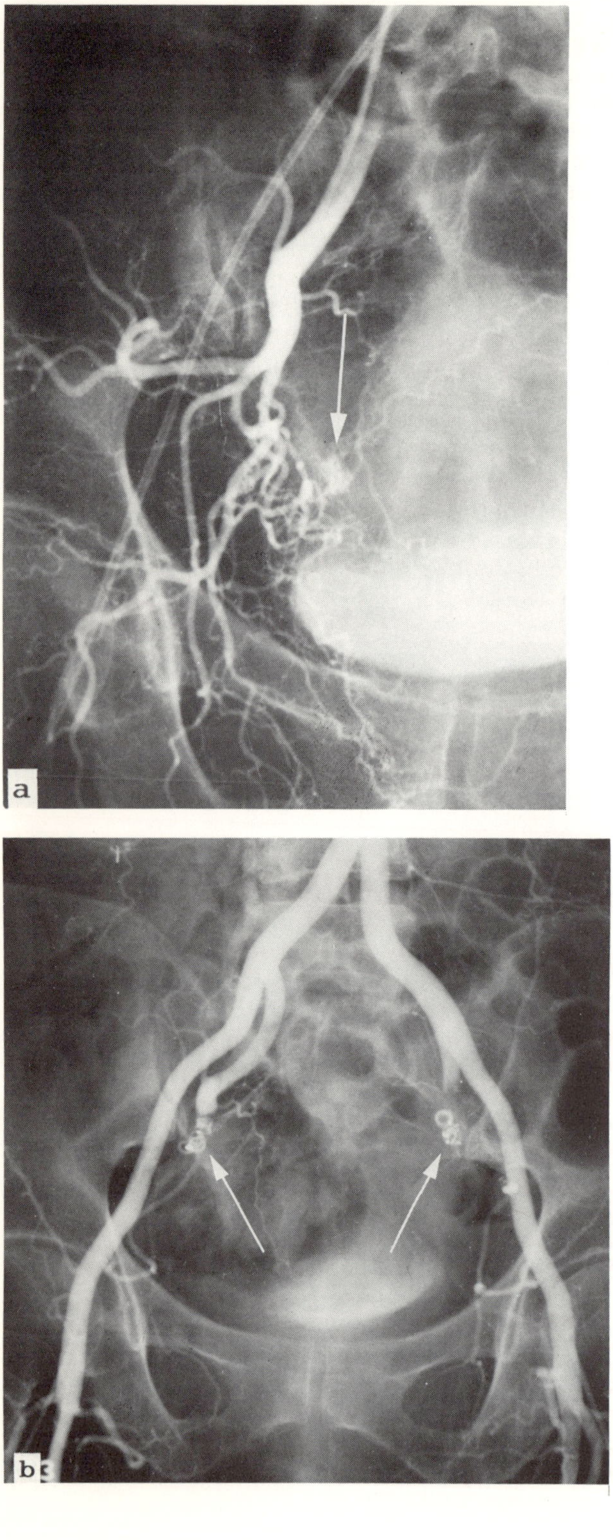

Figure 27: *Chronic bleeding from recurrent cervical carcinoma.* **a.** *Right hypogastric arteriogram shows tumor vascularity (arrow) but no extravasation.* **b.** *Both right and left hypogastric arteries are embolized with Gianturco coils (arrows). Vaginal bleeding stopped.*

satisfactorily controlled using nonpermanent occlusive embolic agents.[31,32] Lang[31] reported two patients with arteriovenous malformations involving the bladder wall in whom Gelfoam embolization was initially successful in eliminating the hemorrhage. One of the two patients, however, developed additional collateral supply to the malformation and re-bled 2½ months later. Recurrence of bleeding has been a frequent problem with particulate therapy for arteriovenous malformations but may well be alleviated by the emergence of newer agents, such as isobutyl-cyanoacrylate or ethanol, which form a cast of the lesion.

Bleeding secondary to genitourinary tract surgery has also been effectively managed with transcatheter vessel occlusion. Mitchell[29] reported control of prostatic bleeding in four patients after transurethral prostatectomy or needle biopsy of the prostate using Gelfoam and autologous clot. Lang[31] reported a series of five such patients, all embolized successfully.

Temporary transcatheter arterial occlusion has been an effective tool for emergency preoperative control of hemorrhage. We employed this technique in one patient with massive renal hemorrhage secondary to a fractured kidney. A Fogarty balloon catheter was inflated in the appropriate renal artery resulting in emergency hemodynamic stabilization. The patient was then taken to the operating suite.[52] Standard angiographic balloon occlusion catheters have been successfully used for this purpose as well.

3. Complications of Embolization

Complications can be divided into three general categories. The first category consists of those complications due to the angiographic portion of the procedure, such as allergic reaction to contrast material or puncture site thrombosis.

The second category of complications includes those due to the reflux of embolic material. Reflux of particulate matter with distal embolization has been reported in the spinal cord,[65,67] the bowel,[68] the liver,[69] and the lower extremity.[70] To prevent such complications, although they occur infrequently, it is imperative that embolic material be injected gently and in small quantities and that frequent monitoring of the extent of embolization be performed using gentle test injections of contrast material. Embolization should be avoided in severely vasoconstricted arteries or in stagnant systems, such as occurs in end-stage renal disease. Double lumen balloon occlusion catheters should be employed when reflux appears possible. Cox et al.[71] reported two cases of infarction of the left colon after ethanol embolization of the kidney without balloon occlusion. We routinely use balloon occlusion catheters during preoperative embolization with ethanol for hypernephromas. Following these guidelines, in 219 embolization procedures performed at the Massachusetts General Hospital, the rate clinical sequelae from reflux was 1%.[72]

Complications with stainless steel coils during renal artery embolization include reports of migration of the coil into the abdominal aorta or the lower extremities[73] or into the contralateral renal artery.[74] Aneurysm formation at the site of the coil has been seen in two cases and was thought to be secondary to the fibrous reaction stimulated by the wool tail that was attached to the coil.[75,76] Dacron tails are now used, and there has been no subsequent report of aneurysm formation. The overall frequency of complications with coils is quite low. In a series of 1,200 coil insertions reported by Chuang,[73] there were eight complications.

The third type of complications includes those due to ischemia or infarction of the target organ. Despite initial concerns that renal artery embolization would inevitably lead to persistent hypertension, this complication is, in fact, quite rare. Hypertension, when it occurs, most probably results from incomplete infarction, either due to a failure of arterial occlusion or due to the formation of collaterals.[74] The latter was seen in a patient who developed hypertension after main renal artery occlusion and was shown to have developed collateral supply to a hypernephroma. Transient hypertension, lasting from hours to several days, does occur, however, in a limited number of patients.[74,77]

Tissue necrosis after embolization has occasionally been reported. Despite extensive collateral supply to the pelvic organs, there are isolated cases of bone necrosis,[72] bladder necrosis,[78] and skin necrosis (in a patient with a positive pressure suit) after hypogastric embolization.[31] Permanent embolic materials that occlude at the arteriolar or capillary level, such as isobutyl-cyanoacrylate or Ivalon granules, are more likely to result in ischemic necrosis. Prior radiation therapy or previous surgery are also predisposing factors because of their devascularizing effect. Gas formation without true abscess formation has been observed in a kidney after embolization.[79]

Sepsis is another rare complication. To avoid this complication, aseptic technique must be maintained and antibiotic coverage provided if appropriate. Because of the demonstrated tendency of Gelfoam to become contaminated when wet, [37] pledgets are routinely soaked in an antibiotic solution prior to insertion.

There have been reports of rupture of false aneurysms in the pancreatic bed during embolization with resultant massive hemorrhage.[80] Because of the thin fragile walls of such aneurysms, it is imperative that catheterization be performed with great care, without wedging of the catheter into the feeding artery, and that minimal pressure be used during the injection of contrast or embolic material.

The post-infarction syndrome consists of pain and/or a mild febrile response and lasts from 24 to 48 hours, and is quite common.[79] This is not a true complication of embolization but is a side effect, and should be treated vigorously with narcotic analgesics. Flank pain may be severe after embolization of large renal masses, but is minimal after branch segmental artery occlusion. Some evidence suggests that the use of 95% ethanol reduces the degree of discomfort.[39] Gluteal pain is common after hypogastric embolization, particularly with agents that occlude at the arteriolar-capillary level. Other frequent but transient post-embolic side effects include nausea and vomiting, paralytic ileus, mild leukocytosis, and elevation of the erythrocyte sedimentation rate.

C. Intra-arterial Chemotherapy Infusion

Intra-arterial chemotherapy can have a role for patients with pelvic malignancy in the adjuvant treatment of low grade bleeding. Intra-arterial chemotherapy delivers a greater concentration of the cytotoxic agent to the malignancy than is possible with systemic chemotherapy at the same dose rate. Chuang[59] reported a series of 21 patients with bladder carcinomas in whom prolonged survival as well as immediate control of pain and hematuria were achieved.

Bilateral internal iliac artery infusions using CDDP (cis-diamminedichloroplatinum) over a 24-hour period were performed every 4 weeks for three courses of chemotherapy in these patients. (Other chapters in this book discuss this approach in greater detail.)

VII. Conclusion

With the emergence of computed tomography and ultrasound, angiography plays less of a diagnostic role than it did in the past in the evaluation of hemorrhagic disorders of the genitourinary tract. Computed tomography can accurately diagnose a renal fracture or intrarenal, subcapsular, or perirenal hematoma, but it is not suggested as a replacement for angiography in an unstable patient in whom surgery is contemplated. Angiography is indicated when other studies are nondiagnostic or equivocal. It remains the most accurate modality for the diagnosis of vascular abnormalities such as traumatic rupture or thrombosis, arteriovenous fistula, aneurysm, or renal vein thrombosis. In addition, angiography may reveal the presence of a previously undiagnosed small renal neoplasm, and it is the only method of obtaining a vascular "road map," which may be vital at the time of surgery.

Angiography has become increasingly important as a therapeutic modality. Transcatheter embolization provides a nonsurgical alternative for both upper and lower urinary tract hemorrhage. Within the kidney, it is particularly efficacious for control of bleeding from benign lesions, such as vascular malformations or post-traumatic bleeding, where preservation of renal tissue and function is paramount. For pelvic trauma, angiographic occlusion has become the therapy of choice, offering a high rate of clinical success with minimal morbidity. The clinical complication rate associated with transcatheter occlusion is low and can be expected to fall even farther with technical improvements, newer embolic materials, and increased experience.

References

1. Nausbaum M, Baum S. Radiographic demonstration of unknown sites of gastrointestinal bleeding. *Surg Forum*. 14:374–375, 1963.
2. Burkholder GV, Dotin LN, Thomason WB, Beach PD. Unexplained hematuria. *JAMA*. 210:1729–1733, 1969.
3. Lee LW, Davis E, Jr. Gross urinary hemorrhage: Symptom, not disease. *JAMA*. 153: 782–784, 1953.
4. Mitty HA, Goldman H. Angiography in unilateral renal bleeding with a negative urogram. *AJR*. 121:508–517, 1974.
5. Jonsson K. Renal angiography in patients with hematuria. *AJR*. 116:758–765, 1972.
6. Beckmann CF, Abrams HL. Renal venography: Anatomy, technique, applications, analysis of 132 venograms, and a review of the literature. *Cardiovasc Intervent Radiol*. 3:45–70, 1980.
7. Goss CM, ed. In: *Anatomy of the Human Body*. Henry Gray. Philadelphia, Lea & Febiger, 1963, p. 642.
8. Hessel SJ, Smith EH. Renal trauma: A comprehensive review and radiologic assessment. *CRC Crit Rev Radiol Nucl Med*. 5:251–293, 1974.

9. Banowsky LH, Wolfel DA, Lackner LH. Considerations in diagnosis and management of renal trauma. *J Trauma*. 10:587–597, 1970.
10. Sandler CM, Toombs BD. Computed tomographic evaluation of blunt renal injuries. *Radiology*. 141:461–466, 1981.
11. Federle MP, Kaiser JA, McAninch JW, Jeffrey RB, Mall JC. The role of computed tomography in renal trauma. *Radiology*. 141:455–460, 1981.
12. Federle MP, Goldberg HI, Kaiser JA, Moss AA, Jeffrey RB, Mall JC. Evaluation of abdominal trauma by computed tomography. *Radiology*. 138:637–644, 1981.
13. Itzchak Y, Adar R, Mozes M, Deutsch V. Occlusion of renal and visceral arteries following blunt abdominal trauma: Angiographic observations. *J Cardiovasc Surg*. 15:383–388, 1974.
14. Lang EK, Trichel BE, Turner RW, Rontenot RA, Johnson B, St. Martin EC. Renal arteriography in the assessment of renal trauma. *Radiology*. 98:103–112, 1971.
15. Almgard L, Fernstrom I. Embolic occlusion of an intrarenal aneurysm: A case report. *Br J Urol*. 45:485–486, 1973.
16. Chang J, Katzen BT, Sullivan KP. Transcatheter Gelfoam embolization of posttraumatic bleeding pseudoaneurysms. *AJR*. 131:645–650, 1978.
17. Messing E, Kessler R, Kavaney PB. Renal arteriovenous fistulas. *Urology*. 8:101–107, 1976.
18. O'Brien DP, Parrott TS, Walton KN, Lewis EL. Renal arteriovenous fistulas. *Surg Gynecol Obstet*. 139:739–743, 1974.
19. Nakamura H, Uchida H, Kuroda C, Yoshioka H, Tokunaga K, Kitatani T. Renal arteriovenous malformations: Transcatheter embolization and follow-up. *AJR*. 137: 113–116, 1981.
20. Johnsride IS, Jackson DC. *A Practical Approach to Angiography*. Boston, Little, Brown, and Co., 1971, p. 174.
21. Stanley JC, Rhodes EL, Gewertz BL, Chang CY, Walter JF, Fry WJ. Renal artery aneurysms: Significance of macroaneurysms exclusive of dissections and fibrodysplastic mural dilations. *Arch Surg*. 110:1327–1333, 1975.
22. Capps JH, Klein RM. Polyarteritis nodosa as a cause of perirenal and retroperitoneal hemorrhage. *Radiology*. 94:143–146, 1970.
23. Beckman CF, Abrams HL. Idiopathic renal vein varices: Incidence and significance. *Radiology*. 143:649–652, 1982.
24. Sacks BA, Gomori J, Lerner M, Masters R, DeWolf W. Left renal venous hypertension in association with the nutcracker phenomenon. *Cardiovasc Intervent Radiol*. 4: 253–255, 1981.
25. Navani S, Bosniak MA, Shapiro JH, Kaufman S. Varied radiographic manifestations of urinary tract bleeding. *J Urol*. 100:339–343, 1968.
26. Ring EJ, Waltman AC, Athanasoulis CA, Smith JC, Baum S. Angiography in pelvic trauma. *Surg Gynecol Obstet*. 139:375–380, 1974.
27. Stock JR, Harris WH, Athanasoulis CA. The role of diagnostic and therapeutic angiography in trauma to the pelvis. *Clin Ortho Related Res*. 151:31–40, 1980.
28. Smith JC, Kerr WS, Athanasoulis CA, Waltman AC, Ring EJ, Baum S. Angiographic management of bleeding secondary to genitourinary tract surgery. *J Urol*. 113:89–92, 1975.
29. Mitchell ME, Waltman AC, Athanasoulis CA, Kerr WS, Dretler SP. Control of massive prostatic bleeding with angiographic techniques. *J Urol*. 115:692–695, 1976.
30. Athanasoulis CA, Waltman AC, Barnes AB, Herbst AL. Angiographic Control of pelvic bleeding with angiographic techniques. *J Urol*. 115:692–695, 1976.
31. Lang EK. Transcatheter embolization of pelvic vessels for control of intractable hemorrhage. *Radiology*. 140:331–339, 1981.
32. Heaston DK, Mineau DE, Brown BJ, Miller FJ. Transcatheter arterial embolization for control of persistent massive puerperal hemorrhage after bilateral surgical hypogastric artery ligation. *AJR*. 133:152–154, 1979.
33. Abrams HL, Ed. *Abram's Angiography. Vascular and Interventional Radiology*. Third Edition. Boston, Little, Brown, and Co., 1983, p. 6043,

34. Lasser EC, Lang J, Sovak M, et al. Steroids: Theoretical and experimental basis for utilization in prevention of contrast media reactions. *Radiology*. 125:1–9, 1977.
35. Byrd L, Sherman RL. Radiocontrast-induced acute renal failure: A clinical and pathophysiologic review. *Medicine*. 58:270–279, 1979.
36. Wilkins RA, Viamonte M, Eds. *Interventional Radiology*. Boston, Blackwell Scientific Publications, 1982, p. 156.
37. Greenfield AJ. Transcatheter vessel occlusion: Selection of methods and materials. *Cardiovasc Intervent Radiol*. 3:222–228, 1980.
38. Kauffman GW, Rassweiler J, Richter G, Hauenstein KH, Rohrbach R, Friedburg H. Capillary embolization with Ethibloc: New embolization concept tested in dog kidneys. *AJR*. 137:1163–1168, 1981.
39. Ellman BA, Parkhill BJ, Curry TS, III, Marcus PB, Peters PB. Ablation of renal tumors with absolute ethanol: A new technique. *Radiology*. 141:619–626, 1981.
40. Patterson FP, Morton KS. The cause of death in fractures of the pelvis: with a note on treatment by ligation of the hypogastric (internal iliac) artery. *J Trauma*. 13:849–856, 1973.
41. Matalon TS, Athanasoulis CA, Margolies MN, Waltman AC, Novellini RA, Greenfield AJ, Miller SE. Hemorrhage with pelvic fractures: Efficacy of transcatheter embolization. *AJR*. 133:859–864, 1979.
42. Kadish LK, Stein JM, Kotler S, et al. Angiographic diagnosis and treatment of bleeding due to pelvic trauma. *J Trauma*. 13:1083–1085, 1973.
43. Kerr WS, Jr, Margolies MN, Ring EJ, Waltman AC, Baum SN. Arteriography in pelvic fractures with massive hemorrhage. *J Urol*. 109:479-482, 1973.
44. Gerlock AJ. Hemorrhage following pelvic fracture controlled by embolization. Case report. *J Trauma*. 15:740–742, 1975.
45. Barlow B, Rottenberg RW, Santulli TV. Angiographic diagnosis and treatment of bleeding by selective embolization following pelvic fracture in children. *J Pediatr Surg*. 10:939–942, 1975.
46. Bookstein JJ, Goldstein HM. Successful management of postbiopsy arteriovenous fistulae with selective arterial embolization. *Radiology*. 109:535–536, 1973.
47. Rosen RJ, Feldman L, Wilson AR. Embolization for post-biopsy renal arteriovenous fistula: Effective occlusion using homologous clot. *AJR*. 131:1072–1073, 1978.
48. Silber SJ, Clark RE. Treatment of massive hemorrhage after renal biopsy with angiographic injection of clot. *N Engl J Med*. 292:1387–1388, 1975.
49. Richman SD, Green WM, Kroll R, Casarella WJ. Superselective transcatheter embolization of traumatic renal hemorrhage. *Am J Roentgenol*. 128:843–846, 1977.
50. Chuang VP, Reuter SR, Walter J, Foley WD, Bookstein JJ. Control of renal hemorrhage by selective arterial embolization. *AJR*. 125:300–306, 1975.
51. White RI, Jr. Arterial embolization for control of renal hemorrhage. *J Urol*. 115: 121–122, 1976. (Editorial.)
52. Athanasoulis CA, Greene RE, Pfister RC, Roberson GH, Eds. *Interventional Radiology*. Philadelphia, WB Saunders, 1982.
53. Wilkins RA, Viamonte M, Eds. *Interventional Radiology*. Boston, Blackwell Scientific Publications, 1982, p. 155.
54. Cho KJ, Stanley JC. Non-neoplastic congenital and acquired renal arteriovenous malformations and fistulas. *Radiology*. 129: 333–343, 1978.
55. Wallace S, Gianturco C, Anderson JH, et al. Therapeutic vascular occlusion utilizing steel coil technique: Clinical applications. *AJR*. 127:381–387, 1976.
56. White RI, Jr, Barth KH, Kaufman SL, Decaprio V, Strandberg JD. Therapeutic embolization with detachable balloons. *Cardiovasc Intervent Radiol*. 3:229–241, 1980.
57. McAlister DS, Johnsrude I, Miller MM, Clapp J, Thompson WM. Occlusion of acquired renal arteriovenous fistula with transcatheter electrocoagulation. *AJR*. 132: 998–1000, 1979.
58. Kerber CW, Freeny PC, Cromwell L, et al. Cyanoacrylate occlusion of a renal arteriovenous fistula. *AJR*. 128:663–665, 1977.

59. Chuang VP, Wallace S. Current status of transcatheter management of neoplasms. *Cardiovasc Intervent Radiol.* 3:256–267, 1980.
60. Hlava A, Steinhart L, Navratil P. Intraluminal obliteration of the renal arteries in kidney tumors. *Radiology.* 121:323–329, 1976.
61. Chuang VP, Soo CS, Wallace S. Ivalon embolization in abdominal neoplasms. *AJR.* 136:729–733, 1981.
62. Freeny PC, Bush WH Jr, Kidd R. Transcatheter occlusive therapy of genitourinary abnormalities using isobutyl 2-cyanoacrylate (Bucrylate). *AJR.* 133:647–656, 1979.
63. Lang EK, Deutsch JS, Goodman JR, Barnett TJ, Lanasa JA Jr, Duplessis GH. Transcatheter embolization of hypogastric branch arteries in the management of intractable bladder hemorrhage. *J Urol.* 121:30–36, 1979.
64. Kobayashi T, Kusano S, Matsubayashi T, Uchida T. Selective embolization of the vesical artery in the management of massive bladder hemorrhage. *Radiology.* 136: 345–348, 1980.
65. Carmignani G, Belgrano E, Puppo P, Cichero A, Giuliani L. Transcatheter embolization of the hypogastric arteries in cases of bladder hemorrhage from advanced pelvic cancers: Follow up in 9 cases. *J Urol.* 129:196–200, 1980.
66. Hald T, Mygind T. Control of life-threatening vesical hemorrhage by unilateral hypogastric artery muscle embolization. *J Urol.* 112:60–63, 1974.
67. Gang DL, Dole KB, Adelman LS. Spinal cord infarction following therapeutic renal artery embolization. *JAMA.* 237:2841–2842, 1977.
68. Mukamel E, Hadar H, Nissenkorn I, Servadio C. Widespread dissemination of Gelfoam particles complicating occlusion of renal circulation. *Urology.* 14:194–197, 1979.
69. Trojanowski JQ, Harrist T, Athanasoulis CA, Greenfield AJ. Hepatic and splenic infarctions as complications of therapeutic transcatheter embolization: A report of two cases. *Am J Surg.* 139:272–277, 1980.
70. Stock JR, Athanasoulis CA, Harris WH, Waltman AC, Novellini RA, Greenfield AJ. Transcatheter embolization for the control of wound hemorrhage following hip surgery. *J Bone Joint Surg.* 62A:1000–1003, 1980.
71. Cox GG, Lee KR, Price HI, Gunter K, Noble MJ, Mebust WK. Colonic Infarction following ethanol embolization of renal-cell carcinoma. *Radiology.* 145:343–345, 1982.
72. Feldman L, Greenfield AJ, Waltman AC, Novelline RA, van Breda A, Luers P, Athanasoulis CA. Transcatheter vessel occlusion: Angiographic result vs. clinical success. *Radiology.* 147:1–5, 1983.
73. Chuang VP, Wallace S, Gianturco C, Soo CS. Complications of coil embolization: Prevention and management. *AJR.* 137:809–813, 1981.
74. Mazer MJ, Baltaxe HA, Wolf GL. Therapeutic embolization of the renal artery with Gianturco coils: Limitations and technical pitfalls. *Radiology.* 138:37–46, 1981.
75. Jhaveri HS, Gerlock J. Jr, Ekelund L. Failure of steel coil occlusion in a case of hypernephroma. *AJR.* 130:556–557, 1978.
76. Struthers NW, Samu P, Chalvardjian A. Renal artery aneurysm: A complication of Gianturco coil embolization of renal adenocarcinoma. *J Urol.* 123:105–106, 1980.
77. Goldstein HM, Medellin H, Beydoun MT, Wallace S, Ben-Menachem Y, Bracken RB, Johnson DE. Transcatheter embolization of renal cell carcinoma. *Am J Roentgenol Rad Ther Nucl Med.* 123:557–562, 1975.
78. Hietala SO. Urinary bladder necrosis following selective embolization of the internal iliac artery. *Acta Radiol Diagn.* (Stockh) 19:316–320, 1978.
79. Rankin RN. Gas formation after renal tumor embolization without abscess: A benign occurrence. *Radiology.* 130:317–320, 1979.
80. Lina JR, Jaques P, Mandell V. Aneurysm rupture secondary to transcatheter embolization. *AJR.* 132:553–556, 1979.

Chapter 9

Surgical Hemostasis in Upper Urinary Tract and Retroperitoneal Surgery

Leonard Zinman, M.D., and John A. Libertino, M.D.

I. Introduction

Prevention and control of bleeding in the presence of normal hemostatic mechanisms are of fundamental importance to the success of any surgical procedure. Loss of blood from damaged bleeding vessels comprises the majority of intraoperative and postoperative hemorrhages, an aspect of hemostasis which should be the primary focus in the management of surgical bleeding. Hemostasis in urologic operations requires safe and reliable application of instrumental methods such as occluding clamps suited to the specific anatomic problems, compression, cautery, ligatures, intraluminal balloon catheters, hypothermia, and absorbable topically applied hemostatic agents appropriate for the pelvic and retroperitoneal spaces.

A. History

The history of surgical hemostasis is linked to the wounds of warfare and to the techniques used to stop bleeding. Styptic agents, cautery, and ligatures were inspired by such events. The first widely practiced method of surgical hemostasis was cautery introduced in the 7th century by Paul of Aegina.[1] and promoted by Avicenna, the Persian surgeon of the 10th century. From the beginning of surgery and well into the 19th century, the cautery heated over a bed of coals was used to control hemorrhage. The anguish the patients must have experienced with cautery inspired the great French surgeon, Ambrose Pare, to develop the ligature, a method he described in 1564.[2] Pare remarked that other surgeons

From Bern MM (ed.): *Urinary Tract Bleeding: Diagnosis and Control by Medical, Radiologic, and Surgical Techniques*. Mount Kisco, NY, Futura Publishing Co., Inc., 1985.

before him had ligated bleeding vessels,[3] but his was a lasting contribution substituting the ligature for the cautery in control of bleeding from large vessels. The ligature was then established as the most reliable mode of hemostasis. Pare often ligated large vessels in continuity before severing them, a practice that illustrated his careful attention to the details of surgical control of hemorrhage. He even developed an instrument to expose and draw out the cut vessel before passing ligatures about it with a curved needle.[3] This instrument was the predecessor of the modern hemostat, which is an essential tool in the management of surgical hemostasis today. After four centuries of phenomenal accomplishments in surgical care, the prevention of bleeding from extensive renal, renovascular, retroperitoneal, and pelvic surgery still continues as a major concern for the contemporary urologic surgeon.

II. Basic Principles of Vessel Control for Hemostasis

A basic principle of blood vessel surgery is avoidance of unnecessary or uncontrollable bleeding. To accomplish this, there should be enough assistants to assure complete freedom of the surgeon and there should be wide enough retraction for exposure of deep incisions. The incisions should be large enough to provide easy access to the regional major vessels in order to allow precise proximal and distal control of vessels during dissection. Careful planning of each operation will allow the operating team to fulfill their primary mission.

A. Materials and Techniques

1. Sutures and Ligatures

To perform delicate, meticulous point ligation of bleeding vessels while avoiding mass tissue clamping with its attendant tissue necrosis has become the hallmark of good surgical technique. In the absence of infection, small randomly disrupted vessels are clamped with fine delicate-tipped hemostats and ligated with fine silk ligatures. Absorbable ligatures, such as catgut and polyglycolic acid, should be used in the lumen of the urinary tract to avoid the calculi that are likely to develop on nonabsorbable sutures. The renal artery and vein, however, should be secured individually with ligatures proximally, followed by suture ligatures distally, usually using nonabsorbable sutures. When the fixed renal pedicles are fibrous and inflamed, this may not be possible. Placing the sutures blindly should be avoided because traumatic arteriovenous fistulae can be produced in the renal pedicle. This type of pathologic condition does not occur when only the mass ligature itself is employed. Suture ligatures should be used to secure any large vessel that has a relatively short stump. The suturing should always be preceded by placing a secure ligature proximal to where the needle will penetrate the vessel in order to avoid tearing arteries that are distended with blood or arteries that are atherosclerotic. Precarious thin-walled veins, such as lumbar and adrenal veins, should be ligated in continuity before they are divided, without preliminary application of the hemostat so as to prevent their tearing in the deep, inaccessible, poorly exposed recesses of the retroperitoneum. Lateral tears in the iliac vessels, aorta, vena cava, or renal vessels should always be secured with running, permanent, nonbiodegradable, fine, monofilament arterial sutures. (Arterial suture lines never heal and are always dependent on the original closure material used.) If the ends of a severed vessel retract from view, leaving an edge of the vessel visible, the edge should be grasped with a hemostat and rotated. This technique will occlude the vessel, and bleeding may decrease sufficiently to gain visibility and allow subsequent ligation.

2. *Vascular Clamps*

For all retroperitoneal and pelvic surgery, the instrument table should include vascular forceps, vascular needle holders, fine no. 5-0 and no. 6-0 monofilament vascular sutures, straight vascular clamps, partial lateral occlusion clamps, soft-jaw Fogarty clamps, and adjustable low-tension bulldog clamps for small vessels.[4,5] The most secure clamps with the least trauma are the Fogarty clamps, which occlude even the most fragile vessels with a minimal lock setting.[6] The jaws of this clamp consist of removable pads that cause no detectable changes in the arterial wall when closed lightly, but which produce a small grooved defect when fully closed. This defect can be visible for up to 60 days, but causes minimal damage to the intima. Careful inspection of instruments to identify faulty clamps before beginning surgery can avoid serious hemorrhage during surgery. Vascular clamps that are defective usually have either catches that are sprung or jaws that do not come together, thus allowing the faulty instrument to slip off the vessel.[7]

3. *Tourniquets*

The Rummel tape tourniquet is the lest traumatic vascular occlusive technique and is ideally suited for control of vena caval or renal veins. This clamp can be made by drawing the two ends of a medium-size umbilical arterial tape through a 4-inch length of a no. 22 Fr or no. 24 Fr soft red rubber catheter and securing the catheter against the vein with a clamp on the tape as it emerges from the distal end of the catheter. The advantage of a tourniquet clamp is that it can be placed outside of the immediate surgical field where exposure may be limited and where instrument handles might interfere with the completion of the tasks. A modified tourniquet tape method that gently controls bleeding from similar vessels without excess tension was reported by Baker.[8] This consists of placing a double loop of rubber of Silastic band around the vessel proximal and distal to the segment to be worked on. Gentle tension is applied to the ends of the band and is adjusted so that just enough compression is applied to stop the flow of blood. A medium-sized metal hemostatic clamp is then applied across the elastic bands to maintain the occluding pressure. This technique allows the vessel to lie in its normal position without undue stretching or twisting, and can be used on pelvic and extremity vessels where anatomic exposures may be limited.

4. *Hemostatic Clips*

The hemostatic metal clip, another commonly employed instrument in retroperitoneal surgery, was introduced by Cushing[9] in 1908 for intracranial procedures, but did not provide consistently secure results until Samuels et al.[10] introduced the biologically inert tantalum clip in 1966. This material was malleable, stable, and as strong as the stainless steel clip.[11] The occlusive surface of the hemostatic clip has a centered longitudinal groove crossed at intervals by transverse depressions. The clips are available in various sizes and have the advantage of being able to accomplish rapid, relatively secure control of blood vessels in deep recesses where ligatures would be difficult to place or where bulky accumulation of hemostatic clamps would be awkward.

Hemostatic clips are not secure on the tributaries from large vessels because they can be easily dislodged during the dissection. However, in performing a cystectomy in men, where the pelvis is narrow and the vessels are poorly exposed, the clip technique for hemostasis is especially helpful. In this situation, two medium-sized hemoclips are placed proximally and two are placed distally for double reinforcement, and the vessel is cut between the inner clips. The clip technique is also useful in adrenal surgery. In resecting a pheochromocytoma, rapid rlease of catecholamines following tumor manipulation is prevented by clipping the adrenal vein before exposing the tumor. Also, a subtotal adrenalectomy can be accomplished using the clips by placing a row of clips across the vascular and fragile glandular tissue, after which the adenoma is resected. Otherwise this procedure can produce considerable oozing from the cut surface of normal gland. The large clips are especially useful in *en bloc* resections for transplantation of donor organs.[12]

The least tissue reaction is achieved with tantalum clips, a metal which is too expensive to produce. Most commercially available clips today are made of stainless steel and are used with a multiple-clip applicator. The applicators that are now mass produced and are disposable, are either straight or right-angle, with a single or double-clip system, and allow simultaneous application of two clips in a sequence followed by automatic separation of the vessel between the clips.

The greatest use of clips in urologic surgery is in retroperitoneal node dissection for tumor of the testes. Here small vessels are often inaccessible. They also can be placed as a guide for future radiotherapy or to obtain repeat biopsies during second-look procedures.[13] The clips can outline an organ or masses that need to be followed as evidence for neoplastic enlargement or position shift.

A disadvantage of this technique, however, is that the metal produces a low-density streaked artifact in computed tomography (CT). Depending on the number of clips used, this can produce confusion when postoperative CT imaging is required, as when monitoring the retroperitoneum after excision of testicular, renal, or bladder carcinoma. The radiologic interference, known as the sparkler effect, often blurs out the silhouette of tumor nodules,[14] a situation that has been improved somewhat by the development of a new synthetic nonopaque polydioxane polymer (PDS) hemostatic clip with locking jaws.[15] Unfortunately, however, these polymer clips are not as easy to apply nor are they as secure as the stainless steel clips.

5. Intraluminal Catheters

An important but often overlooked hemostatic instrument is the intraluminal Fogarty balloon or Foley catheter. This tool is particularly useful during secondary or tertiary vascular procedures in which vena cava, aorta, or renal and pelvic vessels are encased with fibrosis. Here laceration of a vessel would require tedious and time-consuming dissection to control hemorrhage.[16] The catheter can be used to replace a vascular clamp when life-threatening hemorrhage has occurred and when sufficient distal or proximal control cannot be obtained. The balloon catheter can be passed through a rent in the blood vessel into the retrohepatic or inferior vena caval lumen during the difficult right nephrectomy or vena cava resection. The catheter, when needed for hemostasis, is passed through the bleeding site for 1 to 2 inches, and the balloon is inflated until bleeding halts. Bleeding from iliac arteries, veins, or tributaries can be controlled with a no. 6 Fogarty catheter or a no. 8 to 16 Foley catheter with 2- to 10-ml balloon, depending on the size and pliability of the vessel. The balloon should remain securely in place if its pressure is about 100 mmHg.[17,18] Vascular occlusion using this method can be invaluable in the management of pelvic bleeding secondary to trauma, or in the removal of large renal tumors that have acquired hemangiomatous surfaces. When a renal artery catheter is placed preoperatively by the percutaneous route, the renal artery can be occluded by means of a Gianturco steel wire coil (Cook, Inc, 925 South Curry Pike, Bloomington, IN 47401), by Gelfoam particles, or by a detachable balloon so as to achieve relative ischemia during the course of nephrectomy (Fig. 1).

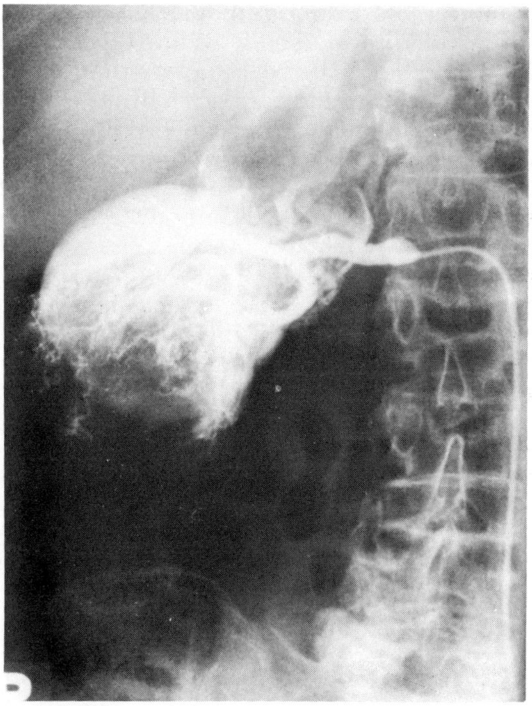

Figure 1: *Renal artery catheter placed preoperatively to be used to achieve ischemia during nephrectomy for renal carcinoma.*

6. *Electrocautery*

Another common instrument that has become a routine tool for surgical hemostasis is electrocautery, which has now been incorporated in a variety of surgical instruments.[19] The method is fast, effective, and convenient with low complication rates. When used properly, the electrocautery causes less tissue necrosis than do most ligatures. The incidence of postoperative wound sepsis after using electrocautery and ligature for hemostasis was studied by Arnott et al.[20] This study randomly assigned 240 "clean" wounds and 308 potentially contaminated wounds to hemostasis by either technique. The incidence of wound sepsis in clean wounds was not influenced by the method used. However, secondary sepsis after formation of a hematoma was more common when ligatures were used. When an adequate topical antibiotic was applied in the potentially contaminated wounds, the method of hemostasis did not influence the incidence of infection. When a systemic antibiotic was not given, the ligature technique was associated with less sepsis than was diathermy (21% versus 31.5%).

Because cautery plays such a major role in wound hemostasis, the principles that are the basis for its tissue damage should be understood.[21] Devices in use today are radiofrequency generators, which supply 500,000 to 2,000,000 Hz AC to the active tip of the electrode. This causes local heating which in turn creates the hemostatic effect. The current density falls rapidly as it is dissipated through the body. The current is returned to the instrument through the dispersive electrode or ground plate, which provides a large surface for contact and, therefore, a low current and power density. While the entire body is a conductor of electricity, some tissues are better conductors than others. Thus, this technique does not constitute a hazard to cardiac rhythms because the myocardium is not sensitive to this frequency range. However, this frequency range can produce extraneous burns at points of contact with ECG leads or at other alternative return pathways if the ground plates are defective or poorly applied. The ground electrodes should not be placed on bony prominences or on irregular surfaces, but are best located over heavy muscle masses which are more conductive.

The most common system for open surgical hemostasis uses monopolar electrodes and incorporates a variety of instruments for contact with bleeding vessels and metal hemostats. The most efficient technique is the use of diathermy forceps. Here the surgeon actually uses dissecting forceps for grasping tissues, and simultaneously achieves hemostasis by adapting a diathermy electrode to the proximal end of the forceps. This technique allows pinpoint coagulation with the vessel grasped between the tips of the forceps and prevents indiscriminate cautery and excess tissue necrosis. The lowest generator setting required for effective hemostasis should be used during the procedure, in order to keep heat production low adjacent to the forceps tips and to prevent creation of a fluid vapor that will desiccate the cells. Sudden increases in generator power cause a massive electrical arc with high temperatures and excessive tissue burns. If this occurs in a closed space, such as the lumen of the bladder or renal pelvis, explosive gases are produced from split-vapor components of hydrogen and oxygen with the potential for traumatic explosion. Massive electrical arcs produced by higher power settings can also generate a certain amount of DC power, which may stimulate muscle contraction and disturb the surgical field.[22–23] The surgeon who uses electrocautery for both cutting and hemostasis learns over a period of time the amount of current or power that will be needed for dissection in each specific region. In plastic and reconstructive surgery in which tissue flaps are created and optimal healing is desired, very low intensity settings should be employed, whereas with mediastinal dissections, more power may be required to stop surface oozing.

7. Lasers

With the development of laser beam technology, the carbon dioxide (CO_2) laser scalpel has emerged as a tool for excision of lesions that may lead to appreciable blood loss. The CO_2 laser has wavelengths in the infrared range. This allows it to react with cellular water so as to vaporize cells, giving it a hemostatic property that can be directed to very fine points. Tissue can be incised precisely, while achieving simultaneous coagulation in vessels that are 2 mm in diameter. Usually the operative field is dryer with use of the laser. It does seal off lymphatics and produces less thermal damage to adjacent tissue than does electrocautery or cryosurgery.[24,25]

Because the larger vessels will bleed when divided using this tool, the CO_2 laser scalpel has limited use in surgery on the renal parenchyma or in prostrate surgery. It also takes longer to make an incision with the laser instrument than it does with the scalpel, and requires considerable practice in its use so as to prevent excess tissue damage while achieving maximal hemostasis.

At the present time, the CO_2 laser is ideally suited for excision of lesions of the penis, scrotum, and perineum; for debridement of infected abscess in patients with low platelet counts; and for the excision of recurrent tumors of the groin or lower abdominal wall.

Presently, the neodymium-yttrium aluminum garnet (Nd-YAG) laser has no particular advantage in surgery in the renal parenchyma for either partial nephrectomy or nephrolithotomy. As for the CO_2 laser, brisk bleeding can occur from the relatively high-pressure arteries. Also, the deep-tissue penetration of the Nd-YAG laser may necrotize needlessly otherwise functional renal parenchyma.

8. Ultrasonic Dissector

Another promising hemostatic tool presently being used in urology is the ultrasonic dissector (Cavitron Ultrasonic Surgical Aspirator, Cavitron Surgical Systems, 1902 McGraw Ave, Irvine, CA 92714), especially for incising renal parenchyma in renocortical surgery. The instrument consists of a water-cooled handpiece connected to a console by a 15-ft. cable. A hollow tantalum tip is continuously irrigated as it vibrates at a frequency of 23,000 c/s. A suction line connected to this tip aspirates irrigant, blood, and tissue fragments using adjustable negative pressure. The instrument selectively fractures tissues in proportion to its water content.[26] At low settings, the instrument fragments and suctions away the renal parenchyma leaving individual blood vessels intact to be secured separately with ligatures. Higher vibratory settings will tear blood vessels and parenchyma and will produce excessive hemorrhage from the torn vessels before they are controlled. Since the consistency of tissue varies, the vibratory setting must be selected in each patient in order to achieve an efficient dissection with minimal damage to structures. Tissues of older patients tend to sonicate more easily than do those of younger patients.

The ultrasonic dissector is not hemostatic within itself, but it does remove the parenchyma, exposing vessels for control by conventional means. Thus, a major advantage of the instrument is for dissection of parenchyma, leaving larger vessels and calices exposed and preserved if desired. Moreover, since important vessels and calices can be detected before damage occurs, true intersegmental planes need not be followed strictly when performing nephrotomy. This allows an anatrophic nephrolithotomy or tumor resection along any convenient location on the renal surface with little additional risk.[27] The ultrasonic dissector is especially useful in resection of large tumors under conditions of controlled hemostasis. After completion of the transection, the cut surface of the kidney is smooth and dry to a degree unattainable with dissection by finger or scalpel.

A true learning curve is present when beginning to use this instrument. The procedures require practice in the laboratory and a familiarity with the vibratory settings, which must be readjusted frequently during the course of any procedure.

9. Compression and Packing Techniques

Compression techniques are important in the temporary control of troublesome bleeding. Simple gauze packing can be an invaluable hemostatic aid in controlling pelvic, prostatic, perineal, and flank hemorrhage. For serious bleeding in a confined space that cannot be controlled by a hemostat, a gauze roll soaked in ice saline solution will give the surgeon time to replace blood platelets and other plasma factors while planning more definitive approaches. Occasionally, patients who have undergone salvage cystectomy or who had pelvic trauma and who now have an oozing surface may benefit from placing a saline-soaked or a dry laparotomy pad firmly in the recesses of the wound, which is held under considerable pressure for hours or even up to several days. These packs may promote local sepsis and cause tissue ischemia. Therefore, the disadvantages must be weighed against the benefits of tamponade or hemorrhage. This packing technique is applicable in procedures where bleeding is occurring from small branches of the aorta, vena cava, or pelvic vessels that have eluded ligatures and clamps.

Packing should never be employed when a renal artery is the source of hemorrhage. This situation requires aortic compression by the transperitoneal route combined with finger compression of the transected arterial lumen, with proper subsequent exposure of the renal pedicle, and hemostatic occlusion of the vessel.

Bleeding from the prostatic fossa, the pelvic cavity, the perirenal area, and the retroperitoneum can respond to a variety of packing techniques. Bleeding after prostatectomy may be controlled by a pressure pack deep in the fossa so as to halt residual oozing. The pack should be placed by a method that allows its painless atraumatic removal. A simple technique we have employed is to gently place warm, moist, 4 × 4 inch gauze pads firmly into the prostatic fossa for 15 to 20 minutes. A small no. 10 red rubber catheter is then passed through a no. 36 cystostomy tube and tied to a 1-inch iodoform gauze strip, which then replaces the previous plain gauze packs. A no. 24 Foley catheter with a 30-ml bag is passed into the bladder through the urethra. After the packing is distributed evenly, the balloon is inflated and pulled against the fossa, exerting additional pressure on the pack. The cystostomy tube with the small red rubber catheter in its lumen can be then used to irrigate the bladder postoperatively even in the presence of the pack. In 48 to 72 hours, the small catheter can be used to extract the gauze pack all through the lumen of the cystostomy tube, leaving the tube in place after deflating the urethral Foley balloon.[28]

Thin soft rubber dam draping is another material that can be packed into the prostatic fossa or perirenal areas; it is also easily removed with minimal trauma through a small opening of a drain site. Patients with tears in the renal parenchyma and expanding subcapsular hematomas in whom coagulopathy has developed are particularly good candidates for this rubber dam packing. Before this technique is applied, all active bleeding of identified large vessels must be stopped by direct ligation. In order to prevent subsequent sepsis, most of the packs should be removed within 48 to 60 hours after operation. The cavity should then be irrigated copiously and drained with soft Penrose drains through different drain sites to reduce the risks of sepsis.

Laparotomy pads are the most effective tamponading agent for retroperitoneal or perirenal hemorrhage. However, they require a second operation for removal. Such a second operation, however, has the added advantages of allowing further debridement of nonviable tissue, irrigation, and insertion of clean drains.[29]

In severe trauma, or for surgical procedures in the presence of a heretofore unrecognized coagulopathy, or for extensive bleeding from inoperable retroperitoneal tumor, packing techniques may save a patient's life and should not be looked on as a reflection of inadequate surgical skill. Walt[30] has stated, "The judicious surgeon who chooses this method should in no way fear the whispered loss of his surgical manhood."

10. G-Suits

Description of mechanical hemostatic adjuncts for traumatic or troublesome surgical bleeding would not be complete without a discussion of the G-suit or external circumferential counterpressure to control hemorrhage (see Chapters 10 and 11). The G-suit, a plastic inflatable envelope, applies external counterpressure in a circular manner by wrapping the abdomen and lower extremities starting at the costal margin. Pressure is regulated by a bubble valve at the outlet of the water column. For therapeutic purposes, the G-suit is inflated with air to a pressure of 20 to 30 cm of water during the period of hypotension before fluid and blood replacement begins. All patients are intubated with endotracheal tubes for ventilatory assistance since there is often interference with diaphragmatic excursion. The G-suit technique decreases the volume of a vascular bed and circulating blood below the diaphragm and redistributes it to the vitally important organs, such as the heart and the brain.

A select group of patients with diffuse bleeding from the retroperitoneum and pelvis may benefit from use of the G-suit if conventional surgical methods fail. It has been successful for short-term use preoperatively in patients with a ruptured aortic aneurysm. In this latter situation, there was an increased survival rate of 40% to 65% in patients waiting to be transported for mechanical control of the aorta.[31] The method is also ideal for control of pelvic bleeding after traumatic fractures in patients who are awaiting transport for angiographic occlusion of bleeding vessels.[32] It provides a smooth control for resuscitating a patient with an unstable pelvic fracture and offers a margin of safety while moving the patient at a time when severe hypotension or cardiac arrest has commonly been observed. Flint et al. achieved hemostasis in nine of ten patients with extensive pelvic fractures with no deaths by using the Jobst antishock trouser on the extremities and lower torso.[33]

The major complications of externally applied circumferential counterpressure involve the pulmonary system and skin. Atelectasis, pneumonia, and pulmonary edema with or without respiratory distress syndrome are common but can be diminished by positive pressure ventilatory assistance. The skin lesions usually seen are blistering and superficial pressure necrosis, which can be kept to a minimum by applying proper padding before applying the G-suit. Periods of external counterpressure greater than 24 hours greatly increase these skin complications. Generally this procedure should be employed only as a last resort in the control of pelvic and retroperitoneal bleeding, and only in desperate situations.

11. Absorbable, Topically Applied Hemostatic Agents

Urologic surgery consists, for the most part, of extirpative and reconstructive operations of the retroperitoneum and pelvis. These procedures create large, oozing, raw surfaces for which topically applied hemostatic agents may at times have their widest application.[34–36] These are not procoagulants in themselves but are a framework upon which the thrombus of platelets and fibrin settles. They play no role in primary arterial bleeding and are in no way a substitute for traditional hemostatic techniques. Their use is not intended to obviate the necessity for major vessel ligation or hemostatic sutures in renal or bladder surfaces. Their principal value is in diffuse surface bleeding where the material can come into contact with a large area very quickly or in renal artery reconstruction when hemostasis is needed during the first few minutes after restoration of blood flow from the anastomotic suture line. The most popular compounds employed are absorbable gelatin sponges (Gelfoam®), a gauze of oxidized regenerative cellulose (Surgicel®), and microfibrillar collagen or purified corium collagen (Avitene®).

A new product from Europe that has shown great promise as a topically applied hemostatic agent in renal surgery is fibrin sealant. However, it has not been used long enough to warrant its release in this country. It is a fibrinogen-thrombin solution that results in a fibrin polymer, which is strengthened by the addition of aprotinin, (an antifibrinolytic agent), factor XIII, and calcium chloride. When applied to the cut surfaces of liver, spleen, and kidney, this enhanced fibrin "glue" gives an excellent hemostatic effect and an adherent tissue bond without foreign body reaction.[34]

Gelfoam usually requires the addition of thrombin and does not adhere adequately to most bleeding surfaces. It has common usage in radiology as an embolic agent because of its convenience of administration in performing percutaneous angioinfarction. (See Chapter 8.)

Surgicel is the most common topical hemostatic compound used. It is prepared by dissolving pure cellulose or lint in an alkalized organic solvent and regenerating the cellulose as a continuous fiber, which is then knitted into gauze-like strips of various sizes and oxidized. The active resultant chemical in the gauze-like material is polyanhydroglucuronic acid, which is hydrolyzed by normal tissue. The material is easy to handle and does not adhere to gloves. It turns black when it comes in contact with blood because of its low pH, which produces acid hematin. The material becomes gelatinous, and controls bleeding by its adherence to tissue surfaces and by its acidic nature, which causes local fibrin deposition, platelet adherence, and vessel contraction. It produces very little foreign body reaction and is absorbed after several weeks. It must be applied to a dry surface under pressure to be effective. If the bleeding is not completely controlled after removal of pressure, then a second layer of this material and 10 minutes of sustained pressure is required. Surgicel is helpful when applied to a vascular anastomosis if it is applied carefully to the suture line using a wet gauze sponge while pressure is applied before the vascular clamps are released. This will control the oozing from the needle holes while the tension of the arterial pressure on the suture line stabilizes. Surgicel may also have some antibacterial activity against common bacterial pathogens by virtue of its low pH.

Avitene may be used as a single agent or may be combined with oxidized cellulose. This material is a water-soluble hydrochloric acid salt of collagen derived from bovine hide, and produced in submicron size. It is a fluffy, white, hydrophilic, flour-like powder or a cloth-like web. Its hemostatic effect is believed to be related to the known affinity of platelets for collagen and for its ability to initiate platelet aggregation and release. It forms a tenacious adhesive mass with these platelets and adheres very effectively to moist surfaces. It must be applied carefully in clumps using dry forceps and must be held in place using a dry surgical sponge. It must be applied quickly so as to prevent premature gelling in unclotted blood. It remains effective in the presence of heparin and thrombocytopenic states. It is an inert substance that is biodegradable and does not increase in size as it absorbs blood.[36]

The major drawback of Avitene is the difficulty in handling the material and in placing it on poorly exposed bleeding sites. These problems can be overcome on occasion by wrapping Avitene in an oxidized cellulose sheet and applying it to the bleeding area in a sandwich-like form. This is especially true for hemorrhage at a renal surface or in a parenchymal crevice created by external or surgical trauma.

B. Specific Problems

1. Splenic Bleeding

Splenic injury is unfortunately a common technical complication of left upper quadrant operations, where the urologic surgeons perform such procedures as radical nephrectomy, adrenalectomy, splenoral arterial bypass grafts, and removal of large retroperitoneal sarcomas. In the latter situation, splenic laceration is at times unavoidable. Splenic injury can also occur as capsular avulsion injuries during complacent mobilization of the omentum, during an exploratory evaluation of the left upper abdominal quadrant, and during the course of mobilization of the splenic flexure in construction of a transverse or sigmoid conduit. A poorly padded intraperitoneal or extraperitoneal abdominal retractor is the usual cause for the splenic injury. Also, rough, impatient handling of the spleen during radical transabdominal nephrectomy or adrenalectomy produces a 15–20% incidence of splenectomy in most well-recorded series.[37] Rarely a laceration develops during an extraperitoneal left renal procedure. This is particularly hazardous since it may go unrecognized and may be identified only after the patient has experienced significant loss of circulatory volume. Splenic tears may also occur during right nephrectomy with the patient in the lateral flank position. This is a result of compression from the elevated kidney bar on the contralateral side, and may also go as an unrecognized source of blood volume loss.

Management of these tears of the splenic surface and parenchymal tears has changed over the past decades from the inevitable splenectomy to the present, almost routine, practice of splenic repair.[38] This new approach is particularly compelling for younger patients where salvaging the spleen can reduce the risks linked to bacteremia. Minor capsular avulsion can be managed frequently by using topically applied hemostatic agents without mobilizing the entire spleen. A minor superficial laceration near the hilum, where suture repair is hazardous, is also a suitable situation for topically applied hemostatic agents. The most effective agent for splenic bleeding is oxidized cellulose wrapped around Avitene in a sandwich applied with continued external pressure. This requires careful application with dry instruments and should be pressed quickly with a dry sponge to the injured surface where it is held for a minimum of 10 minutes. This will form a firm flexible coagulum with good adherence and will effectively penetrate the interstices of the splenic parenchyma. If there is premature gelling of the cellulose-Avitene sandwich due to improper application, the coagulum is removed, and a fresh preparation is reapplied. More can be added to the first application. In superficial transverse lacerations in which sufficient capsule has been preserved, hemostasis may be effected by suturing the edges under slight pressure with a no. 3-0 chromic suture on an atraumatic fine needle. This is best accomplished by gently placing running locked sutures sited accurately at 0.5-cm intervals without exerting too much tension on the suture line. The keys to the successful repair of splenic tears are good exposure of the injury and gentle handling of suture material. The splenic parenchyma is readily capable of holding sutures.

Deep splenic lacerations may be treated by partial resection. The spleen is similar to the kidney in that it possesses a segmental circulation that permits excision of isolated fragments. This should be considered only in younger patients in whom complete isolation of the blood supply has been achieved and after all peritoneal and omental attachments have been separated. Still the risk of splenic salvage is appreciable, and splenectomy should be the primary approach in the older or poor-risk patient in whom an extensive injury has occurred. The risk of morbidity from such an injury outweighs that of future bacterial sepsis. Hemorrhage after splenectomy is rare in a normal-sized spleen. Hemorrhage, when it occurs, usually arises from the raw surface of the diaphragm or splenic bed, and less commonly from the surface of the pancreas or from a dislodged ligature. Obviously meticulous hemostasis of the splenic bed should be an integral part of all routine splenectomies.

2. *Retroperitoneal Hemorrhage*

The most common bleeding problems in urologic surgery occur during retroperitoneal and pelvic operations. Technically difficult procedures that not infrequently can lead to severe hemorrhage include excision of large renal and retroperitoneal tumors, secondary renal and ureteral procedures, partial nephrectomy, operations for staghorn calculi, renal trauma, renovascular reconstruction, and radical cystectomy and prostatectomy (Fig. 2). The most challenging technical procedure in urology is to operate on a kidney that has undergone numerous previous surgeries. These renal operations can involve all kinds of potential injuries to adjacent organs and serious uncontrolled hemorrhage if not performed in a most careful manner.

Adequate visualization and exposure can be achieved only with an appropriately generous incision that gives good access. The optimal incision should be extendable if the pathologic condition warrants, and should not be governed by any cosmetic factors. The approach chosen should allow medial access to the renal pedicle, adrenal gland, aorta, vena cava, and upper ureter. For most secondary renal surgery limited to the renal parenchyma and renal collecting system, the supracostal 11th interspace extraperitoneal incision with division of the costovertebral ligament and insertion of a large rib-spreading retractor is satisfactory. On occasion, the 9th interspace thoracoabdominal transdiaphragmatic incision is preferable, especially in the obese patient in whom the kidney is large, or where possible splenic or pancreatic injury may be incurred. This is especially true in patients with large left upper quadrant masses where the kidney may be located high under the diaphragm. Either incision, however, can be extended by division of the ipsilateral and contralateral rectus abdominis muscles to allow entry into the peritoneal cavity.

3. *The Previously Operated Kidney*

The previously operated kidney often lies subfascially and is at high risk of being lacerated during the initial exposure. Thus, mobilization requires sharp

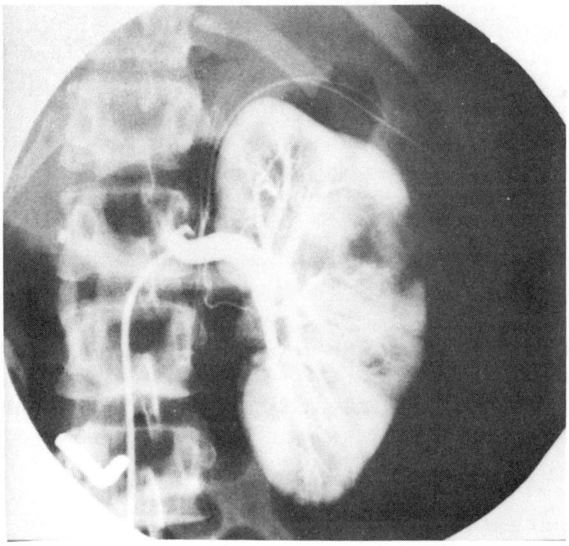

Figure 2: *Renal artery angiogram demonstrating a fractured kidney. (From the Learning File of the Center for Devices and Radiological Health, FDA, case GU608.)*

dissection of the scar tissue formed by Gerota's fascia, by sclerosed perirenal fat, and from the renal capsule on the one hand, and the lateral abdominal wall, posterior psoas, and quadratus fascia on the other. The minor bleeding that occurs here is usually limited to the collateral vessels and to the lacerated psoas muscle. This can be controlled easily with sponge compression. Both renal poles should be initially mobilized laterally where it is safe from the diaphragm to the lower renal margin. The peritoneum is usually loosely adherent and can be separated by blunt dissection at the lower medial portion of the kidney. The psoas muscle usually forms an avascular cleavage plane and, when followed, leads to the ureter and gonadal vessels. These vessels can at times bleed vigorously but are easy to control. The gonadal vessels should be ligated, and a large segment resected to avoid confusing them with the ureter. This approach also allows improved exposure of the ureteropelvic junction and aorta. In order to expose the renal pelvis, the ureter is followed proximally, dividing the surrounding scars, including those between the renal sinus and the parenchymal edge. By staying close to the renal pelvic wall, it is possible to avoid the overlying connective tissues with its plexus of veins. If the dissection is carried too far cephalad, the segmental branch of the posterior lower or midsagittal renal artery can be injured. The peritoneal fold of the right and left colon then must be identified by opening the peritoneal cavity in order to mobilize the remaining portion of the kidney. This maneuver also allows good exposure of the spleen, duodenum, vena cava, and mesenteric vessels, and simultaneously aids in developing exposure of the upper polar surfaces. Some peritoneum should be left on the renal surface in order to avoid disrupting the renal capsule. Disruption, when it occurs, can be a source of continued oozing. Exposure of the upper pole is also a hazardous dissection because the adjacent vascular structures can be injured readily. As an example, there is risk of adrenal laceration; however, this can be prevented by staying close to the rim of the renal surface. The angle between the psoas muscle, the diaphragm, and the renal vein, which covers the renal artery, is then exposed by lifting the upper renal pole outward to where it can be palpated dorsally and cephalad. It can then be detached from the diaphragm and the tenuous adrenal fascia. The maximal exposure is achieved at the surface of the incision by avoiding the cone effect which requires blind dissection in the areas adjacent to the renal pedicle, vena cava, and aorta. Unexpected hemorrhage may still occur from these sites despite having good access to these vessels. Thus, the surgeon should be prepared for each potential event by having available vascular forceps, fine-tipped needle holders, no. 5-0 and no. 6-0 vascular monofilament sutures, bulldog clamps for renal vessels, partial and total occlusion clamps for aorta and vena cava, umbilical tapes and Silastic loops, tourniquet clamps for veins, long Babcock and Allis clamps for vessel lacerations, a source for local hypothermia, a Cell Saver® (Haemonetics®, Inc, 400 Wood Road, Braintree, MA 02184) for autotransfusion, and soft-surface Fogarty clamps of various sizes.

Control of hemorrhage in this setting requires a calm, deliberate approach. Small lacerations or avulsions of the renal and adrenal veins can be managed by temporarily controlling the bleeding site with finger pressure. Vascular rents 4 to 5 mm long may be closed with vascular clips. Small openings in the vena cava or aorta should be secured with a Babcock clamp and closed with a running no. 5-0 or no. 6-0 vascular suture. Topical pressure will diminish or stop most bleeding while the surgeon is assessing the problem, improving lighting, and preparing the field with proper exposure. If small vessels, such as lumar or gonadal veins, retract from view leaving only part of the lumen visible, the edge of the vessel wall can be grasped with a long narrow hemostatic clamp and rotated. This maneuver twists the entire vessel so as to occlude the lumen, allowing the vessel to be ligated in a dry field.[39]

For larger rents in the renal vein, partial occlusion is desirable so that blood flow is not completely stopped. Repair then can be approximated with a large, long DeBakey forceps held by an assistant, an Allis or Babcock clamp, or a short-beak, right-angle clamp with a serrated atraumatic surface. The surgeon must avoid placing the needle through the fenestrated portion of the in-place Babcock clamp, fixing it to the vessel wall.

Arterial bleeding can be handled by gaining proximal and distal control of the vessel with atraumatic clamps or a Fogarty balloon placed in the lumen proximally and applying pressure distally. Lacerations in the renal artery can be secured with interrupted fine no. 6-0 sutures or by placing a venous patch so as to prevent compromise of the arterial lumen.

One of the most difficult aspects of secondary kidney operation is exposure of the renal pedicle. If the adhesions between the renal pelvis and the renal vein are dense, normal planes cannot be achieved. One must then concentrate on dissecting the renal artery, which usually is a palpable identifiable structure. Even though it may also be encased in adhesions, the thicker, tougher wall more readily allows separation from its contiguous structures. If neither structure can be isolated adequately, a large vascular clamp, such as a Satinsky or a DeBakey aortic clamp, should be used to cross-clamp the entire pedicle creating surgical ischemia.

When the secondary operation is for renal calculi, there may be a capacious renal pelvis. Here, mobilization of the ureter is best accomplished after placement of a palpable ureteral catheter by cytoscopy before exposing the retroperitoneum. The ureter is then followed carefully up to the renal pelvis where an avascular surface can usually be found on its posterior wall. Care must be taken to identify first the site of the pyelotomy by aspirating the renal pelvis in order to identify urine.

4. Renal and Adrenal Tumors

Neoplasms of the kidney and the adrenal gland are particularly prone to develop extensive engorged venous and arterial collateral vessels on their surface, often obliterating the normal avascular plane (Fig. 3). The larger the tumor the more extensive will be the neovascularity, and the more likely it is that extensive bleeding will be encountered during the initial portion of renal mobilization. Here the most important technical aspect in obtaining good anatomic control of bleeding is to have wide exposures and unimpeded access to the vena cava, aorta, and renal vessels. Inadequate limited incisions invite potential disasters in any operation for renal tumors. The renal pedicle can have a variety of anatomic configurations with renal tumor, depending on whether the tumor is located centrally, anteriorly, or is in polar position. The amount of perivascular fat and fibrous tissue and length of the pedicle will be major factors that can impede the safe isolation of each of the vessels.

In this situation, the best exposure of the renal artery is achieved by mobilizing the lower pole and the lateral portions of the upper pole, and by turning the kidney and its fatty envelope medially. This is especially useful when a

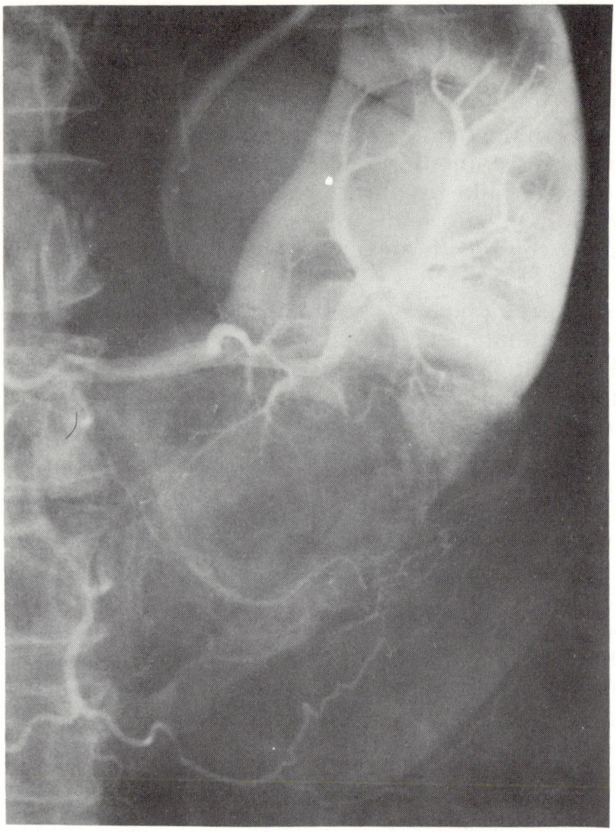

Figure 3: *Renal artery angiogram demonstrating extensive neovascularization surrounding a renal carcinoma. Multiple small arterial collateral vessels are seen.*

tumor is centrally and anteriorly located with shelf-like projection over the hilum. The vein is then anterior and the pelvis inferior to the posterior segmental branch, which is often the first artery thus identified. By following this vessel proximally, one can readily gain access to the main stem. In essence, this is a posterior approach allowing simultaneous exposure of the aorta and some of the medially located adrenal vessels on the left side. When on the right side, this posterior approach affords a good view of the posterior and lateral vena cava below the adrenal gland. Some of the lateral lymphatics can then be dissected from the surface of the vena cava and the aorta, and good control can be gained of the right lumbar veins.

The renal artery should be the first structure to be ligated for a nephrectomy, especially when the operation involves excision of a renal tumor. If there is an initial ligation of the renal vein, there will be a massive engorgement of the organ and tumor, followed by excessive bleeding from the renal surface. The artery should be ligated in continuity using a no. 0 silk ligature followed by a distal suture ligature of the same material after dividing the vessel. This will prevent delayed slipping of the ligature with attendant hemorrhage.

Rents in the renal artery can be produced during this dissection from tearing of small branches, from penetration of the tip of a needle during the application of a suture ligature, or by forcing the points of a right-angle clamp behind the vessel. In the event of any of these injuries, the bleeding can be controlled by compression with a proximally placed finger or sponge stick, or by lateral tangential partial occlusion with a Babcock clamp. Compression also can sometimes be achieved if both renal poles have been mobilized, and by compressing the proximal artery between the forefingers of both the right and left hands. The assistant can then sharply or bluntly dissect the vessel with the help of the end of a tonsil suction tip, or directly apply an atraumatic microvascular bulldog clamp. Small bulldog clamps gently applied proximally combined with a distal Silastic loop tourniquet ligature also can control the bleeding. Because the renal artery has a fragile intima, large clamps or rough handling of the vessel during the scramble to control the bleeding from the laceration can result in a traumatic thrombosis.

In the event the kidney is not being removed and a renal preserving procedure is being performed, the distal vessel should be irrigated copiously with a heparin solution of 10,000 U/L of saline. The edges of the vessel should be approximated meticulously using interrupted no. 6-0 monofilament sutures including full-thickness vessel wall. The intima must be identified if it has been separated and be incorporated into the closure. The arterial wall can be patched with autogenous vein when it appears that the renal arterial lumen will be compromised by a vertical arteriotomy closure.

An uncommon complication of nephrectomy for tumor occurs when the artery attains a disproportionately large size. Delayed hemorrhage can occur if the ligature has slipped away or cut through an arteriosclerotic wall. This may occur even after closure of the wound,[29] and this possibility must be taken into consideration when designing the arterial closure.

5. *Management of Pathologic Conditions of the Vena Cava*

The increasingly radical management of renal cell carcinomas involving the vena cava and testicular salvage surgery after chemotherapy have expanded the urologist's responsibility in operations of the infrahepatic and suprahepatic portions of the vena cava.[40–45] During the past two decades, a variety of aggressive surgical approaches have been adopted for removal of renal tumor thrombi. With improved preoperative methods of assessing the cranial extent of any tumor thrombus in the vena cava, the appropriate surgical procedure for recovery of the venous extension of the tumor can be planned and troublesome bleeding prevented. Procedures now used for extraction of vena caval tumor thrombus include cavotomy, partial mural cavectomy, segmental suprarenal cavectomy and atriotomy, usually in conjunction with cavotomy (Figs. 4, 5).

Cavotomy, the most widely used method for extracting tumor thrombus from the vena cava, consists of extending the caval incision from the renal vein orifice cephalad, and removing the free floating thrombus in continuity with the tumor. Partial mural cavectomy involves removing variable lengths of the lateral caval wall with attached thrombus and kidney en bloc followed by vascular reconstruction of the suprarenal portion of the vena cava leaving a narrow but patent lumen. In segmental cavectomy, a cylindric portion of the inferior vena cava is excised because it has been invaded by tumor. Successful suprarenal vena caval resections, except for two cases,[46] have been in patients with the

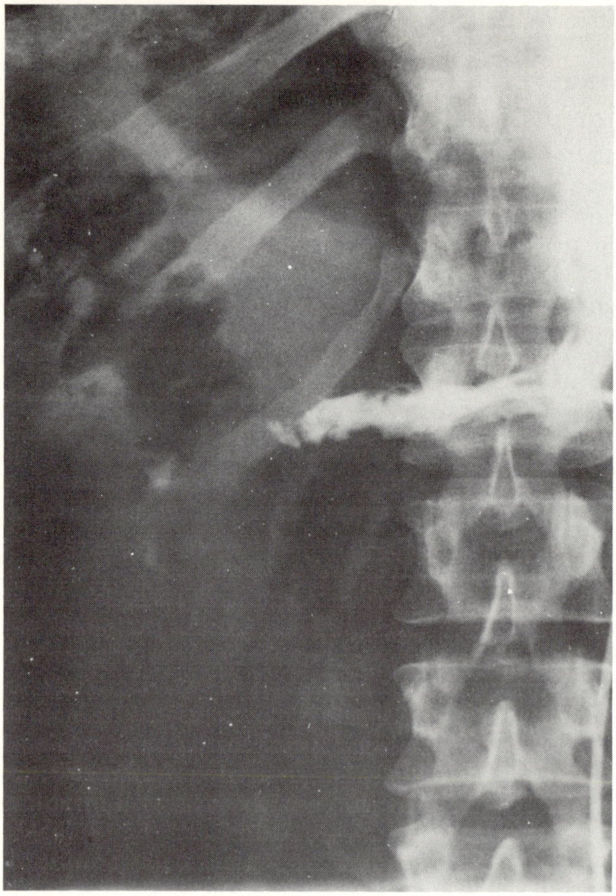

Figure 4: *Venogram of renal vein demonstrating tumor extending into the renal vein.*

tumor arising from the right kidney. The left kidney, unlike the right kidney, possesses alternate collateral vein pathways for return to the superior vena cava. Even segmental resection with removal of the right renal tumor and ligation of the left kidney renal vein has resulted in a few incidences of temporary renal shutdown necessitating dialysis and a more troublesome prolonged postoperative course.[41,47] Because this tumor rarely invades the wall of the vein, vena caval resection is seldom justified, and a major effort should be made to maintain a conduit between the left renal vein and the vena cava.

Blood losses incurred during dissection of a large renal tumor with simultaneous thrombectomy can be copious with reported figures[43,44] ranging from 1.5 to 15 L. The sources of blood loss include the cavotomy incision and the delicate perirenal retroperitoneal venous collaterals that are under high pressure and are vulnerable to lacerations. Much of this bleeding can be prevented by preliminary placement of vascular tourniquets on the infrarenal portion of the vena cava, the left renal vein, and the infrahepatic and suprahepatic portions of the vena cava in an unclamped state. Depending on the cephalad level of the

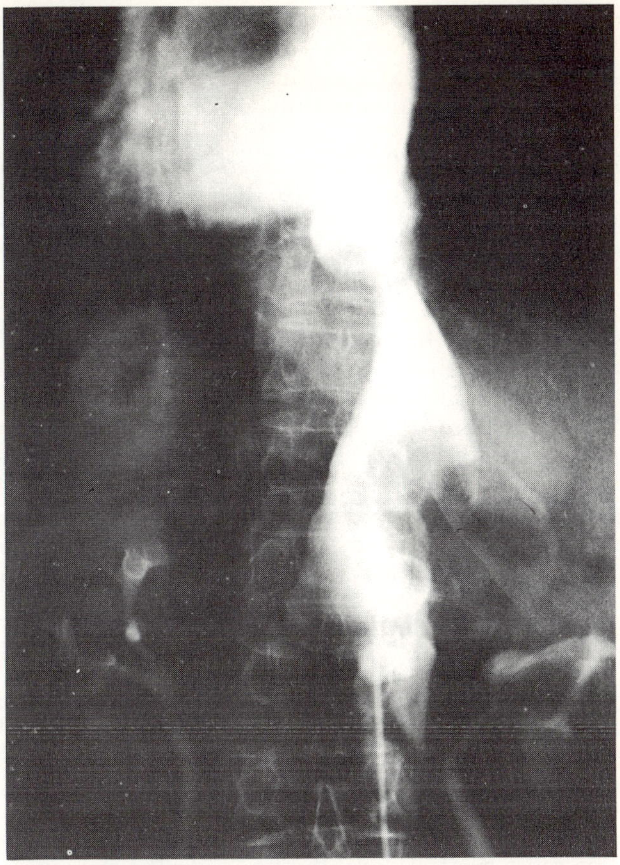

Figure 5: *Venogram of the vena cava demonstrating a bulky tumor extending from a renal carcinoma into the vena cava.*

tumor thrombus, a fenestrated clip or intracaval umbrella filter is placed before dissection begins to prevent pulmonary tumor emboli. The vena cava then is usually mobilized through a right thoracoabdominal or midsternal-splitting incision to provide optimal exposure.[48] Early ligation of the renal artery will usually diminish the bleeding from the perirenal venous collaterals and from the caval inflow derived from the tumor-bearing kidney. All branches of lumbar, gonadal, and adrenal veins are then secured after retracting the ascending colon, duodenum, and small bowel and pancreas, elevating them on the pedicle of the superior mesenteric artery. The four or five inferior minor tributaries of the hepatic vein are then ligated and divided so as to allow proximal placement of the tourniquet below the liver. This tourniquet will also help to block movement of dislodged embolic fragments. The kidney, its fascia, and adrenal and perihilar nodes then are detached leaving the renal vein and thrombus as the only structures still to be managed. If the thrombus extends into the retrohepatic or intracardiac portion of the vena cava, further hemostatic control will be required, including compression of the portal vein and hepatic artery in the porta hepatis by the Pringle maneuver, clamping of the superior mesenteric artery and the aorta, and placement of a Rummel tourniquet loosely around the intrathoracic inferior vena cava through a vertical pericardiotomy. For tumors on the left side, a soft Fogarty vascular clamp is placed on the right renal artery to avoid occluding the right renal vein.

The sequence of securing the vessels is important in order to prevent engorging the liver and the vena cava. The superior mesenteric artery and porta hepatis are clamped first, after which the Rummel tourniquets on the distal vena cava, contralateral renal vein, and intrathoracic cava are tightened, thus isolating the suprarenal vena cava segment from all venous inflow. At this point the splenic surface should be noted since by clamping the portal vein high intrasplenic venous pressures can be produced with possible rupture. This catastrophe can go unnoticed in patients with the right chest elevated. A vertical incision is made then in the anterolateral portion of the vena cava cephalad to allow inspection for the thrombus. A caudal and circumferential extension is made distal to the involved renal vein. If persistent troublesome bleeding from the liver occurs, a right-angle, long, soft Fogarty clamp sometimes can be placed across the pedicle of the hepatic vein in a retrohepatic position between the vena cava and the liver.[44] The tumor thrombus can then be extracted by blunt enucleation or dissection from the intima of the vein wall. If a Foley catheter is used to loosen the thrombus proximally, it can be left *in situ*, and the balloon is inflated to reduce bleeding. The patient should be placed in the head-down position during this maneuver to prevent subsequent air embolism. If the precavotomy trial of clamping of all these structures causes the blood pressure to fall and sufficient intravascular volume replacement is inadequate, the surgeon must resort to extracorporeal circulation.[45]

The principles described here for managing intracaval tumor thrombus also apply to excision of retroperitoneal tumors that are adherent to or compressing the vena cava. The inadvertent laceration of the vena caval wall or avulsion of venous tributaries are potential complications of all extensive retroperitoneal dissections even in the hands of the most skilled surgical anatomist. Again, it is good to gain proximal and distal control of the segment of the vena cava involved. Careful dissection in the proper tissue planes at some distance from the tumor or inflammatory condition are important factors in preventing uncontrolled bleeding. It is particularly important to be very gentle with dissection of the thin-walled tributary branches and to have a detailed understanding of the normal and the anomalous anatomies of the region between the right gonadal vein and the diaphragm. The lumbar veins on the posterolateral aspect and those veins entering the left renal vein or entering the vena cava near the origin of the right renal vein are the common locations for creating troublesome vena caval lacerations. When removing tumor thrombi or large tumors, these tributaries should be ligated in continuity with silk ligature and carefully divided between ligatures leaving sizable proximal and distal stumps. No greater challenge exists in surgical hemostasis then dissection of suprahilar vena caval structures involved with neoplasm.

6. Renal Artery Reconstruction

Surgery for renovascular hypertension constitutes a major challenge in surgical hemostasis. To prevent bleeding during management of the renal artery requires an adequate incision so as to avoid the cone effect that occurs following the standard flank or midline abdominal approaches. It is necessary to have easy access to the proximal main renal artery, aorta, and the vena cava above the renal veins in order to have good hemostatic control. A transverse incision from the lateral borders of the contralateral rectus muscle extending across the midline into the ipsilateral flank between the 11th and 12th ribs provides adequate access and greater technical freedom to the high-lying retroperitoneal aortorenal junctions. The pedicle and great vessels are exposed by reflecting the colon and duodenum after incising the lateral peritoneal gutter. The cecum, hepatic flexure, and small bowel are then elevated on the right side, and the splenic flexure and descending colon are raised on the left side. Gerota's fascia is not entered so as not to disturb the collateral circulation, which affords protection of the kidney during long ischemic periods.

Bleeding may be troublesome during the dissection of the hilar fat due to the large collateral vessels that are uniquely present in chronic occlusive renal artery disease. As exposure of the artery progresses, meticulous control of these structures with clips and ligatures is necessary. Heparin should not be administered until the dissection is complete, thus preventing extensive hemorrhagic oozing from the perihilar vessels.

The extent of the dissection depends largely on the type of reconstructive procedure required. Bypass techniques require less exposure of the hazardous suprarenal portion of the aorta, while transaortic endarterectomy requires large exposure to insure suprarenal control, and this may invite potentially serious injury to the inaccessible lumbar vessels. Serious bleeding from a disrupted anastomosis is fortunately a rarely reported event and is usually associated with approximation of a diseased vessel or with an error in surgical technique. The use of monofilament polypropylene sutures in renal and aortic anastomoses has helped to avoid bleeding from suture lines in the presence of systemic heparinization.[49]

False aneurysms may occur at the site of any vascular anastomosis, including those involving the renal arteries.[50] They result in the intermittent, delayed, and often life-threatening hemorrhage into the gastrointestinal tract or retroperitoneal space. The likelihood of this complication occurring is minimized by giving meticulous attention to the anastomosis, by avoiding silk suture lines, and by using an end-to-side or end-to-end tension-free graft onto a normal undiseased portion of the renal artery. On rare occasions after a splenorenal bypass graft when pancreatic injury has liberated digestive enzymes over the anastomosis, there has been a delayed arterial leak. Delayed bleeding also has been reported[50] from an aortoduodenal erosive fistula after the placement of a prosthetic bypass graft between the aorta and the right renal artery. This kind of intestinal hemorrhage is most likely to occur in prosthetic replacements when silk sutures are used. The most common site for this bleeding is in the third portion of the duodenum, which often lies on the proximal aortic anastomosis. This type of complication can be prevented by using autogenous graft material with synthetic sutures and by interposing a portion of the peritoneum or omentum between the graft and the duodenum.

7. Intrarenal Cortical Incisions

Intrarenal parenchymal operations for calculi and other localized conditions require a spectrum of cortical incisions that become a potential source of intraoperative and postoperative hemorrhage. Partial nephrectomy is the most common renal parenchymal procedure performed and is primarily employed for calculus disease and a lower abnormal calix, an abnormal duplicated collecting system with damaged parenchyma, renal trauma with destroyed segments, vascular abnormalities, or renal cell carcinoma in association with a solitary kidney or bilateral tumors. A variety of techniques are employed depending on the pathologic condition, but they are all designed to remove abnormal tissue while achieving good hemostasis of the remaining cortical surface.

For these procedures, the kidney is completely mobilized and the hilum and polar vessels are carefully identified. If a polar resection is planned, the vessel going to that pole is ligated and the avascular area is identified by injecting the distal portion with methylene blue dye (Fig. 6). This ensures that no necrotic tissue is left behind after the resection. The main renal artery is mobilized and a soft gentle Silastic loop is placed around it in the event of uncontrolled hemorrhage. The capsule is then stripped back and a transverse resection of the pole of the kidney is achieved with a sharp guillotine type of incision through the parenchyma proximal to the diseased portion.

Hemostasis is achieved by an assistant applying broad pressure to the kidney between thumb and forefinger while the surgeon places fine shallow figure-of-eight sutures on the pulsating cut vessels. Open veins require less suturing if the pedicle is unobstructed. The cut edge of the parenchyma is then closed by bringing forward the previously peeled-back capsular flaps and holding them in place with horizontal mattress sutures.[51] If the cortical edge is still oozing, the main renal artery is temporarily clamped with a soft noncrushing clamp to stop the bleeding, and the cut surface is carefully scrutinized for open vessels. Placing a free fragment of fat from Gerota's fatty capsule onto the exposed cortex may aid hemostasis in partial resections for tumor when the capsule has been sacrificed and when surface compression is difficult to

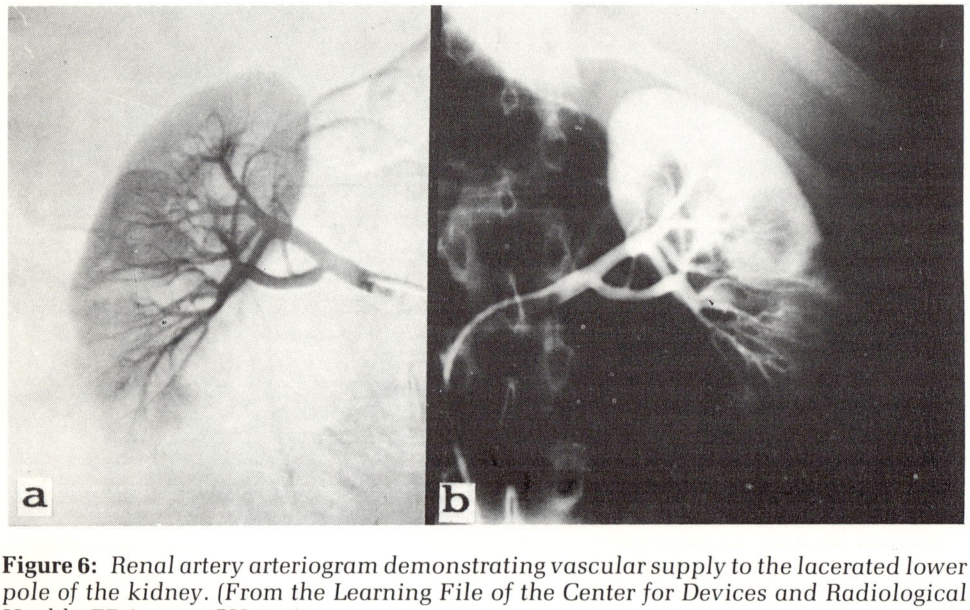

Figure 6: *Renal artery arteriogram demonstrating vascular supply to the lacerated lower pole of the kidney. (From the Learning File of the Center for Devices and Radiological Health, FDA, case GU609.)*

achieve. Horizontal mattress sutures are essential for good hemostasis in a midsegmental partial nephrectomy or with polar resections for tumor. Here the hilar structures must be dissected before only parenchymal incisions are made. This is necessary in order to identify the arterial branches so that no cortical sutures inadvertently trap any vital segmental blood flow. These procedures require complete ischemia using safe atraumatic main stem arterial clamp and external hypothermia to achieve a blood-free field and to protect hilar vessels during cortical incisions.

Midsagittal resections require especially meticulous suture ligation of the arcuate vessels on the cut surface because there is almost no tamponade effect from surrounding tissue after closure of the wound. In resecting a large midrenal tumor in a patient with a solitary kidney and complex arteriovenous malformations, long periods of ischemia are required for good hemostatic control. Resection should be carried out on the bench with extracorporeal reconstruction to achieve ideal exposure and well-controlled intrarenal hypothermia. The kidney can then be autotransplanted into the iliac fossa after the disease has been managed with a good renal salvage.

III. Conclusion

Performing surgery of the upper urinary tract and the retroperitoneal spaces is an invitation to potentially serious bleeding. An adequate well-planned exposure for the pathologic condition involved, a detailed knowledge of the regional anatomy and its variations, a careful gentle dissection of the major vessels, and a calm disposition of the surgeon are the critical factors in preventing intraoperative hemorrhage. Nevertheless, unexpected bleeding is at times unavoidable. The urologic surgeon should have well-thought out methods for managing hemorrhage during each procedure. Temporary control with gauze packs, sponge sticks, or the surgeon's finger should be the initial steps in the control of serious hemorrhage. The surgeon should communicate with the anesthesiologist who must replace the blood already lost and forewarn the blood bank of future needs. The surgeon is then obligated to improve exposure of the bleeding site, dissect out the vessel(s) involved, obtain any additional necessary lighting and suction equipment, and call for a colleague to help secure the vascular rent while applying continued proximal and distal tamponade. Because serious intraoperative hemorrhage can be encountered by even the most skilled surgeon, consultation with an experienced colleague should be looked on as an integral part of the armamentarium in the optimal care of the urologic patient.

References

1. Paul of Aegina. *The Seven Books of Paulus Aeginega*. Vol. 2, book 6, section 84. Adams F (trans.). London, Sydenham Society, 1846, p. 409.
2. Pare A, cited by Thompson J. *Lectures on Inflammation*. 2nd ed. (American). Philadelphia, Carey & Lea, 1831.
3. Zimmerman L, Veith I. *Great Ideas in the History of Surgery*. Baltimore, Williams & Wilkins Co., 1961, pp. 130–134.

4. Hickman GA, Mortenson JD. A comparative evaluation of vascular clamps. *J Thorac Cardiovasc Surg.* 44:561–569, 1962.
5. Henson GF, Rob CG. A comparative study of the effects of different arterial clamps on the vessel wall. *Br J Surg.* 43:561–569, 1956.
6. Fogarty TJ, Raible DA, Krippaehne WW. A new vascular clamp. *Am J Surg.* 112:967–968, 1966.
7. Banowsky LH. Basic principles and techniques of vascular surgery. In: *Vascular Problems in Urologic Surgery.* Novick AC, Straffon RA, Eds. Philadelphia, WB Saunders Co., 1982, pp. 3–15.
8. Baker JD. A simple method for atraumatic control of small vessels. *Am J Surg.* 38:336–337, 1979.
9. Cushing H. The control of bleeding in operations for brain tumors: With the description of silver "clips" for the occlusion of vessels inaccessible to the ligature. *Ann Surg.* 54:1–19, 1911.
10. Samuels PB, Roedling H, Katz R, Cincotti JJ. A new hemostatic clip: 2-year review of 1007 cases. *Ann Surg.* 163:427–431, 1966.
11. Reynolds W Jr.. Metal clip techniques utilizing pistol grip appliers. *Am J Surg.* 143:274–276, 1982.
12. Geelhoed GW. Radiopaque clips: The special applications. *Contemp Surg.* 11(3):9–14, 1977.
13. Helmkamp BF, Beecham JB, Knauf SS. Diaphragmatic peritoneal biopsy. *Surg Gynecol Obstet.* 157:372–373, 1983.
14. Marks WM, Callen PW. Computed tomography in the evaluation of patients with surgical clips. *Surg Gynecol Obstet.* 151:557–558, 1980.
15. Schaefer CJ, Colombani PM, Geelhoed GW. Absorbable ligating clips. *Surg Gynecol Obstet.* 154:513–516, 1982.
16. Foster JH, Morgan CV, Threlkel JB. Proximal control of aorta with a balloon catheter. *Surg Gynecol Obstet.* 132:693–694, 1971.
17. Thomas TV. Control of bleeding in complicated peripheral vascular lesions. *Surg Gynecol Obstet.* 132:1015–1018, 1971.
18. Monro JL, Weaver EJM. A use for the Fogarty embolectomy catheter in hemostasis. *J Thorac Cardiovasc Surg.* 65:897–898, 1973.
19. Pollock AV, Evans M. Surgical-wound sepsis and methods of hemostasis. Letter. *N Engl J Med.* 302:970,1980.
20. Arnot RS, Evans M, Pollock AV. The influence of two methods of haemostasis on the rate of wound sepsis: A random controlled trial of ligature and diathermy, abstracted. *Br J Surg.* 62:655, 1975.
21. Neufeld GR. Principles and hazards of electrosurgery including laparoscopy. *Surg Gynecol Obstet.* 147:705–710, 1978.
22. Flachenecker G, Fastenmeier K. Die Transurethrale Prostataresektion mit Hochfrequenzstromen aus elektrotechnischer Sichte. *Urologe* [A]. 15:167–172, 1976.
23. Ning TC, Jr., Atkins DM, Murphy RC. Bladder explosions during transurethral surgery. *J. Urol.* 114:536–539, 1975.
24. Fidler JP. Technology of laser burn surgery. In: *The Biomedical Laser.* Goldman L, Ed. New York, Springer-Verlag, 1981, pp. 199–218.
25. Slutzki S, Shafir R, Bornstein LA. Use of the carbon dioxide laser for large excisions with minimal blood loss. *Plast Reconst Surg.* 60:250–255, 1977.
26. Hodgson WJB, Poddar PK, Mencer EJ, Williams J, Drew M, McElhinney AJ. Evaluation of ultrasonically powered instruments in the laboratory and in the clinical setting. *Am J Gastroenterol.* 712:133–140, 1979.
27. Putnam CW. Techniques of ultrasonic dissection in resection of the liver. *Surg Gynecol Obstet.* 157:475–478, 1983.
28. Grabstald H. Prostatic fossa packing via cystostomy tube: An aid to hemostasis in selected cases. *J Urol.* 103:200–201, 1970.
29. Feliciano DV, Mattox KL, Jordan GL, Jr. Intra-abdominal packing for control of hepatic hemorrhage: A reappraisal. *J Trauma.* 21:285–290, 1981.

30. Walt AJ. The mythology of hepatic trauma—or Babel revisited. *Am J Surg.* 135:12–18, 1978.
31. Burdick JF, Warshaw AL, Abbot WM. External counterpressure to control postoperative intra-abdominal hemorrhage. *Am J Surg.* 129:369–373, 1975.
32. McLaughlin AP III, McCullough DL, Kerr WS Jr., Darling RC. The use of external counterpressure (G-suit) in the management of traumatic retroperitoneal hemorrhage. *J Urol.* 107:940–944, 1972.
33. Flint LM Jr, Brown A, Richardson JD, Polk HC. Definitive control of bleeding from severe pelvic fractures. *Ann Surg.* 189:709, 1979.
34. Brands W, Haselberger J, Mennicken C, Hoerst M. Treatment of ruptured kidney by gluing with highly concentrated human fibrinogen. *J Pediatr Surg.* 18:611–613, 1983.
35. Wahlstrom E, Yadegar J, Amodeo P, O'Connell M, Morgenstern L. Comparative tissue reactivity to topical hemostatic agents in the periureteral area. *Arch Surg.* 118:1375–1377, 1983.
36. Morgenstern L, Michel SL, Austin E. Control of hepatic bleeding with microfibrillar collagen. *Arch Surg.* 112:941–943, 1977.
37. Swanson DA, Borges PM. Complications of transabdominal radical nephrectomy for renal cell carcinoma. *J Urol.* 129:704–707, 1983.
38. Cooper MJ, Williamson RCN. Splenectomy: Indications, hazards and alternatives. *Br J Surg.* 71:173–180, 1984.
39. Novick AC, Straffon RA (eds). *Vascular Problems in Urologic Surgery.* Philadelphia, WB Saunders Co, 1982.
40. McCullough DL, Gittes RF. Vena cava resection for renal cell carcinoma. *J Urol.* 112:162–167, 1974.
41. Cherrie RJ, Goldman DG, Lindner A, de Kernion JB. Prognostic implications of vena caval extension of renal cell carcinoma. *J Urol.* 128:910–912, 1982.
42. Clayman RV, Gonzalez R, Fraley EE. Renal cell cancer invading the inferior vena cava. Clinical review and anatomical approach. *J Urol.* 123:157, 1980.
43. Beck AD. Renal cell carcinoma involving the inferior vena cava. Radiologic evaluation and surgical management. *J Urol.* 118:533–537, 1977.
44. Bihrle R, Libertino JA. Renal cell cancer with extension into the vena cava. In: *Renal Cell Cancer.* de Kernion J, Ed. Baltimore, Williams & Wilkins Co. (In press).
45. Lieskovsky G, Pritchett R, Skinner DG. Surgical management of renal cell carcinoma. *Monogr Urol.* 5:98–125, 1984.
46. Schechter DC. Cardiovascular surgery in the management of malignant renal neoplasms: Survey of 187 cases in the literature. *Tex Heart Inst J.* 10:163–175, 1983.
47. Alexander F, Zinman LN, Braasch JW. Safe division of the renal vein with a solitary left kidney. *Surgery.* 93:598–599, 1983.
48. Libertino JA, Zinman L. Surgery for renovascular hypertension. In: *Renovascular Hypertension.* Breslin DJ, Swinton NW Jr. Libertino JA, Zinman L, Eds. Baltimore, Williams & Wilkins Co., 1982, pp. 166–212.
49. Nerstrom B, Engell HC. Operative treatment of renovascular hypertension: A study of 60 consecutive patients with follow-up findings between 1 and 7 years postoperatively. *Ann Surg.* 176:590–596, 1972.
50. Cerney JC, Fry WJ, Gambee J. Koyanki T. Aorto-duodenal fistula. *J Urol.* 107:12–14, 1972.
51. Montie JE. Partial nephrectomy. In: *Vascular Problems in Urologic Surgery.* Novick AC, Straffon RA, Eds. Philadelphia, WB Saunders Co., 1982, pp. 109–115.

Chapter 10

Management of Intractable Bladder Hemorrhage

H. David Mitcheson, M.D., and Martin Schiff, Jr., M.D.

I. Introduction

The major causes of prolonged intractable, life-threatening hemorrhage from the urinary bladder are radiation-induced cystitis, cyclophosphamide-induced cystitis, neoplasms, and patients with bleeding or clotting disorders who require bladder surgery. Interstitial cystitis, amyloidosis, and purpura or telangiectasis affecting the bladder are rare causes of such bleeding. Infection-induced cystitis causes bleeding that is usually quite easily managed, but on rare occasions it can be difficult to control. Hematuria is judged to be significant and requires control if it necessitates hospitalization or blood transfusion or if it persists for more than 24 hours.

Hemorrhage from these causes is difficult to manage and it is often necessary to use several of a variety of techniques to achieve control. These techniques are applicable to bleeding due to any of the aforementioned causes. This chapter will concentrate on the methods that can be used, and when and in which order to apply them.

Hemorrhage due to acute trauma is managed in a quite different way. Hemorrhage from the bladder without bladder or urethral disruption can usually be managed with Foley catheter drainage and bladder irrigation. Hemorrhage associated with bladder rupture or urethral disruption demands surgical intervention and the bleeding is usually readily controlled. The techniques described in this chapter are rarely needed in the management of this type of bleeding. For a full discussion of the management of hemorrhage due to acute trauma, please see Chapters 8 and 9.

From Bern MM (ed.): *Urinary Tract Bleeding: Diagnosis and Control by Medical, Radiologic, and Surgical Techniques*. Mount Kisco, NY, Futura Publishing Co., Inc., 1985.

II. Immediate Treatment of Intractable Bladder Hemorrhage

The patient's vital signs are recorded and good intravenous access obtained. Serum is sent to the blood bank for cross-matching and crystalloid solutions are infused at an appropriate rate. Plasma is sent for determination of the hemoglobin, hematocrit, white cell count, platelet count, prothrombin time, partial thromboplastin time, creatinine, and blood urea nitrogen. If the bladder is distended, a 22 Fr. Foley catheter is inserted, the bladder irrigated with saline to remove as many clots as possible, and the catheter is placed to straight drainage. A three-way catheter with continuous bladder irrigation may be used if desired. Often the clots are tenacious or organized, cannot be removed in this fashion, and may require insertion of a cystoscope or resectoscope sheath to facilitate their removal. If there is severe bladder pain, intramuscular analgesics should be given. The urine sediment should be gram-stained and examined under the microscope and the urine cultured. Blood should be transfused as clinically indicated.

III. Diagnosis

The diagnosis of the cause of the bleeding may be suggested by the history—for example, if there has been radiation treatment to the bladder, uterus, or cervix, or by previous treatment with cyclophosphamide. Bleeding or clotting disorders should be revealed by the coagulation screen. Acute bacterial cystitis will be detected by urinalysis and culture. Tuberculous cystitis must be considerd when sterile pyuria exists. Cystoscopy should be performed and general or spinal anesthesia should be used.

A. Cystoscopy

Evacuation of a Clot

A large cystoscope (24 Fr.) or resectoscope sheath should be inserted into the bladder and the bladder examined. All blood clots must be removed and their total removal must be confirmed by inspection. This is for two reasons. First, the bladder cannot be adequately examined if part is obscured by clot. Second, residual clot will prevent complete contraction of the bladder, thus inhibiting the vasoconstriction element of hemostasis and thereby predisposing to subsequent recurrent bleeding. The blood clot is often extremely tenacious and it may be laminated and adherent. Such clot will not be removed by simple irrigation and it is necessary to break up the clot by a combination of maneuvers. The beak of the sheath can be used to tease the clot or the resectoscope loop can be used to disrupt it. The clot can be broken up hydrodynamically using an Ellik's evacuator or a catheter-tipped glass Toomey syringe. The optimal method of syringing is to fill the bladder with about 200 ml of saline if the capacity is normal and, using a 60 ml syringe full of saline, repeatedly inject and withdraw about 40 ml of fluid in a rapid push-pull fashion.

B. Cystoscopic Appearance and Histologic Changes

1. *Radiation-induced Cystitis*

Radiation-induced cystitis can occur in three stages. The first is primary erythema occurring within 24 hours of the treatment. The second is secondary erythema appearing within 3 or 4 weeks. The third is the most common and occurs at any time between 3 months and 10 years after radiation. The early stages are characterized by bullous edema, hyperemia, and epithelial desquamation. In the late reaction, there is induration of the bladder wall, reduction of luminal capacity, and encrustation of the mucosa with salts (the "Panzerblase" of German authors). Raspberry-like granulations radiating tortuous ectatic blood vessels may be seen. The surrounding mucosa may be blanched and ischemic, or may be hyperemic. Ulcers may occur and are sharply outlined, surrounded by bullous edema and radiating the same tortuous blood vessels.

These changes may occur regardless of whether the bladder is the primary target of radiation therapy or incidentally included in the field of radiation. The histologic features of acute radiation change in the normal bladder incidentally included in the field of radiation are seen in the epithelium and in the stroma (Fig. 1). The epithelial cells show variable enlargement accompanied by nuclear enlargement and pyknosis. The stroma is markedly edematous and contains giant fibroblasts. The latter may become multinucleated and are probably the basis for the diagnosis of "giant cell cystitis." With the passage of time following completion of radiotherapy, the changes subside but may never vanish com-

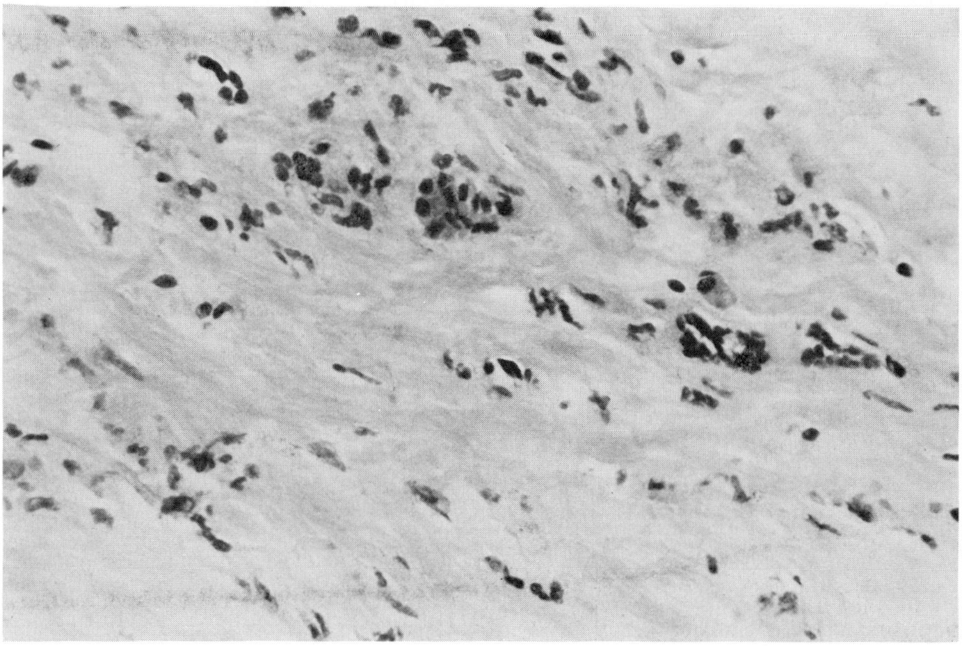

Figure 1: *Radiation cystitis showing subendothelial edema and a perivascular inflammatory reaction (original magnification × 400).*

pletely. Shields Warren[1] stated that the bladder epithelium is moderately resistant to ionizing radiation and is able to withstand up to 8,400 rads in divided doses. However, the incidence of late radiation-induced cystitis reportedly ranges between 3% and 12% in patients who received pelvic irradiation,[2,3] and because late complications can present up to 10 years after the irradiation, this is probably an underestimate since some patients presumably died before developing late complications. Pool[4] commented that there was no correlation between the irradiation dose and the intensity of the bladder reaction, but he opined that small doses of irradition administered over a longer time were less likely to cause a reaction than larger doses administered over a shorter time.

2. *Cyclophosphamide-induced Cystitis*

The alkylating agent, cyclophosphamide, has a major effect on the bladder. It can cause a hemorrhagic cystitis with marked bullous edema of the mucosa, generally increased vascularity, areas of telangiectasia, and multiple areas of hemorrhage. The urinary sediment may contain abnormal cells in large numbers and their differentiation from cancer cells may be extremely difficult. Significant epithelial abnormalities in the form of nuclear enlargement and hyperchromasia may be observed in the biopsies. The effects of cyclophosphamide have been reproduced experimentally in rats and dogs; the drug causes necrosis of bladder epithelium followed by an atypical regeneration hyperplasia. The latter is the source of the markedly atypical cells observed in the urinary sediment. Cyclophosphamide can also cause necrosis of the smooth muscle of the bladder. Fibrosis of the bladder wall resulting in a sharp curtailment of bladder capacity is probably the result of repair of the damaged muscle. The incidence of bladder toxicity following cyclophosphamide treatment has been reported to be between 2% and 40%.[5] Oppers and Gerhartz[5] stated that the increasing use of high doses of cyclophosphamide has been accompanied by instances of massive hemorrhage, which may be far worse than the degree of hemorrhage more commonly seen with prolonged courses of low-dose cyclophosphamide. In every case of hematuria, during cyclophosphamide therapy distinction should be made between acute transient cystitis and bladder wall fibrosis. This can be done during cystoscopy under anesthesia by measuring the capacity of the bladder and by observing the mucosal appearances. The acute hemorrhagic cystitis usually clears if treatment is stopped. Bladder wall fibrosis is irreversible. Johnson and Meadows[6] found that bladders exhibiting the most advanced fibrosis were from patients who had received the largest quantities of cyclophosphamide. However, bladders exhibiting moderate but definite fibrosis were from patients who had received little more total quantity of cyclophosphamide than many others in whom bladder fibrosis did not occur. In a series of 50 children treated with a combination of pelvic irradiation and cyclophosphamide, Kumar et al.[3] found that 17 (34%) had bladder toxicity. Eight of the 17 had transient hematuria and dysuria, which cleared completely after the treatment was stopped. Nine had chronic or intermittent hematuria. No relationship was found between the total amount of therapy and the development of severe hematuria. Acute hemorrhagic cystitis usually clears when treatment is stopped and drug administration can be safely reinstated later. Patients with chronic bladder toxicity can continue to receive treatment with cyclophosphamide but full protective measures must be taken. These are diuresis and frequent voiding or bladder drainage (details are given below). It would seem sensible to use these precautions in all patients treated with cyclophosphamide.

Prevention of Cyclophosphamide-Induced Hemorrhagic Cystitis: The occurrence of hemorrhagic cystitis with the use of high-dose cyclophosphamide is thought to be a toxic effect of cyclophosphamide metabolites directly on the bladder mucosa.[7] To decrease both the concentration of metabolites in contact with the bladder mucosa and the time of such contact, Droller et al.[8] instituted a regimen of diuresis and frequent voiding, or indwelling catheterization, with a dramatic decrease in the incidence of hemorrhage. The diuresis was produced by intravenous infusion of 4–5 liters of D5/0.5 NS with 20 mEq KC1 every 24 hours beginning 24 hours before infusion of cyclophosphamide. Urine output was maintained at 150–200 ml/hour, using furosemide if necessary. Patients voided every hour, even at night. A catheter was placed if there was evidence of residual urine.

Acetylcysteine irrigation of the bladder of patients has also been employed to control cyclophosphamide-induced cystitis,[9] but it appears to be no more effective than the regimen of diuresis and frequent voiding.

3. *Neoplasms*

Neoplasms may be intrinsic to the bladder (Fig. 2) or encroach the bladder from the prostate, uterus, cervix, or rectum. Muscle involvement causes a

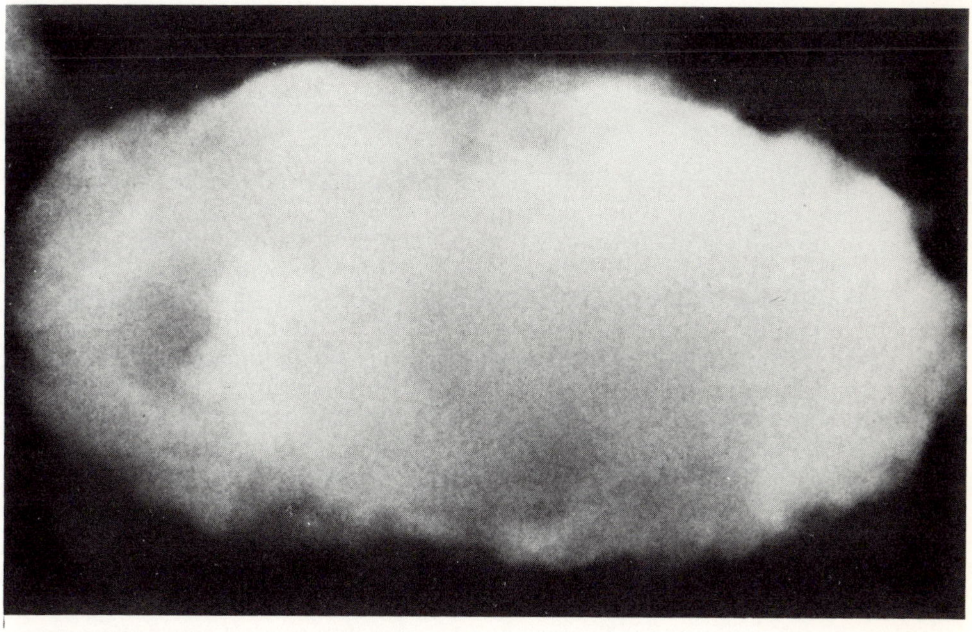

Figure 2: *Intravenous pyelogram x-ray depicting the bladder from a patient with recurrent bladder tumor following definitive radiation for an original primary tumor several years previously. The bladder is small and contracted and shows an area of poor filling at the bladder base and right lateral wall.*

reduced luminal capacity. The cytoscopic appearances vary from the obvious papillary or sessile tumor to the inflammation, hypervascularity, and bullous edema of a carcinoma-in-situ or extrinsic invading growth. Tumor necrosis with ulceration may occur. The massive bleeding that occurs in tumor patients is often after radiation treatment and the cystoscopic appearances can be a combination of tumor recurrence and radiation changes. The histologic features of the effect of radiation on invasive cancer of the bladder comprise necrosis and sometimes a giant cell reaction of foreign body type. It can be extremely difficult to differentiate radiation effect and persistent or recurrent tumor either by gross or histologic appearances. In such a situation, cystologic examination of the urinary sediment may be most helpful. After the acute radiation effect has abated, the presence of cancer cells in the urinary sediment indicates the presence of persistent or recurrent bladder cancer.

4. *Bleeding and Clotting Disorders*

Hemophilia and Christmas disease occur almost invariably in males, while other disorders such as hereditary hemorrhagic thrombasthenia can occur in either sex. Severe intractable hematuria can occur in these patients after surgery, accidental trauma, infection, or even without any apparent precipitating cause. Most patients will have had previous problems but for some this might be the initial presentation. Detailed and precise assessment of the appropriate defect is needed and this demands the services of an expert hematological laboratory. Once known, the appropriate treatment can be given. Even with the appropriate treatment, the control of hematuria in these patients is difficult and will usually require the use of the methods described in this chapter (see Chapters 1 and 2).

5. *Interstitial Cystitis*

Patients with interstitial cystitis usually present with intermittent or continuous suprapubic or retropubic pain of long-standing, and urinary frequency, dysuria, or hematuria occurring in the absence of demonstrable urinary tract infection. At cystoscopy, findings include erythematous areas that blanch or split during filling, linear scarring, ulceration, and free or petechial bleeding. The petechiae may sometimes be seen when the bladder is first examined but more often become apparent when the bladder is distended, subsequently emptied, and then refilled. The histological features in early cases are edema and an inflammatory infiltrate punctuated by prominent numbers of mast cells. In late cases, ulceration (Hunner's ulcers) and bladder wall fibrosis with diminished bladder capacity are common. Hematuria in interstitial cystitis is usually mild, rarely heavy, but it is often resistant to treatment.

6. *Amyloidosis*

Amyloidosis is a rare disease characterized by the extracellular deposition of a homogenous eosinophilic fibrillar protein in various tissues. Both primary and secondary amyloidosis can involve the lower genitourinary tract. Primary amyloidosis occurs de novo in the absence of chronic disease and can either be of the systemic form with multiple organs involved or be localized to one organ. Secondary amyloidosis is found in association with chronic granulomatous disease, rheumatoid arthritis, decubitus ulcers, multiple myeloma, and other tumors. McDonald and Heckel[10] reviewed 11 cases of primary amyloidosis affecting the bladder. The cystoscopic findings are of a solid circumscribed elevated sessile mass with a hemorrhagic irregular surface oozing blood. Mucosal ulceration can occur. Almost invariably the mass appears as an infiltrating neoplasm. The histologic findings are of irregular areas of hemorrhage in the submucosa associated with large discrete, amorphous eosinophilic masses. Amorphous material is also found in between the muscle fibers. Crystal violet and Congo red stains give characteristic reactions for amyloid in these amorphous deposits. Painless gross hematuria is characteristic and is often difficult to control. The hemorrhage occurs from perforation of the blood vessels, their walls having been weakened by amyloid infiltration.

7. *Purpura or Telangiectasis Affecting the Bladder*

Patients with diseases characterized by or associated with purpura or telangiectasis may rarely have bladder involvement. Bleeding from these lesions can be difficult to control. The diagnosis may be suspected when purpura or telangiectasis is seen in the bladder in the absence of prior treatment with cyclosposphamide or irradiation.

8. *Infection-induced Cystitis*

Infection-induced cystitis of sufficient severity to cause massive bleeding has the cystoscopic appearances of gross inflammation, with pronounced hyperemia, bullous edema, and generalized oozing with increased contact bleeding. Gross hematuria is occasionally seen in children and a viral etiology is proposed. Adenovirus type 11 and occasionally type 21 have been recovered from the urine in these children.[11] The disease is usually self-limiting over a 3–14-day period. Herpes zoster affecting the bladder can cause persistent hematuria, but this is usually mild and pain is much more of a problem. Bleeding from infection-induced cystitis may require catheterization and bladder irrigation. It is unusual that additional measures are required to control bleeding from this etiology.

The cytoscopic appearances may be very similar for all these diseases and it is tempting to perform biopsies to make a histologic diagnosis. However, this temptation must be resisted since the primary need is to control the bleeding and performing a bladder biopsy may worsen the problem. At the end of the procedure the patient should be catheterized with a 22 or 24 Fr. Foley catheter. Our preference is to use a three-way catheter and continuous bladder irrigation with saline at a rate sufficient to keep the urine a rose color. Others prefer a two-way catheter to straight drainage. In either case, intermittent irrigations may be used on a regular basis, e.g. every 6 hours and also as required to dislodge fresh clots. Catheters with spirally running wire or nylon reinforcement in the wall are available and are especially useful since they will not collapse during irrigation. An antispasmodic such as oxybutynin (Ditropan) or propantheline (Pro-Banthine) should be administered to prevent bladder spasms.

IV. Treatment of Hemorrhagic Cystitis

Surgery to control severe bladder bleeding may be necessary in the last resort. However, the poor general medical condition of these patients may preclude major surgery, while urinary diversion in previously irradiated patients may be poorly tolerated, and cystectomy may be technically impossible. The surgical mortality rate is great. For this reason, we prefer to use conservative measures to attempt to control the bleeding. The conservative measures that are available are detailed in the following section. They are listed in our order of preference.

A. Light Electrocoagulation

Lapides reported four patients with intractable hematuria treated successfully with light fulguration of the bleeding points.[12] He used a ball-tip electrode and an intensity of current barely sufficient to produce searing of the capillaries. Subsequently, others have used this technique but did not find it very effective.[13–15] We suggest that this technique should be used during cystoscopy if specific bleeding points are seen.

B. Hydrostatic Balloon

If bleeding persists after cystoscopy and light electrocoagulation of specific bleeding points, we favor the use of the intravesical hydrostatic pressure balloon. The use of intravesical hydrostatic pressure was first described by Helmstein as a treatment for carcinoma of the bladder.[16] He noted that bleeding following treatment was minimal, and heavy pretreatment bleeding was often arrested. Holstein used the intravesical pressure balloon in six patients for control of intractable hemorrhage: three stopped bleeding after a few days, two had temporary relief, and one continued to bleed.[17] Schiff and McGuire[18] reported 11 patients with intractable hemorrhage treated using this method. Marked improvement occurred in eight patients, three of whom required a second hydrostatic treatment, in that significant bleeding ceased for a minimum of 3 months. They noted that the volume of the bladder increased with repeated treatments and that the symptoms of urgency and strangury were eased. Hammonds et al. treated eight patients using this method and seven stopped bleeding.[19]

Reported complications of the procedure are rupture of the musculature with intact mucosa,[16] complete rupture of the bladder,[20] and temporary urinary incontinence.[19]

Technique

The initial proponents of this technique devised a pressure balloon from a condom or rubber party balloon attached to a Foley catheter. Fortunately, a hydrostatic catheter with a capacity of 500 ml is now commercially available (Warne Surgical Products, Andover, England; distributed in the US by International Hospital Products, Inc., Little Silver, New Jersey). Regional epidural anesthesia is administered through an epidural catheter. The bladder can be examined with a cystoscope but a biopsy must not be performed at the time of dilatation because of the risk of rupture. The hydrostatic catheter is inserted into the bladder and the small retention balloon is inflated with 20 ml of saline and gently pulled against the bladder neck. The hydrostatic balloon is then inflated using a solution of normal saline containing two bottles of 50% diatrizoate (Hypaque). A radiograph of the pelvis is obtained to insure correct positioning of the intravesical balloon. The patient is taken to the recovery room for the remainder of the procedure. A central venous pressure line is used to connect the infusion solution and the hydrostatic balloon, and the T-limb with a three-way stopcock is connected to a water manometer (Fig. 3). The height above the pubis of the fluid line in the infusion bag is determined by first measuring the height at which flow begins, which is the pressure necessary to overcome resistance in the catheter and balloon. To this height is added the diastolic blood pressure expressed in centimeters of water (millimeters of mercury × 4/3). The intravesical pressure is maintained at this pressure for 6 hours. The intravesical pressure is also measured directly by using the three-way stopcock to disconnect the infusion bag and connect the T-limb water manometer. An acceptable alternative is to connect the T-limb of the central venous pressure line to a mercury or anaeroid manometer and maintain the intravesical pressure between the systolic and diastolic blood pressure. The blood pressure, intravesical pressure, and drip rate of the infusion solution are monitored at frequent intervals. A sudden increase in

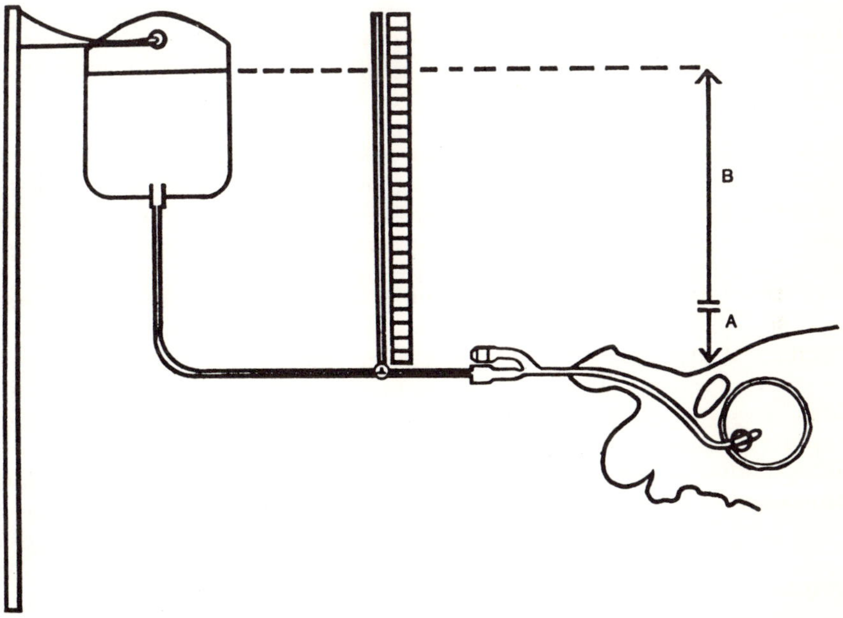

Figure 3: *Schematic drawing showing the hydrostatic balloon catheter inflated in the bladder and connected to the infusion solution. The height above the pubis of the fluid line in the infusion bag (A+B) is determined by first measuring the height at which flow begins (A) and adding to this the diastolic blood pressure expressed in cm of water (B) (mmHg × 4/3). The intravesical pressure is also measured directly by using the three-way stopcock to disconnect the infusion bag and connect to the T-limb water manometer.*

the drip rate may indicate bladder rupture. To avoid sudden intra-abdominal pressure rises, the patient is not moved and may be gently sedated. Anti-emetics are given. Since the urinary output will be obstructed during the procedure, large volumes of intravenous fluids should not be administered. A small dose of furosemide may be given afterwards. The hydrostatic catheter is removed and replaced by a Foley catheter for 48 hours.

If the bladder is heavily trabeculated or there are saccules or diverticula, certain areas will be protected from the pressure effect. In this case, the bladder is filled with 100 ml of fluid before the hydrostatic balloon is inserted. During treatment, a fluid layer is maintained between the bladder wall and the balloon. The fluid is pressed into the diverticula and other irregularities, resulting in constant pressure all over the bladder wall.

If significant bleeding continues after 48 hours, necessitating continued hospitalization or blood transfusion, we repeat the treatment with the intravesical hydrostatic pressure balloon.

C. Intravesical Formalin

Should significant bleeding continue despite two treatments with the hydrostatic balloon, we then instill 1% formalin into the bladder. We find better success when these techniques are combined, rather than when each is used alone.[13] When applied to living tissues, formalin has a desiccating effect that hydrolyzes protein and coagulates the tissue on a superficial level. It is this effect that seems to control the hemorrhage from telangiectatic capillaries in the mucosal and submucosal layers. The urothelium sloughs. Regeneration of the urothelium occurs in approximately 3 weeks. The ingrowth proceeds from the ureteral orifices and bladder neck.

This treatment was effective in 93 of 104 cases reported in the literature (89% effective) although many patients required repeated treatments.[21−33]

There is confusion in the literature about the concentration of formalin or formaldehyde used. Formaldehyde in the natural state is a gas and in solution its greatest concentration is 37.8%. This is known as a 100% solution of formalin. Therefore, for example, a 10% solution of formalin will contain 3.8% formaldehyde, a 4% solution will contain 1.5% formaldehyde, and a 1% solution will contain 0.38% formaldehyde. Various authors have recommended formalin solutions of 1% to 10% in volumes of 10 to 300 ml for a duration of 10 to 30 minutes. Following treatment, some drain the bladder but do not rinse it while others rinse copiously using normal saline, distilled water, 10% ethyl alcohol, or 10% ethyl alcohol followed by normal saline.

Brown[28] originally described the technique of intravesical instillation of formalin using a 10% solution. Subsequently, severe complications have been recorded following the use of a 10% solution. These include severe reduction of bladder capacity, ureterovesical obstruction with hydronephrosis or anuria or both, the development of vesicoureteral reflux, ureteral fibrosis, papillary necrosis, and fatal intraperitoneal extravasation.[13,22,24,25,34] Existing vesicoureteral reflux must be looked for with a cystogram before using formalin because reflux of formalin will lead to severe upper tract complications. Since the edema and inflammation of the formalin treatment can cause ureterosvesical obstruction and subsequent vesicoureteral reflux,[22,24] it is obligatory to do a cystogram immediately prior to each and every instillation of formalin. A post-treatment IVP will demonstrate any ureterovesical obstruction.

The use of lower concentrations has led to essentially equal success with far fewer complications although ureterovesical obstruction has occurred after the use of a 4% solution.[25] Fair has reported excellent results with no complications using a 1% solution and increasing to a 2% solution if the weaker solution was infective.[22]

Technique: Formalin instillation is very painful and general or regional anesthesia should be used. In patients too ill for general or regional anesthesia, topical intravesical anesthesia has been used with success using 100 ml of 2% viscous lidocaine left indwelling for 15 minutes.[32] All clots are removed from the bladder. The bladder is inspected and any large bleeding vessels are fulgurated using light diathermy. An 18 Fr. Foley catheter is inserted into the bladder and the balloon inflated and snugged down onto the bladder neck to prevent extravasation of the formalin into the urethra or leakage onto the external genitalia. A cystogram is performed to exclude reflux, and 1,000 ml of 1% formalin solution in water (i.e. a 0.38% solution of formaldehyde gas in water) is passively irrigated in and out of the bladder for a total time of 15 minutes in the following way (Fig. 4). The plunger is removed from a catheter-tipped asepto syringe and the barrel connected to the Foley catheter. The syringe is held 15 cm

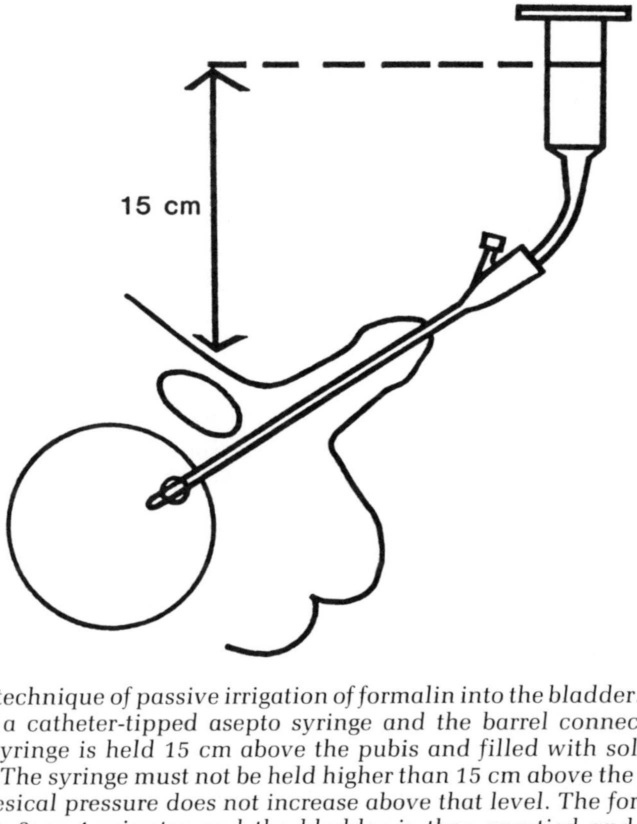

Figure 4: *The technique of passive irrigation of formalin into the bladder. The plunger is removed from a catheter-tipped asepto syringe and the barrel connected to a Foley catheter. The syringe is held 15 cm above the pubis and filled with solution until the bladder is full. The syringe must not be held higher than 15 cm above the pubis to insure that the intravesical pressure does not increase above that level. The formalin is left in the bladder for 3 or 4 minutes and the bladder is then emptied and the procedure repeated. The irrigation is stopped after 15 minutes.*

above the pubis and filled with the solution until the bladder is full. The formalin is allowed to stay in the bladder for 3 or 4 minutes and the bladder is then emptied by gravity and the procedure repeated. At no time is the catheter clamped. Holding the syringe no higher than 15 cm above the pubis will insure that the intravesical pressure will not increase above the level. After instillation of the formalin for 15 minutes, the bladder is washed with 1 liter of distilled water. The Foley catheter is left in place for 24 hours.

If bleeding continues after 24 hours, we repeat the procedure again using 1% formalin solution. If this is still not effective, we then use a 2% formalin solution. Although Fair[22] has given up to five treatments without problems, we stop after three treatments since additional benefit is unlikely to accrue with subsequent treatments. We do not advise using formalin solutions stronger than 2%, except when the treatment is for bleeding from defunctionalized bladders in patients who have supravesical urinary diversions.

Patients with reflux can be treated provided either of the following precautions are taken. Fair[22] and Shrom et al.[21] use low spinal anesthesia with the patient placed in marked Fowler position (semi-erect) so that the level of the kidneys is higher than the level of the formalin irrigation. A brisk diruesis is maintained to lower the concentration of formalin delivered into the refluxing system (Fig. 5). Gottesman and Ehrlich[27] and Bright et al.[26] have used Fogarty catheters to occlude one or both ureters while the formalin is instilled (Fig. 6). The technique is to insert a 4 or 5 Fr. Fogarty catheter into the ureter and advance it 3–5 cm up the ureter. The balloon is then filled with 1.5–2 ml of normal saline and the plunger of the attached syringe taped to keep the balloon inflated. The hub of the Fogarty catheter will not pass through the cystoscope so the formalin has to be instilled through the cystoscope. The lens is removed to prevent damage by the formalin and the lens opening in the cystoscope is occluded by a small caliber (10 Fr.) Foley catheter inserted through the opening into the bladder, its balloon inflated and pulled back against the barrel of the cystoscope. A cystogram is performed through the Foley catheter to confirm that the ureter is totally occluded by the Fogarty balloon. After instillation of the formalin through the Foley catheter and irrigation with distilled water, the Fogarty is deflated and removed.

D. Alum

Intravesical hydrostatic pressure and instillation of formalin comprise the mainstays of our treatment, but a recent report enthusiastically recommends bladder irrigation with alum solution.[35]

Continuous closed bladder irrigation with a 1% alum solution (either aluminum ammonium sulfate or aluminum potassium sulfate) has been used successfully to control bleeding in six patients. The patients were treated at bedside without anesthesia and all responded, over various periods, with cessation of bleeding. There were no complaints and no side effects. Alum is an astringent whose mechanism of action is protein precipitation. The cell penetrability is so low that action is limited to the cell surface and the cell remains viable. Systemic absorption does not occur.

Technique: A 1% solution of alum is made by dissolving alum in a 3-liter sterile water container used for transurethral procedures. Continuous bladder irrigation is performed through a 22 Fr. three-way Foley catheter.

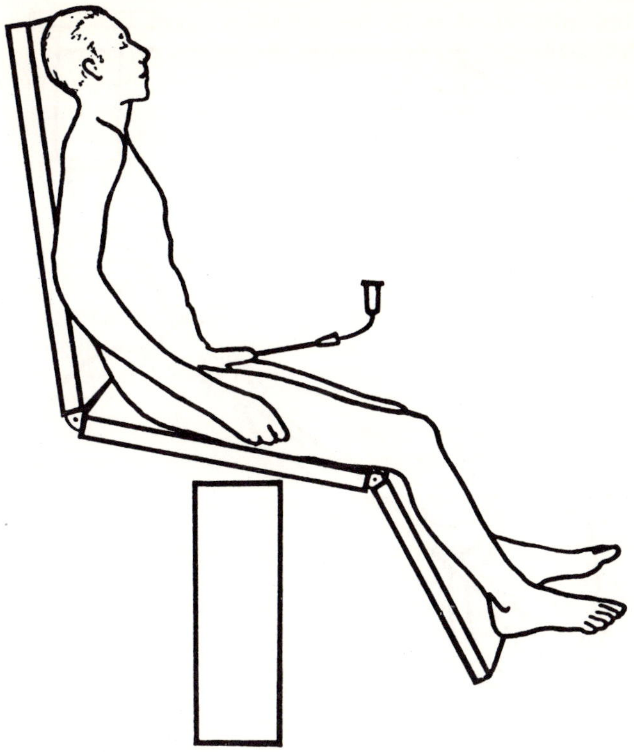

Figure 5: *Schematic drawing of a patient with vesicoureteral reflux being treated with passive irrigation of formalin into his bladder. After low spinal anesthetic, he is placed in marked Fowler positon so that the level of the kidneys is higher than the level of the formalin in the syringe. A brisk diuresis is maintained to lower the concentration of formalin delivered into the refluxing system.*

This treatment appears promising and has the special advantages of being apparently safe and painless, which allows it to be administered at bedside without anesthesia. Since its use has only been reported in six patients, it is too soon to be able to recommend it before the previously described more established methods of controlling bleeding. Nevertheless, it seems reasonable that this technique should be further evaluated.

E. Silver Nitrate

Silver nitrate bladder irrigation can occasionally be effective when the previous methods have failed. It is easy to obtain and use and side effects are relatively mild.

Its use to stop intractable hematuria has been reported by Kumar et al.[3] and Pool.[4] The cessation of bleeding was temporary but recurrent episodes were controlled with further silver nitrate irrigations. Post-treatment bladder spasms were common.

Technique: General or regional anesthesia is used. The bladder is evacuated of clots and electrocautery is used for specific bleeding points. An 18 Fr. Foley

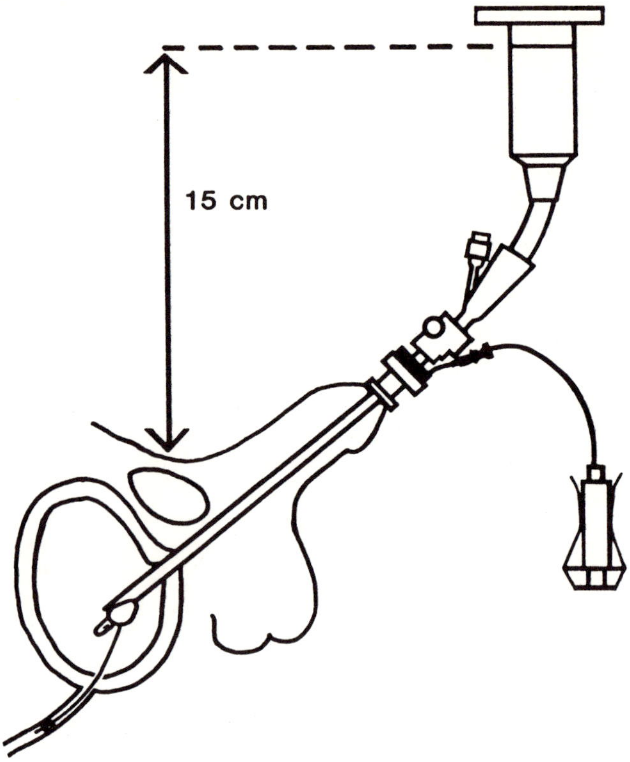

Figure 6: *An alternative technique of passive irrigation of formalin into the bladder of a patient with vesicoureteral reflux. A 4 Fr. Fogarty catheter has been inserted into the ureter and its balloon inflated with 1.5 ml of saline. The plunger of the attached syringe is taped to keep the balloon inflated. The lens has been removed and the lens opening in the cytoscope occluded by a 10 Fr. Foley catheter. A cystogram has confirmed the ureter to be totally occluded. Formalin irrigation of the bladder is performed through the Foley catheter. The syringe must not be held higher than 15 cm above the pubis.*

catheter is inserted into the bladder and the balloon inflated and snugged down onto the bladder neck to prevent extravasation of the silver nitrate into the urethra. Two hundred milliliters of a 1% silver nitrate solution is instilled into the bladder for 15 minutes. The bladder is then emptied and irrigated with saline. Continuous bladder irrigation with saline through a three-way Foley catheter is maintained for 48 hours postoperatively.

F. EACA

The fibrinolytic enzyme system, or plasminogen-plasmin system, has an important physiological role in maintaining the patency of the vascular tree. Plasminogen, which is an inert plasma globulin, is converted by activators to plasmin, a proteolytic enzyme. Plasmin causes fibrinolysis and suppresses fibrin formation from fibrinogen. Activators of plasminogen are found in most human tissues and body fluids. The prostate has an especially high concentration of tissue activator and urine contains a powerful activator called urokinase.

There are also plasma activators and bacterial activators, e.g. streptokinase (see Chapters 3, 4 and 5).

Epsilon-aminocaproic acid (EACA) is a synthetic inhibitor of fibrinolysis acting by inhibition of plasminogen activation and inhibition of plasmin (see Chapters 5 and 6).

Primary or local fibrinolysis is a process localized to the tissue that is damaged. Locally formed fibrin clots are dissolved leading to prolongation of bleeding. There is no abnormal fibrinolytic activity demonstrable in the circulating blood. EACA treatment effectively inhibits this fibrinolysis and stops or suppresses the bleeding.[36–38] Secondary or generalized fibrinolysis is seen in patients with disseminated intravascular coagulation (DIC). Fibrinolytic activity is demonstrable in the circulating blood. In DIC, the fibrinolytic activity is possibly a protective mechanism. Treatment should be aimed at eliminating or controlling the cause of the DIC. EACA therapy given systematically in such a patient may predispose to widespread thrombosis.[39–40]

Local fibrinolysis probably occurs frequently after surgery to the prostate or other parts of the urinary system, and one concern is whether EACA might also increase the incidence of thromboembolism in patients with local fibrinolysis. Although case reports have been recorded,[38] in several large series of patients treated with EACA the incidence of thromboembolism was not increased when compared to appropriate control groups.[38,41–43] Although these series do not show an increased incidence of thromboembolism, Gollub[44] suggested that the incidence of thrombotic complication was increased if doses greater than 12 grams/day were given. Nilsson et al.[38] achieved good control of urinary bleeding with a dose of 3 grams given three to four times a day. Even this dose may be more than required since control of fibrinolytic activity in the circulating blood can be obtained with doses of EACA as low as 2–3 grams/day.[44] Moreover, EACA is concentrated 50–100 times in the urine indicating that the dose required to inhibit fibrinolysis in the urinary tract is even less than that required to suppress the activity in the circulating blood (see Chapter 6).

Nilsson et al. found that EACA effectively reduced severe and prolonged bleeding after bladder surgery in 19 of 23 patients but its effect on bleeding from bladder cancer was less marked: in only 13 of 35 cases did it control bleeding.[38] They also tried EACA without success in two patients with bladder bleeding due to radiation-induced hemorrhagic cystitis. McGuire et al.[13] and Hammonds et al.[19] also found that EACA was not effective in controlling the bleeding from radiation or tumor-induced cystitis.

Other side effects of EACA include hypotension, cardiac arrhythmias, and rhabdomyolysis. Upper urinary tract obstruction by tenacious blood clots has been described in patients with hematuria of renal origin, e.g. due to sicklemia or hemophilia.[37,43]

Technique: EACA is well absorbed orally and can be given as a tablet or syrup, as well as intravenously. The duration of action is about 4 hours. It is given orally in six divided doses or intravenously by constant infusion. Most commonly used schedules administer more EACA than is required for inhibition of fibrinolysis and good control can be obtained in an adult with a loading dose of 3 grams followed by continuous infusion at a rate of 3 grams/8 hours. The dose should be decreased in patients with renal failure. For bladder hemorrhage, where it is desired to inhibit the fibrinolytic activity of the urine in the bleeding region, treatment may also be given by continuous instillation of EACA into the bladder using a solution of 4 grams of EACA in 1 liter of normal saline. Generalized fibrinolysis must be excluded by a negative DIC screen before EACA is administered.

Although EACA administration is not very effective in controlling bladder bleeding, we suggest that it be tried if light electrocoagulation, hydrostatic pressure, formalin, alum, and silver nitrate have not stopped the bleeding. We administer it by continuous bladder irrigation, although it can be given orally or intravenously instead.

G. G-Suit (Circumferential Pneumatic Compression)

In 1903, Crile described external counterpressure as a method to maintain the blood pressure in hypovolemic and hypotensive surgical patients.[45] Although the pressurized rubber suits suggested by him were very effective, they were plagued by frequent and untimely air leaks. With the advent of blood transfusion, this method was abandoned. External counterpressure became widely used in aviation during World War II as a means of reducing the gravitational stress on pilots. The counterpressure was applied using an anti-gravity suit (G-suit). In 1966, Gardner and Storer[46] called the technique circumferential pneumatic compression (CPC), a term that more accurately describes the mode of action but is interchangeable with external counterpressure, pneumatic pressure, circumferential pressure, and G-suit pressure. Chapters 9 and 11 contain descriptions of the materials and styles. Each G-suit has unique advantages.

CPC has been used successfully to treat patients with hypotension caused by fluid or blood loss or redistribution of fluids, as in spinal or septic shock.[47] The garment can be applied in less than a minute and when inflated, it provides an estimated autotransfusion of approximately 1,000 ml of blood.[47]

CPC has been used successfully to tamponade intra-abdominal or intrapelvic bleeding, intractable postoperative bleeding from renal surgery or retropubic prostatectomy, and hemorrhage following percutaneous needle biopsy[48–52] (see Chapter 11).

The mechanism of action of the G-suit is discussed in Chapter 11. Briefly, it increases peripheral resistance, shunts blood away from hemorrhagic areas, and elevates blood pressure to supradiaphragmatic organs. It decreases the caliber of the blood vessels beneath it, including the vena cava and aorta, and the smaller vessels.

The CPC procedure is not without potential complications. Glomerular filtration rate may fall, with an increase in filtration fraction. However, the renal tubular metabolic function does not fall.[53] There can be a reduction of vital capacity and a slight increase in respiratory rate.[54] Tidal volume, expiratory and inspiratory reserve, and maximum breathing capacity are not affected uniformly.

Chapter 11 discusses the contraindications to using CPC. CPC should be used with caution in patients with suspected underlying renal or pulmonary disease and is generally contraindicated in patients with cerebral or pulmonary edema, congestive heart failure, and bleeding from above the diaphragm.

The patient must be prepared before being placed in the CPC garment. The lower limbs and bony prominences must be protected by light cotton padding material. Peroneal nerve injury is avoided by padding over the head of the fibula with Reston foam (3M Company, Minnesota). A nasograstic tube and a urethral catheter are inserted. The pressure needs to be carefully applied and maintained between 15 and 30 mmHg. The urinary output is to be monitored. Patients may be disturbed by not being able to move their lower limbs in the suits and because of this, sedation is often needed. The treatment can be maintained for up to 72 hours and should continue for 24 hours after the bleeding has stopped. When the treatment is discontinued, the pressure should be reduced slowly over a 30-minute period. The deflation should stop if the blood pressure falls by 5 mmHg. Intravenous fluids are then administered until the blood pressure returns to the former level.

H. If the Above Measures Fail, What Next?

If bleeding persists despite the above measures, then various other conservative measures can be attempted. Some success has been claimed for each, but we regard them as last-ditch attempts.

1. *Phenol*

Phenol cauterization of bladder mucosa for management of hemorrhagic cyclophosphamide cystitis has been successful in controlling bleeding in five patients.[55,56] General anesthesia and surgery are required. Since phenol is extremely toxic to tissue, extreme care must be exercised to protect the surrounding normal structures. There is destruction of the epithelial layer of the bladder with preservation of the muscle. The bladder capacity at first is diminished, but later is adequate.[57]

Technique: An 18 Fr. Foley catheter is inserted into the bladder and the balloon inflated and snugged down onto the bladder neck to prevent the phenol from entering the urethra. The bladder is exposed through a suprapubic approach. The edges are grasped with Allis forceps and walled off with packs to absorb any spill of the agents used. A mixture of 30 ml of 100% phenol and 30 ml of glycerin is instilled into the bladder and painted around the wall with a stick sponge. The mixture is allowed to stay in contact with the mucosa for 1 minute and is then suctioned out. It is wise to have two suction apparatuses working and on the table. Sixty milliliters of absolute alcohol is instilled for 1 minute and then removed by suction. Copious amounts of saline are used to irrigate the bladder and surrounding tissues. Phenol should not enter the urethra. The bladder is closed with suprapubic drainage.

2. *Transcatheter Embolization*

Transcatheter embolization is more effective when used to control major vessel bleeding secondary to pelvic trauma rather than the diffuse bleeding from many submucosal vessels that occurs in hemorrhagic cystitis (see Chapter 8). However, Gelfoam embolization of the internal iliac arteries or their branches has been used for chronic intractable bleeding.[58,59] The bleeding was markedly reduced immediately and stopped after 24 hours. This may have been due to the

Gelfoam inducing a localized intimal inflammatory reaction leading to further occlusion of the vessels that were not totally blocked in the process of embolization. Transcatheter embolization is much more effective than surgical ligation because ligation is a proximal procedure that cannot control the collateral vascular supply, while embolization is a peripheral procedure. The level of the arterial occlusion with embolization depends on the size of the emboli and this size must be tailored with care. Very small emboli may embolize at the capillary level and irreversible bladder infarction may occur.[60]

Technique: A straight red Keifka catheter is advanced from the contralateral side via the femoral artery. A Cook deflecting wire directs the catheter into the internal iliac artery. Gelfoam blocks 1–3 mm in size are mixed with Renografin 76. The mixture is injected through the catheter, which is placed in the distal part of the internal iliac artery or its branches. Care must be taken not to inject too quickly since an overflow can cause escape of the emboli into the iliac and femoral arteries. After embolization, an arteriogram is obtained to assess the adequacy of the vascular occlusion. More emboli may be injected if needed (see Chapter 8 for further details).

3. *Cyrosurgery*

Cyrosurgery, using low temperatures, produces rapid intracapillary thrombosis. This method has been used on five patients with intractable bladder hemorrhage and produced immediate cessation of bleeding.[61] The techniques of freezing varied. In one case, a cryoprobe was introduced through a preexisting cystotomy and in another patient enlarged bleeding areas were coagulated under direct supervision. In three patients, a cystotomy was used to pour liquid nitrogen into the bladder through a funnel. Care was taken to monitor adjacent structures and precautions were taken to prevent their being damaged by the freezing process.

Technique: The bladder is exposed through a suprapubic approach. Structures neighboring the bladder are dissected away from the bladder and protected from freezing damage by interposed laparotomy packs and sterile wooden spatulas. A metal funnel is placed into the bladder and liquid nitrogen is poured in. A warm solution of saline is available to spray or drip onto the outside of the bladder if it becomes whitened. Rectal temperature is monitored by a rectal temperature probe. If the rectal temperature falls, the rectal mucosa is protected by inserting a condom filled with warm water into the rectum. Once the liquid nitrogen has vaporized, the congelated tissue is allowed to thaw spontaneously since slow thawing is itself necrotising. The freeze-thaw cycle is repeated. A suprapubic catheter is maintained for about 3 weeks.

4. *Vasopressin*

There is considerable experience in controlling upper gastrointestinal hemorrhage by either selective arterial or peripheral intravenous infusion of vasopressin. It acts by causing contraction of the smooth muscle of all parts of the vascular bed, especially the capillaries, small arterioles, and venules. Intravenous vasopressin has been used in one patient to control bleeding from cyclophosphamide-induced hemorrhagic cystitis.[62] The vasopressin was administered at a rate of 0.4 units per minute by peripheral intravenous infusion. Bladder irrigation with vasopressin to control bleeding has been attempted but was ineffective.[26]

5. *Hyperthermic Irrigation of Bladder*

Ludgate et al.[63] used hyperthermic irrigation of the bladder in the treatment of bladder cancer. This treatment arrested uncontrollable hematuria in a group of six patients. The mechanism of action appeared to be acute vascular thrombosis in the mucosal and muscular layers.

Technique: Epidural anesthesia is used. The bladder capacity is measured and the bladder is perfused through a three-way Foley catheter with normal saline heated by passing through a heating coil inserted in a waterbath. The outflow is made to ascend over a gradient to an overflow tank, the height of which is adjusted so that slightly less than the known bladder capacity causes overflow. This is usually 15–20 cm above the symphysis pubis. The inflow and outflow temperatures are monitored constantly. Perfusion is at a constant rate of 3 liters per hour, and the inflow temperature is adjusted to give an outflow temperature of 44°C. The apparatus required and the many and frequent adjustments that are needed make this technique burdensome.

6. *Tocopherol*

Wojewski and Roessler[64] described the use of tocopherol (vitamin E) in patients with radiation-induced cystitis. The patients were classified into three groups according to whether their changes were of medium degree, extensive, or very extensive. The treatment improved the symptoms and stopped bleeding in those with medium-degree changes but was much less effective in more severely affected patients. The best results occurred after the daily use of 150 mg intramuscularly and 800 mg orally for a 14–21 day period. The success of these investigations has not been duplicated.

7. *ACTH*

ACTH has been used in patients with radiation cystitis but it was given to assess its effects on dysuria and bladder capacity and not for intractable hematuria.[65] In these patients, there was no marked cystoscopic change except for a slight diminution in the area of ulceration. There was relief of dysuria that was rapid in onset, but it was of variable and unpredictable duration. The bladder capacity doubled.

I. Surgery

If severe bladder hemorrhage cannot be controlled by any other means, it is necessary to resort to surgery. Urinary diversion, internal iliac artery ligation, and cystectomy have all been tried. Extirpative surgery, however, is often precluded by the poor general medical conditions of these patients. Moreover, urinary diversion in previously irradiated patients may be poorly tolerated, and cystectomy may be technically impossible.

Urinary diversion using bilateral ureteral catheters placed cystoscopically has been documented by a review by Berkson et al.[14] Seven patients were treated in this manner and four gradually stopped bleeding. In two of the other three patients, the ureteral catheters had to be removed because of obstruction and sepsis.

Supravesical urinary diversion alone can be effective in stopping the bleeding. Berkson et al. described four patients that stopped bleeding after diversion.[14] One had bilateral nephrectomies plus ureteral ligation, one had cutaneous ureterostomies, and two had ileal conduits.

Bilateral internal iliac artery ligation has been combined with supravesical urinary diversion. Spiro et al.[25] treated one patient in this way and the bleeding stopped. McGuire et al.[13] treated three patients and one stopped bleeding. Goldstein et al.[15] treated three patients; two stopped bleeding but all three died soon after surgery from related complications.

Suprapubic cystotomy and internal iliac artery ligation considerably diminished the bleeding in one patient.[15] Suprapubic cystotomy and packing the bladder without supravesical urinary diversion did not control bleeding in five patients.[14]

Bilateral internal iliac artery ligation alone did not control bleeding in four patients.[13,66] Ravitch has made the point that the arterial collateral to the iliac arteries is so enormous that one would not expect ligation to have much effect.[66]

Cystectomy and urinary diversion can be effective,[14] but the mortality rate of this procedure is great. Higgins[67] reported a mortality rate as high as 60% in 1967 but with improvements in postoperative management, and, in particular, with parenteral hyperalimentation, the operative mortality has fallen. Blandy reported a mortality rate of 22% in 1975 and a rate of 11% in 1980.[68] A 1966 review of 182 postoperative fatalities in urology[69] showed that the causes of death were, in descending order, infection, including pneumonia (29%), renal failure (23%), carcinomatosis (12%), cardiac disease (14%), cardiac arrest (5%), pulmonary emboli (5%), cerebrovascular accident (2%), hemorrhage (2%), and miscellaneous (7%). At present, the major causes of postoperative death are cardiopulmonary disease, infection, and thromboembolism.

To summarize: Eleven of the 23 patients reported by Berkson et al., McGuire et al., and Goldstein et al. died after surgical intervention to control the bleeding.[13–15] Four died from infection, three from cardiac disease, one with renal failure, one with multiple pulmonary emboli, one with carcinomatosis, and one did not have a post-mortem.

Because of the high mortality, we prefer nonsurgical means to control the bleeding and only if these fail do we proceed to surgery. We suggest initially performing bilateral ureteral catheterization. Size 6–8 Fr. Stamey ureteral stents are passed through a cytoscope up the ureters into the pelvis of each kidney. A 22 Fr. three-way Foley catheter is passed into the bladder and its balloon inflated. This catheter can be used for bladder irrigation. The ureteral stents are securely taped to the Foley catheter to prevent their being dislodged. If ureteral catheterization fails, supravesical urinary diversion should be performed. Placement of bilateral percutaneous nephrostomies can be tried but these are usually unable to prevent some urine from passing down the ureters into the bladder and so may not be effective. Surgical diversion is then necessary either by ileal conduit or cutaneous ureterostomy or even nephrostomy; we prefer ileal conduits. Suprapubic cystotomy and bladder tamponade can be done at the same time or subsequently if necessary. Suprapubic cystotomy and tamponade without urinary diversion is not effective, nor is internal iliac artery ligation.

V. Summary

Severe, prolonged and life-threatening hematuria due to hemorrhagic cystitis is commonly caused by pelvic irradiation, cyclophosphamide, bladder neoplasms, and bleeding and clotting disorders. Hematuria in these patients is significant if it necessitates hospitalization, blood transfusion, and persists more than 24 hours. The primary aim of treatment is to control the bleeding via conservative measures since the general medical condition of the patients is often poor. Surgery may be poorly tolerated or technically impossible and the mortality rate is unacceptably high.

The initial treatment is to stabilize the general medical condition of the patient. Cystoscopy is performed to evacuate blood clot, to examine the bladder, and to lightly fulgurate specific bleeding points. The bladder is then continuously irrigated through a three-way Foley catheter.

If significant bleeding persists, then various conservative measures can be used in an attempt to control it (Table I). We advocate initially using an intravesical hydrostatic pressure balloon for 6 hours under regional epidural anesthesia. If this is not successful, we repeat the treatment after 48 hours. If the bleeding continues, we then instill 1% formalin into the bladder under general anesthesia and are prepared to repeat this twice more, for a total of three treatments, using 1% formalin again for the second treatment, and 2% formalin for the third treatment. It is mandatory to perform a cystogram before each and every formalin treatment since the treatment can cause vesicoureteral reflux, and reflux of formalin into the upper urinary tract has disastrous and sometimes fatal consequences. We do not use formalin solutions stronger than 2% unless the treatment is for bleeding from defunctionalized bladders, in patients with supravesical urinary diversions. Patients with vesicoureteral reflux can be cautiously treated with formalin provided certain precautions are taken. These are described above. Continuous bladder irrigation with a 1% solution of the astringent alum appears promising, but so far its use has been reported in only one small series of six patients. Alum treatment has the advantages of being safe and painless, allowing it to be administered at the bedside without anesthesia. It is too soon to recommend its use before more established techniques, but it seems reasonable that the technique should be further evaluated. Bladder irrigation with a 1% silver nitrate solution can occasionally be effective when the previous methods have failed. It is easy to obtain and use and its side effects are mild. When light electrocoagulation, hydrostatic pressure, formalin, alum, and silver nitrate have not stopped the bleeding, we use EACA. This agent is a synthetic inhibitor of fibrinolysis and it is effective in reducing bleeding in situations where there is local fibrinolysis. It is useful in controlling bleeding from the prostate but not very effective in controlling bleeding from the bladder. We administer it by continuous bladder irrigation although it can be given orally or

Table I
Control of Intractable Bladder Hemorrhage

Conservative Measures:

1. Cytoscopy under general anesthesia. Evacuation of clots and light electrocoagulation of bleeding points. Catheterization with a 22 Fr. three-way Foley catheter and continuous bladder irrigation.
2. Hydrostatic intravesical balloon catheter inflated to diastolic blood pressure for 6 hours under epidural anesthesia. Subsequent Foley catheter drainage for 48 hours. Repeat once after 48 hours if bleeding continues.
3. Intravescial instillation of formalin under general anesthesia. Do cystogram beforehand to exclude vesicoureteral reflux. Use 1 liter of 1% formalin solution (i.e. 0.38% solution of formaldehyde gas in water). Instill by passive irrigation for 15 minutes with pressure not exceeding 15 cm of water. Rinse with liter of distilled water. Foley catheter drainage for 24 hours. Repeat twice after 24-hour intervals if bleeding continues. Use 1% formalin for the second instillation, and 2% formalin for third instillation.
4. Continuous bladder irrigation with 1% solution of alum. Can be performed at bedside.
5. Intravesical instillation with 200 ml of 1% solution of silver nitrate for 15 minutes under general anesthesia. Subsequent continuous bladder irrigation with saline for 48 hours.
6. Continuous bladder irrigation with EACA solution. Use 4 gm of EACA in 1 liter of N/S. Oral or intravenous EACA can be used instead. Dose is then 3 gm as loading dose and thereafter 3 gm every 8 hours.
7. Circumferential pneumatic compression (G-suit). Wrap lower limbs with cotton padding and use Reston foam over fibula heads. Insert nasogastric tube and urethral catheter. Sedate patient. Inflate to 15–30 mmHg. Monitor urine output. Deflate slowly.

Last-Ditch Conservative Measures:

1. Phenol
2. Transcatheter embolization
3. Cryosurgery

Surgery

1. Bilateral ureteral catheterization using 6–8 Fr. Stamey catheters.
2. Bilateral percutaneous nephrostomy.
3. Supravesical urinary diversion (ileal conduit, cutaneous ureterostomy, nephrostomy) ± suprapubic cystotomy and bladder tamponade.

intravenously. EACA can cause thromboembolism if there is generalized fibrinolysis and it is important to insure that a DIC screen is negative before using EACA. It has been suggested that it may predispose to thromboembolism in situations of local fibrinolysis also, and although there are case reports of thromboembolism in patients treated with EACA, these patients were in a high-risk group for developing thromboembolism. Several large series of patients did not detect any increased incidence of thromboembolism in patients treated with EACA.

Circumferential pneumatic compression using a G-suit has been used to stop successfully intrapelvic and retroperitoneal bleeding. We have used this method to stop intractable hemorrhage from the bladder and prostate and enthusiastically endorse its use. We believe this technique can be life-saving. The CPC garments can usually be obtained from the Emergency Room.

If the above methods all fail to control the bleeding, there are various other measures that can be attempted. Some success has been claimed for each but we regard them as last-ditch attempts. These methods are outlined below. Phenol cauterization of the bladder mucosa can be used, but extreme care must be taken because phenol is toxic to tissue. Transcatheter embolization has been tried but it is more applicable to major vessel bleeding secondary to pelvic trauma rather than the diffuse bleeding from many submucosal vessels that occurs in hemorrhagic cystitis. Cryosurgery, using liquid nitrogen poured into the bladder through a cystotomy incision, has been used but it is difficult to control the degree of freezing damage. Techniques using vasopressin, hyperthermic irrigation of the bladder, tocopherol, and ACTH have been included in the text for completeness but they do not seem effective in controlling bleeding and we do not recommend them.

In the last resort, surgery may be necessary. We initially perform bilateral ureteral catheterization at cystoscopy. Size 6–8 Fr. Stamey catheters are used and secured to a 22 Fr. three-way Foley catheter, which can be used to irrigate the bladder. If ureteral catheterization fails, supravesical urinary diversion should be performed. Bilateral percutaneous nephrostomies can be placed but they will not prevent some urine from getting to the bladder and so may not be effective. Surgical diversion by ileal conduit, which we favor, or cutaneous ureterostomy or even nephrostomy is then required. Suprapubic cystotomy and bladder tamponade can be done at the same time or subsequently. Suprapubic cystotomy and tamponade without urinary diversion is not effective, nor is internal iliac artery ligation.

Finally, the best form of treatment is prevention and in the case of cyclophosphamide-induced hemorrhagic cystitis, it is possible to prevent or reduce the side effects with a regimen of diuresis and frequent voiding or indwelling catheterization.

VI. Conclusion

We have presented our plan of management to control bleeding in patients with severe, intractable, and life-threatening hemorrhagic cystitis. Many of the methods can be described as well established as demonstrated by Boerhaave in 1709 when he wrote, "if much blood doth issue out of the wound occasioned by its causes. . . it is stopped, (1) with a hot iron, (2) with caustics or corrosives, (3) astringents, (4) tying the vessels with a thread, (5) cutting them asunder, (6) with bandages and bolsters upon the vessels, closing their channels."[70]

References

1. Shields Warren. Arch. Pathol. XXXIV:1970, 1942.
2. Watson EM, Herger CC, Sauer HR. Irradiation reactions in the bladder: Their occurrence and clinical course following use of x-ray and radium in treatment of female pelvic disease. *J Urol.* 57:1038–1053, 1947.

3. Kumar AP, Wrenn EL, Jr, Jayalakshmamma B, Conrad L, Quinn P, Cox C. Silver nitrate irrigation to control bladder hemorrhage in children receiving cancer therapy. *J Urol.* 116:85–86, 1976.
4. Pool TL. Irradiation cystitis: Diagnosis and treatment. *Surg Clin N Am.* 39:947–951, 1959.
5. Oppers I, Gerhartz H. Zur Hammorrhagischen Cystitis unter der Chemotherapie min N-Lost-Phosphamidestern. *Klin Wschr.* 44:450–457, 1966.
6. Johnson WW, Meadows DC. Urinary-bladder fibrosis and telangiectasia associated with long-term cyclophosphamide therapy. *N Engl J Med.* 248:290–294, 1971.
7. Philips FS, Sternberg SS, Cronin AP, Vidal PM. Cyclophosphamide and urinary bladder toxicity. *Cancer Res.* 21:1577–1589, 1961.
8. Droller MJ, Saral R. Santos G. Prevention of cyclophosphamide-induced hemorrhagic cystitis. *Urology.* 20:256–258, 1982.
9. Primack A. Amelioration of cyclophosphamide-induced cystitis. *J Natl Cancer Inst.* 47:223–227, 1971.
10. McDonald JH, Heckel NJ. Primary amyloidosis of the lower genitourinary tract. *J Urol.* 75:122–132, 1956.
11. Mufson MA, Belshe RB, Horrigan TJ, Zollar LM. Cause of acute hemorrhagic cystitis in children. *Am J Dis Child.* 126:605–609, 1973.
12. Lapides J. Treatment of delayed intractable hemorrhagic cystitis following radiation or chemotherapy. *J Urol.* 104:707–708, 1970.
13. McGuire EJ, Weiss RM, Schiff M, Jr., Lytton B. Hemorrhagic radiation cystitis. *Urology.* 3:204–208, 1974.
14. Berkson BM, Lome LG, Shapiro I. Severe cystitis induced by cyclophosphamide: Role of surgical management. *JAMA.* 225(6)605–606, 1973.
15. Goldstein AG, D'Escrivan JC, Allen SD. Haemorrhagic radiation cystitis. *Br J Urol.* 40:475–478, 1968.
16. Helmstein K. Treatment of bladder carcinoma by a hydrostatic pressure technique. *Br J Urol.* 44:434–450, 1972.
17. Holstein P, Jacobsen K, Pederson JF, Sorensen JS. Intravesical hydrostatic pressure treatment: New method for control of bleeding from the bladder mucosa. *J Urol.* 109:234–236, 1973.
18. Schiff M, Jr, McGuire EJ. Experience with the use of an intravesical hydrostatic pressure balloon. *Surg Gynecol Obstet.* 150:322–324, 1980.
19. Hammonds JC, Williams JL, Fox M. The control of severe bleeding from the bladder by intravesical hyperbaric therapy. *Br J Urol.* 46:309–312, 1974.
20. Cattolica EV. Hydrostatic bladder distention for bladder tumor. A fatal outcome. *Urology.* 5:115–116, 1975.
21. Shrom SH, Donaldson MH, Duckett JW, Jr, Wein AJ. Formalin treatment for intractable hemorrhagic cystitis. *Cancer.* 38:1785–1789, 1976.
22. Fair WR. Formalin in the treatment of massive bladder hemorrhage: Techniques, results and complications. *Urology.* 3:573–576, 1974.
23. Rao MS, Bapna BC, Chugh KS, Dutta TK, Singhal PC, Vaidyanathan S, Bhat VN, Gupta CL. Fatal complication of intravesical formalin during control of intractable hemorrhage from radiation cystitis. *Urology.* 11:588–590, 1978.
24. Kalish M, Silber SJ, Herwig KR. Papillary necrosis: Result of intravesical instillation of formalin. *Urology.* 2:315–317, 1973.
25. Spiro LH, Hecht H. Horowtiz A, Orkin L. Formalin treatment for massive bladder hemorrhage. *Urology.* 2:669–671, 1973.
26. Bright JF, Tosi SE, Crichlow RW, Selikowitz SM. Prevention of vesico-ureteral reflux with Fogarty catheters during formalin therapy. *J Urol.* 118:950–952, 1977.
27. Gottesman J, Ehrlich RM. Preventing vesicoureteral reflux during intravesical formalin instillation. *Urology.* 3:494–495, 1974.
28. Brown RB. A method of management of inoperable carcinoma of the bladder. *Br J Urol.* 40:489, 1968.

29. Brown RB. A method of management of inoperable carcinoma of the bladder. *Med J Aust.* 2:23–24, 1969.
30. Brown RB. Further experiences with intravesical formalin administration in advanced carcinoma of the bladder. *Br J Urol.* 42:738–739, 1970.
31. Kumar S, Rosen P, Grabstald H. Intravesical formalin for the control of intractable bladder hemorrhage secondary to cystitis or cancer. *J Urol.* 114:540–543, 1975.
32. Firlit CF. Intractable hemorrhagic cystitis secondary to extensive carcinomatosis: management with formalin solution. *J Urol.* 110:57–58, 1973.
33. Shah BC, Albert DJ. Intravesical instillation of formalin for the management of intractable hematuria. *J Urol.* 220:519–520, 1973.
34. Scott MP, Jr, Marshall S, Lyon RP. Bladder rupture following formalin therapy for hemorrhage secondary to cyclophosphamide therapy. *Urology.* 3:364–365, 1974.
35. Ostroff EB, Chenault OW, Jr. Alum irrigation for the control of massive bladder hemorrhage. *J Urol.* 128:929–930, 1982.
36. Nilsson IM. Local fibrinolysis as a mechanism for haemorrhage. *Thrombos Diathes Haemorrh.* 34:623–633, 1975.
37. Griffin JD, Ellman L. Epsilon-aminocaproic acid (EACA). *Semin Thromb Hemostas.* 5:27–40, 1978.
38. Nilsson IM, Andersson L, Bjorkman SE. Epsilon-aminocaproic acid (EACA) as a therapeutic agent based on 5 year's clinical experience. *Acta Med Scand.* (Suppl) 448:1–46, 1966.
39. Bergin JJ. The complications of therapy with epsilon-aminocaproic acid. *Med Clin N Am.* 50:1669–1678, 1966.
40. Naeye RL. Thrombotic state after a hemorrhagic diathesis, a possible complication of therapy with epsilon-aminocaproic acid. *Blood.* 19:694–701, 1962.
41. Vinnecombe J, Shuttleworth KE. Aminocaproic acid in the control of haemorrhage after prostatectomy: A controlled trial. *Lancet.* 1:230–232, 1966.
42. Gordon-Smith IC, Hickman JA, El Masri SH. The effect of the fibrinolytic inhibitor epsilon aminocaproic acid on the incidence of deep vein thrombosis after prostatectomy. *Br J Surg.* 59:522–524, 1972.
43. Black WD, Hatch FE, Acchiardo S. Aminocaproic acid in prolonged hematuria of patients with sicklemia. *Arch Intern Med.* 136:678–681, 1976.
44. Gollub S, in discussion, Deysine M, Cliffton EE. Mechanism of action of epsilon-aminocaproic acid in the control of hemorrhage. *Ann NY Acad Sci.* 115:291–301, 1964.
45. Crile GW. *Blood Pressure in Surgery: Experimental and Clinical Research.* Philadelphia, J.B. Lippincott Co., 1903, pp. 288–291.
46. Gardner WJ, Storer J. The use of the G Suit in control of intra-abdominal bleeding. *Surg Gynecol Obstet.* 123:792–798, 1966.
47. Paris PM. Antishock garments. *N Engl J Med.* 305:960, 1981. (Letter).
48. Pelligra R, Sandberg EC. Control of intractable abdominal bleeding by external counterpressure. *JAMA.* 241:708–713, 1979.
49. Batalden DJ, Wichstrom PH, Ruiz E, Gustilo RB. Value of the G suit in patients with severe pelvic fracture: Controlling hemorrhagic shock. *Arch Surg.* 109:326–328, 1974.
50. Burdick JF, Warshaw AL, Abbott WM. External counterpressure to control postoperative intra-abdominal hemorrhage. *Am J Surg.* 129:369–373, 1975.
51. McCullough DL, McLaughlin AP, Warshawsky AB. The gravity suit: A useful device in complicated urologic hemorrhage. *Urology.* 6:468–470, 1975.
52. Cangiano JL, Kest L. Use of a G-suit for uncontrollable bleeding after percutaneous renal biopsy. *J Urol.* 107:360–361, 1972.
53. Shenasky JH, Gillenwater JY. The renal hemodynamic and functional effects of external counterpressure. *Surg Gynecol Obstet.* 134:253–258, 1972.
54. Espinosa MH, Updegrove JH. Clinical experience with the G-suit. *Arch Surg.* 101: 36–69, 1970.

55. Susan LP, Marsh RJ. Phenolization of bladder treatment of massive intractable hematuria. *Urology*. 5:119–121, 1975.
56. Duckett JW, Peters PC, Donaldson MH. Severe cyclophosphamide hemorrhagic cystitis controlled with phenol. *J Pediatr Surg*. 8:55–57, 1973.
57. Vermooten V, Peters PC, Johnson DE. Treatment of papillomatosis of the bladder with phenol and glycerin: A clinical and laboratory study. *J Urol*. 99:588–592, 1968.
58. Higgins CB, Bookstein JJ, Davis GB, Galloway DC, Barr JW. Therapeutic embolization for intractable chronic bleeding. *Radiology*. 12:473–478, 1977.
59. Just HA, Hooshmand I. Transcatheter angiographic control of bleeding. *Urology*. 11:629–632, 1978.
60. Hietala SO. Urinary bladder necrosis following selective embolization of the internal iliac artery. *Acta Rad Diag*. (Stockh), 19:316–320, 1978.
61. Cahan WG, Adam Y, MacKenzie RA, Brockunier A, Clark DG. Intractable bladder hemorrhage treated by cryosurgery: A preliminary report. *J Urol*. 103:606–611, 1970.
62. Pyeritz RE, Droller MJ, Bender WL, Saral R. An approach to the control of massive hemorrhage in cyclophosphamide-induced cystitis by intravenous vasopressin: A case report. *J Urol*. 120:253–254, 1978.
63. Ludgate CM, McLean N, Tulloch WS. Hyperthermic irrigation of bladder in treatment of transitional cell carcinoma: Its effectiveness in controlling persistent hematuria. *J Roy Soc Med*. 72:336–340, 1979.
64. Wojewski A, Roessler R. Treatment of post-irradiation lesions of the urinary bladder. *Bull Pol Med Sci Hist*. 8:110–113, 1965.
65. Persky L, Austen G, Jr. ACTH in radiation cystitis. *J Urol*. 70:724–728, 1953.
66. Ravitch MM (Editorial). Hypogastric artery ligation in acute pelvic trauma. *Surgery*. 56:601–602, 1964.
67. Higgins PM, Hamilton RW, Hope-Stone HF. The hazards of total cystectomy after supervoltage irradiation of the bladder. *Br J Urol*. 38:311–318, 1967.
68. Blandy JP, England HR, Evans SJW, Hope-Stone HF, Mair GMM, Mantell BS, Oliver RTD, Paris AMI, Risdon RA. T3 bladder cancer - the case for salvage cystectomy. *Br J Urol*. 52:506–510, 1980.
69. Sakati IA, Marshall VF. Postoperative fatalities in urology. *J Urol*. 95:412–420, 1966.
70. Boerhaave H. Aphorisms 218. In: *Aphorisms: Concerning the Knowledge and Cure of Diseases*. London, B. Cowse and W. Innys, p. 59, 1715.

Chapter 11

Management of Post-Prostatectomy Hemorrhage

H. David Mitcheson, M.D., and Martin Schiff, Jr., M.D.

I. Introduction

Prostatectomy is an operation which, even in expert hands, can be complicated by bleeding. Because of the nature of the operation, the site, and the tendency to local fibrinolysis, bleeding may be difficult to control during the actual operation, and postoperative bleeding is not uncommon. Postoperative bleeding interferes further with hemostasis by preventing good bladder drainage and causing overdistension of bladder and detrusor spasm. This can lead to sepsis, increased hemorrhage, intractable pain, debility, and occasionally death. This chapter will concentrate on the prevention, recognition, and treatment of hemorrhage from the prostatic fossa occurring after enucleative or transurethral prostatectomy.

Prostatectomy can be performed by transurethral resection (TUR) or by operation through either a transvesical or a retropubic approach. More than 90% of prostatectomies are by TUR. Bleeding at TUR may be arterial or venous. Arteries are easily seen and dealt with by diathermy with the loop electrode and the coagulating current. Small and medium veins also can be coagulated in this way. Large venous sinuses bleed severely when the loop takes a tangential slice out of the wall; these cannot be sealed by electrocoagulation (Fig. 1). Fortunately, most bleeding from these sinuses can be controlled by tamponade with a Foley catheter balloon and light traction (Fig. 2). In a retropubic procedure, the main sources of bleeding are the arteries at 5 and 7 o'clock, which are easily suture-ligated. Hemostasis during a transvesical prostatectomy is more inexact because the vessels that are bleeding are not visualized. Singh et al.[1] reviewed 1,135 men who had prostatectomy, 935 by TUR and 217 by open operation. Of the TUR group, 7.0% were transfused with one or two units of blood and 1.9% with more

From Bern MM (ed.): *Urinary Tract Bleeding: Diagnosis and Control by Medical, Radiologic, and Surgical Techniques.* Mount Kisco, NY, Futura Publishing Co., Inc., 1985.

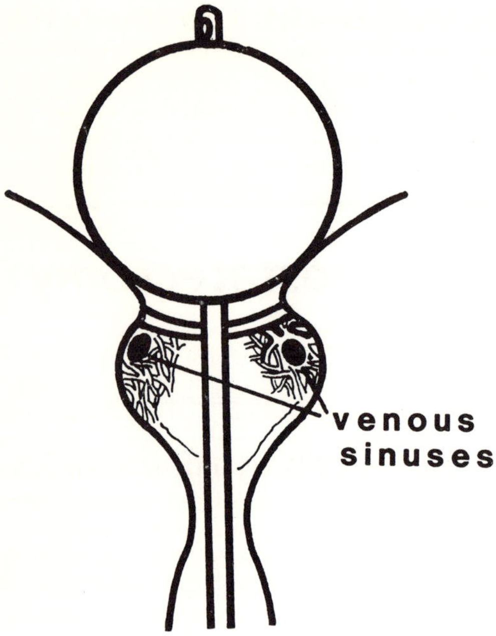

Figure 1: *Transurethral resection of the prostate gland. Severe bleeding can occur from venous sinuses opened via perforation in the capsule.*

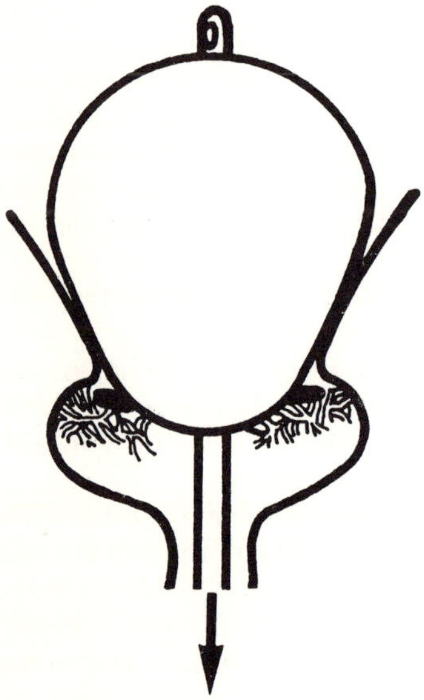

Figure 2: *Bleeding from the venous sinuses is controlled by tamponade of a Foley catheter balloon when light traction is applied to the catheter.*

than two units. Of these cases, 1.6% had postoperative clot retention, and 1.0% required operative clot evacuation. This compares to the open surgery group wherein 40.2% were transfused with one or two units of blood, and 16.0% with more than two units. Here 0.9% had clot retention, and 0.5% required clot evacuation. The hemorrhage-associated mortality rate (MR) was 0.3% in the TUR group and 0.5% in the open group. Similar results have been documented by Bergman et al.,[2] Wines et al.,[3] Perrin et al.,[4] and Lund and Dingsor.[5] When open prostatectomy was the standard operation, morbidity and mortality related to hemorrhage were higher. For example, Salvaris[6] documented that of 1,200 men who had retropubic prostatectomy, 97 had heavy bleeding and 29 died from related complications giving a hemorrhage-associated MR of 2.4%.

II. Preventive Measures

Preventive measures to avoid postoperative bleeding and the prompt recognition and aggressive treatment of hemorrhage when it does occur are essential to minimize the morbidity and mortality.

Before surgery, the patient should be questioned about any abnormal individual or family history of clotting abnormalities. Details of his medications, including aspirin, must be obtained. Blood should be sent for a complete count, platelet count, prothrombin time, and partial thromboplastin time. A bleeding time should be performed if there is any suspicion of bleeding abnormality or if the patient is uremic (see previous chapters). Two units of blood should be available. If there is history of excessive bleeding or if a coagulation test is abnormal, a hematological consultation is required. During surgery it is important to obtain meticulous pinpoint hemostasis and to avoid inadequate resection especially at the apex of the prostate.

III. Medications to Reduce Post-Prostatectomy Hemorrhage

The anesthetic agents used may influence blood loss during the operation but have little effect afterwards. There is conflicting evidence about the values of spinal anesthesia,[7,8] hypothermia, and cooling the irrigation fluid.[9,10] Bruce, Zorab, and Still[11] observed a 50% reduction in pre- and postoperative blood loss with controlled hypotension, but this carries a risk of cerebral and myocardial infarction, especially in older men.[8]

Many drugs have been used to reduce post-prostatectomy hemorrhage (see chapters 1, 2, and 6). Several have had little success, e.g. carbazochrome salicylate,[12] kutapressin,[13] premarin,[9] polyestradiol phosphate,[14] and aprotinin.[15] EACA, on the other hand, substantially reduces postoperative bleeding but with no appreciable effect on bleeding during operation (see below). Diethylammonium 1, 4-dihydroxy-3-benzone sulfate (Dicynone, Dicynene) as used by Symes et al.[16] significantly reduced blood loss during and after TUR for benign prostatic hyperplasia (BPH). It increases platelet adhesiveness, increases the rate of release of intrinsic thromboplastin, improves capillary resistance, and reduces the bleeding time. With its use there is no apparent increase in the incidence of deep vein thrombosis.[17] It should be used selectively. Dicynene has not been used to treat severe post-prostatectomy hemorrhage.

IV. Recognition of Significant Postoperative Hemorrhage

The degree of bleeding is always difficult to assess since after prostatectomy the urine is usually bloody. There should be cautious observation, especially if accurate hemostasis could not be obtained during surgery, if the postoperative bleeding is such that clots form in the drainage tubing, or if continuous irrigation is not able to keep the urine a rose color.

A. Immediate Treatment

The patient's vital signs are recorded. Crystalloid solutions and/or blood are infused to keep the pace with the volume and blood losses. Additional blood is cross-matched, and repeat laboratory evaluations are carried out. Besides the hemoglobin, hematocrit, platelet count, PT, PTT, electrolytes, blood urea nitrogen, and creatinine, studies for fibrinolysis are now needed. These include fibrinogen, FDP, and functional assay such as euglobin lepes or serial thrombin time. The blood clots are removed from the tubing and the bladder using a catheter-tipped bladder syringe. The optimal method is to fill the bladder with about 100 ml of saline and, using a 60 ml syringe full of saline, repeatedly inject and withdraw about 40 ml of fluid in a rapid push-pull fashion. This is continued until all the clots have been evacuated and the patient is comfortable. Traction is then applied to the catheter and output is observed for continued bleeding (see the section in this chapter on use of the hemostatic balloon catheter and traction). If a three-way Foley catheter continuous bladder irrigation is used, the rate of irrigation is adjusted to maintain the urine a rose color. If a two-way Foley catheter is used, the intravenous infusion is maintained at 150 ml/hour and the patient is encouraged to drink copiously to insure a good diuresis. At this point, use of EACA intravenously can be applied (see the section in this chapter on EACA).

B. Cytoscopic Evacuation and Fulguration

If, as is often the case, the clots cannot be removed adequately by syringing, it is necessary to evacuate the clots using endoscopy. Under general or spinal anesthetic, a resectoscopic sheath (24 Fr.) is inserted through the urethra, and the bladder and prostatic fossa are inspected. All blood clots must be removed and cytoscopically reconfirmed as having been removed. This is for two reasons. First, all the bleeding points cannot be adequately identified and fulgurated if there is obscuring clot. Second, residual clot will prevent complete contraction of the prostatic fossa, thus inhibiting the vasoconstrictive component of hemostasis. These blood clots may be extremely tenacious and may not be removed by simple irrigation. In this case, it is necessary to break up the clot with the beak of the cytoscope or the diathermy loop and remove it by using the loop and irrigation. Bleeding points in the fossa are identified and meticulously coagulated. A 22 Fr. hemostatic three-way Foley catheter is inserted and continuous bladder irrigation commenced. Traction is applied if necessary and treatment started.

C. Foley Catheter as a Hemostatic Balloon

When Foley introduced the hemostatic balloon catheter in 1937, he suggested that the bag be inflated in the prostatic urethra.[18] Weyrauch cautioned against positioning the bag at this site except to control bleeding from an exposed sinus and warned that traction on a balloon so situated might result in incontinence.[19] Greene resolved this conflict by evaluating 200 consecutive patients following transurethral resections of prostates (TURP). He inflated the balloon with 30 ml of radiographic contrast material and positioned it in three positions: (1) in the bladder, (2) in the bladder and snugged down on the bladder neck, or (3) in the prostatic fossa. He also compared straight catheter drainage using a two-way catheter to continuous bladder irrigation using a three-way catheter. From these studies, it was found that the balloon was an aid in hemostasis depending on which of several situations pertained at the end of the resection. If acceptable hemostasis had been secured by electrocoagulation and persisted after introduction of the catheter, the balloon played no role in hemostasis, and only retained the catheter in position. However, more difficult were those cases where despite careful electrocoagulation, bleeding became apparent. This may have been the result of bleeding from a perforated venous sinus or from numerous small arteries or veins commonly encountered during resections of large prostates. In such instances, the position of the balloon played a significant role in the hemostasis. Positioning the balloon in the bladder was least satisfactory, while positioning it in the prostatic fossa was usually successful. If bleeding persisted despite inflation of the balloon in the fossa to 30 ml, adding 10 or 20 ml into the balloon frequently resulted in excellent hemostasis. Positioning the balloon in the bladder and snugging it down against the bladder neck was also satisfactory but roentgenograms showed that the balloon entered into the prostate cavity in 73% of the cases and this is likely to be the reason for its effectiveness. Greene also evaluated the objections to inflating the balloon in the prostatic cavity. These objections had been (1) that a balloon in that position actually prevented hemostasis and thereafter increased postoperative bleeding, (2) that a balloon in that position would not remain in place, and (3) that urinary incontinence might result. Greene found that there was no evidence of impaired hemostasis, that the balloon remained in position for 24 hours in 80% of cases, and that increased urinary incontinence did not occur. Straight catheter drainage compared with continuous bladder irrigation revealed no significant difference. Continuous bladder irrigation did not result in increased postoperative blood loss, allowed accurate monitoring of blood loss, and obstruction of the catheter by clot was less likely. The disadvantages of continuous irrigation were the inability to measure urinary output and the need for increased supplies and personnel. Interestingly, cine-radiography of continuous irrigation showed that the fluid egressed from the bladder as quickly as it entered and that the bladder remained contracted around the catheter. The irrigant actually did not enter the prostatic fossa, unless the outflow limb of the catheter was occluded and the bladder became distended.

Technique: After transurethral prostatectomy, a 22 Fr. Foley catheter is passed into the distended bladder and its position confirmed by free egress of fluid through the catheter. The balloon is then inflated with 30 cc of saline and snugged down against the bladder neck, bringing the balloon into the prostatic fossa in most patients. We prefer to use a three-way catheter and continuous bladder irrigation and, by altering the rate of irrigation, assess the degree of post-prostatectomy bleeding. If there is appreciable bleeding, the balloon is further inflated with an additional 10 or 20 ml of saline. If bleeding still continues, the catheter is placed on traction, which can be done in three ways. Salvaris suggested[20] tying a gauze sponge firmly around the catheter and pulling it against the external meatus (Fig. 3). With this there is the danger of pressure necrosis of the glans if the sponge is left in position for more than 30 minutes or so, thus you *must* remove the sponge yourself before the patient leaves the recovery room. A safer method of maintaining the traction is to fasten the catheter to the thigh with adhesive tape applied in a chevron fashion (Fig. 4). This is easy to perform but has the disadvantage that the amount of traction cannot be quantified when the patient moves his leg and thus may be painful. The best method is to fasten a cord to the catheter, run the cord over a pulley at the end of the bed, and attach a 1-pound waterbag weight (Fig. 5). This gives known traction and is comfortable. The traction should be removed after 3–4 hours and the situation is re-evaluated. If bleeding persists, the traction can be reapplied and maintained for up to 24 hours. The catheter is irrigated with normal saline as briskly as it will go for the first 20 minutes, and is then adjusted to keep the outflow just pink. The catheter drainage tube is over the rail of the bed so as to keep a pressure gradient of about 5 cm above the bladder. This will modestly distend the bladder and allow the irrigant to enter the bladder and prostatic fossa. Chips of tissue or blood clots that block the catheter can be forcibly washed out with a bladder syringe. If this does not clear the catheter, it should be changed. Catheters with spiral wire or nylon reinforcement in the wall are especially useful since they will not collapse during irrigation.

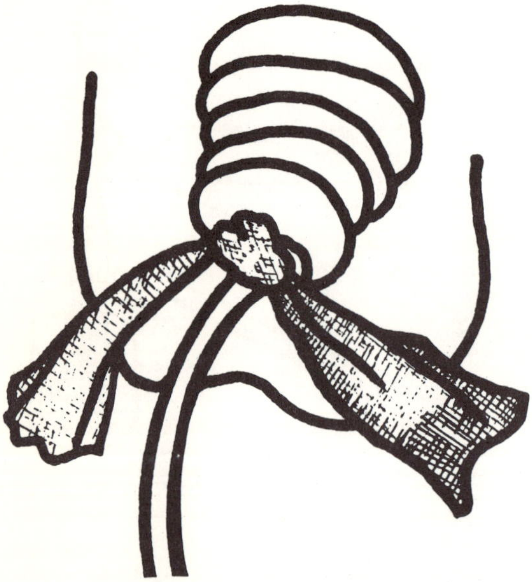

Figure 3: *Traction applied to a catheter by a gauze sponge tied firmly around the catheter and pushed up against the glans penis. This method can be used for no longer than 30 minutes because of the danger of pressure necrosis to the glans.*

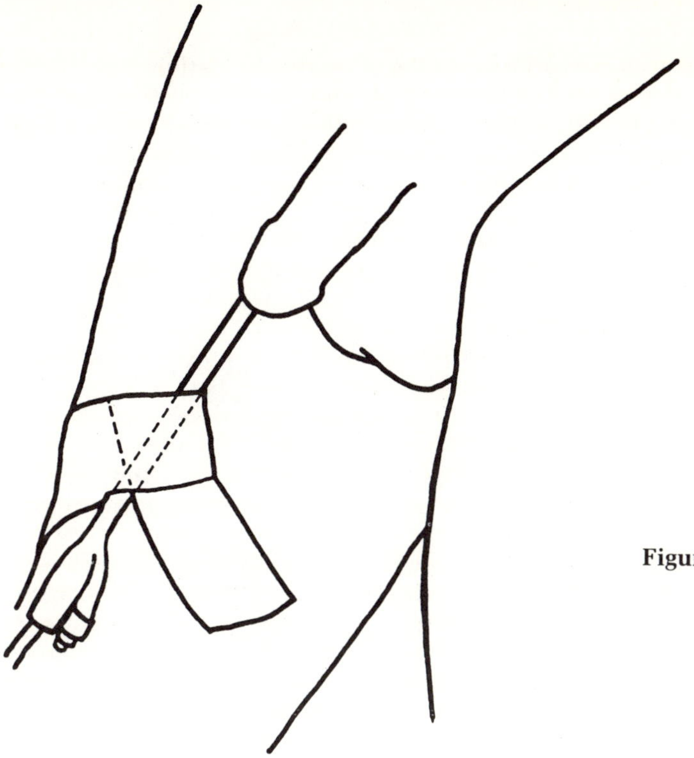

Figure 4: *Traction applied to a catheter and maintained by fastening the catheter to the thigh with adhesive tape applied in a chevron fashion.*

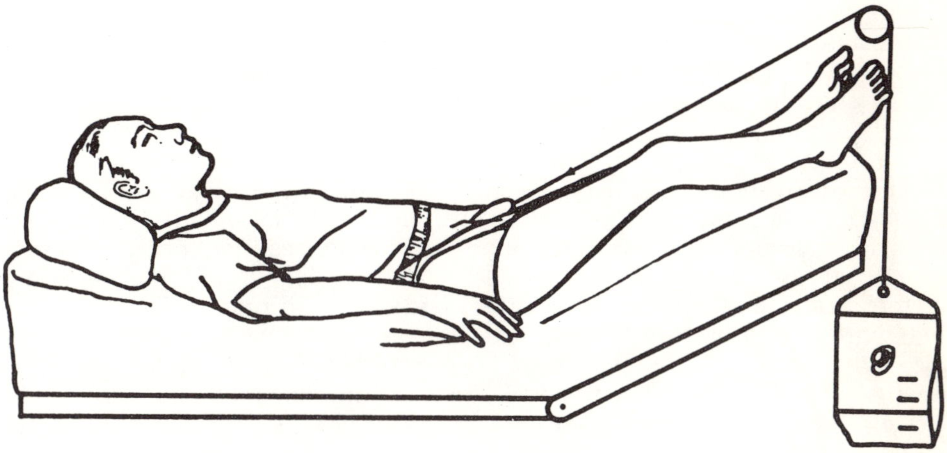

Figure 5: *The favored method of applying traction to a catheter: a cord is fastened to the catheter, run over a pulley at the end of the bed and attached to a 1-pound waterbag weight. This gives known traction in a comfortable fashion.*

D. EACA (Amicar®)

Prostatectomy, like other operations, is often attended by a slight increase in the fibrinolytic activity. The activity returns to normal after about 2 hours[21] (for full discussion of fibrinolysis and its inhibition, see Chapters 5 and 6). The cause of the increase in fibrinolytic activity has not been defined with certainty. The prostatatic parenchyma has a high content of plasminogen activators and it is possible that prostate surgery releases activators into the circulation. However, this need not be the only cause since increased fibrinolytic activity can occur just with anesthesia. While the increased fibrinolysis during surgery can be prevented by the administration of EACA, a synthetic inhibitor of fibrinolysis, the blood loss during surgery is not affected.[21]

EACA treatment before or during prostatectomy does not reduce the blood loss during surgery or soon after surgery since such bleeding is usually due to a bleeding artery or venous sinus, and is only rarely due to fibrinolysis.[21] Nevertheless, some local fibrinolysis probably does occur frequently after surgery to the prostate since the activators of plasminogen are liberated by the surgery. Furthermore, the raw wall of the prostatic cavity is bathed with urine, which contains the plasminogen activator urokinase.

In 1961, McNicol[22] reported the results of a controlled study in which 22 patients received EACA after either a suprapubic or transurethral prostatectomy. Blood loss was markedly reduced when compared with prostatectomy patients who did not receive EACA. Nilsson et al.[23] treated with EACA large numbers of patients who had bleeding from BPH or prostatic carcinoma. Fifty-two patients with carcinoma of the prostate had hematuria, and EACA controlled the bleeding in 48 but failed in four. Three patients with carcinoma of the prostate had generalized bleeding from DIC, and EACA controlled bleeding in all three, but one patient died from a coronary artery thrombosis. Of 130 patients with BPH and hematuria, EACA controlled the bleeding in 115 but had no effect on 15. One patient died of a myocardial infarct. Two patients with BPH had generalized bleeding from DIC and both responded to EACA. Two hundred and fifty patients had prostatectomy, and EACA significantly diminished postoperative bleeding. Fourteen patients had hematuria following perineal biopsy of the prostate; EACA controlled the bleeding in 13 but had no effect on one patient who subsequently required ligation of a bleeding artery at the bladder neck.

Besides plasminogen activators, the prostate also contains thromboplastically active substances.[21] These thromboplastically active substances are also released into the bloodstream from the prostate in association with surgery and may lead to an increased risk of thrombosis.[24] EACA treatment of patients with generalized fibrinolysis may predispose to thrombosis,[25,26] and one concern is whether EACA might also increase the incidence of thromboembolism in patients with local fibrinolysis. Although case reports of serious and even fatal episodes of vascular thrombosis have been recorded,[23] in several large series of patients treated with EACA the incidence of thromboembolism was not increased when compared to appropriate control groups.[23,27-29] Review of the incidence of thromboembolism after prostatectomy shows that it is more common after open prostatectomy with the reported incidence of symptomatic thromboembolism ranging from 8.5–27%,[24,30] and with a 51% incidence of deep venous thromboses detected with radioiodine-fibrinogen scanning.[31] Thromboembolism is much less common after transurethral prostatectomy with a clinical incidence of 1%[2] and a 10% incidence of deep venous thromboses as detected by radioiodine-fibrinogen scanning.[31] Andersson[21] showed that

EACA substantially decreased the blood loss after open prostatectomy and that the incidence of thromboembolism in groups that received high dose EACA or low dose EACA was the same as a control group that did not receive EACA (20% incidence of thromboembolism in each group).

In a subsequent study, Andersson[32] demonstrated that combined treatment with EACA and heparin (15,000 units daily in two divided doses) after open prostatectomy lowered the incidence of thromboembolism to 1% and the blood loss remained low. Heparin anticoagulation without concomitant use of EACA has been used in 15 patients during and after prostatectomy.[33] There were no thromboembolic complications but there were severe bleeding problems. Although the controlled series of patients treated with EACA do not show an increased incidence of thromboembolism, Gollub suggested that the incidence of thrombotic complications was increased if doses greater than 12 grams/day were given. Nilsson et al.[23] achieved good control of urinary bleeding with a dose of 3 grams three to four times a day. Even this dose may be more than required since control of fibrinolytic activity in the circulating blood can be obtained with doses of EACA as low as 2–3 grams/day.[34] Moreover, EACA is concentrated 50–100 times in the urine indicating that the dose required to inhibit fibrinolysis in the urinary tract is even less.

Although these studies demonstrate that EACA can be used to reduce blood loss after prostatectomy, its routine use does not appear to be warranted since blood loss in most cases is minimal. EACA should be reserved for those patients with severe post-prostatectomy hemorrhage, as can occur following surgery for carcinoma of the prostate.[35] Those with diffuse intravascular coagulation (DIC) should not receive the drug under most conditions. Therapy with EACA can also cause hypotension, cardiac arrhythmias, rhabdomyolysis, and tenacious blood clots in the urinary tract.[36] For full discussion of the pharmacology and toxicity of EACA therapy, please refer to Chapters 5 and 6. When being given by continuous instillation into the bladder, a solution of 4 grams of EACA in 1 liter of normal saline can be used until the urine is macroscopically clear.

E. Silver Nitrate

Parton[37] used a 1 in 10,000 solution of silver nitrate to rapidly irrigate the bladder if post-prostatectomy hemorrhage was excessive. He found that control of hemorrhage was rapidly and dramatically achieved within 30 or 60 minutes, after which saline irrigation was resumed.

F. G-Suit (Circumferential Pneumatic Compression)

In 1903, Crile first described external counterpressure as a method to maintain the blood pressure in hypovolemic and hypotensive surgical patients.[38] Although his pressurized rubber suits were effective, they were plagued by frequent and untimely air leaks. With the advent of blood transfusion, this method was abandoned.

External counterpressure was used again in aviation during World War II as a means of reducing the gravitational stress on pilots, using an anti-gravity suit (G-suit). In 1966 Gardner and Storer[39] called the technique circumferential pneumatic compression (CPC), a term that more accurately describes the mode of action. It has been used to treat patients with hypotension caused by fluid or blood loss or redistribution of fluids as in spinal or septic shock.[40] The garment can be applied in less than a minute and, when inflated, it provides an estimated autotransfusion of approximately 1,000 ml of blood.

CPC has been used successfully to tamponade intra-abdominal or intra-pelvic bleeding.[41-43] McCullough et al.[44] used the G-suit to control bleeding in four patients with intractable postoperative bleeding from the urinary tract: three after renal surgery and one after retropubic prostatectomy. The bleeding was controlled with preservation and restoration of vital signs in each case. The suit inflation time varied between 5 and 78 hours. After the bleeding was reduced, the suit was gradually deflated without subsequent hemorrhage. The G-suit has also been used to successfully treat nine patients with uncontrollable renal hemorrhage following percutaneous needle biopsy.[45]

The G-suit provides an artificial peripheral resistance that tends to shunt blood from the subdiaphragmatic areas of the body to the supradiaphragmatic areas (heart, brain, lungs). This autotransfusion elevates systemic blood pressure, lowers the pulse, and increases the central venous pressure. It also decreases the caliber of the blood vessels beneath it. Decreases in the diameter of the inferior vena cava and aorta have been measured, but the reduction in caliber of the smaller vessels such as arterioles, venules, and capillaries (Poiseuille's Law) is more impressive. This may explain why the G-suit has been so successful in the treatment of diffuse small vessel hemorrhage in the retroperitoneum.

There are possible complications of CPC. Shenasky and Gillenwater[46] applied 30 mmHg CPC to anesthetized dogs for 4 hours and found a substantial decrease in urinary output. The glomerular filtration rate fell 23% and was accompanied by an increased filtration fraction, indicating efferent arteriolar constriction. Renal tubular metabolic function was not impaired. Diminished blood flow was noted in one-third of the patients treated with CPC by Burdick et al.[43] No renal impairment was found in other series of patients treated with CPC.[41] Although the problem of impaired renal hemodynamics appears to be of questionable importance, urinary output should be monitored carefully in patients treated with CPC.

Respiratory function can be altered when exposed to 20–30 cm H_20 (20 mmHg) CPC. Espinosa and Updegrove[47] measured an average 18% reduction of vital capacity and a slight increase in respiratory rate in eight healthy volunteers. Tidal volume, expiratory and inspiratory reserve, and maximum breathing capacity were not affected uniformly.

There are contraindications to using CPC. CPC should be used with caution in patients with suspected underlying renal or pulmonary disease. Because of the shunting of blood from the abdomen and lower extremities, CPC is generally regarded as contraindicated when there is cerebral or pulmonary edema, congestive heart failure, or bleeding from tissues above the diaphragm.

There are different CPC devices available. The military "Anti-G Suit" (Air Force Anti-G Garment Cutaway CSU-e/P)can be readily adapted to the therapeutic situation. It is available in small, medium, and large sizes and can be laced snugly to fit the patient. Although it has separate calf, thigh, and abdominal bladders, they cannot be inflated selectively. Filled with either air or water, the suit can be effectively used by the ambulatory patient with orthostatic hypotension. It can be inflated orally to pressures of approximately 100 mmHg, or it can be attached to a simple manometer and air supply system and brought to pressures in excess of 700 mmHg. The G-suit permits access to the perineal area but has the disadvantage of having a small abdominal bladder, which compresses only the pelvic and lower abdominal areas.

The MAST Suit (Armstrong Industries Inc, Northbrook, Ill) made of polyvinyl, wraps around the patient and secures with Velcro fasteners. It contains an abdominal bladder that extends from the xiphoid to the pubis and has two separate leg bladders. Each bladder can be inflated selectively to pressures of 104 mmHg using a foot pump and simple valve system. Manometer attachments for monitoring pressures within the suit are available from the manufacturer.

The Jobst Anti-Shock Airpants suit is also constructed of polyvinyl and is sealed with a polyurethane coating and welded seams. It differs from the MAST suit by having zippers on the legs instead of Velcro fasteners. It has a ventral abdominal bladder that can be fitted snugly to the patient using a belt and ring buckle. There are no relief valves on the individual bladder compartments as in the MAST suit; however, the Jobst suit is provided with a gauge to monitor pressures. The face of the gauge is marked in red above the 30 mmHg, and the user is advised to obtain medical supervision for use of pressures in the red zone. MAST suits and Jobst suits are available in pediatric sizes.

Before fitting the patient in the CPC garments, the lower limbs and bony prominences are protected by wrapping with a light cotton padding similar to that used beneath casts. This prevents skin maceration. Personal nerve injury is avoided by placing Reston foam (3M company, MN) padding over the head of the fibula. A nasogastric tube and a urethral catheter are inserted. When treating hemorrhage and hemorrhagic shock, pressurization to 15–30 mmHg ranges are effective. There appears to be no benefit to using greater pressures; the potential for CPC to compromise respiration, increase hydrostatic pressure in the pulmonary and cerebral circulation, impair renal function, and induce metabolic acidosis and trophic skin changes appears to be directly related to the magnitude of the pressure applied. Patients in inflated CPC garments cannot move their lower limbs, which can cause distress. Sedation is often needed. The treatment can be maintained for up to 72 hours and should continue for 24 hours after the bleeding has stopped. When the treatment is discontinued, the pressure should be reduced slowly over 30 minutes. The deflation should stop if the blood pressure falls 5mmHg. Intravenous fluids are then administered until the blood pressure returns to the former level.

G. Open Surgery

If bleeding persists despite cytoscopic evacuation of the clot, diathermy coagulation of specific bleeding points, use of the hemostatic balloon, EACA, and silver nitrate irrigation, open surgery becomes necessary.

The bladder and prostate are exposed through a suprapubic approach. The capsule of the prostate is opened as in a retropubic prostatectomy. The enucleated prostatic fossa is firmly packed with sponges to stop venous bleeding. The main sources of arterial bleeding are usually the arteries at 5 and 7 o'clock in the corners of the incision made in the capsule. Secure these with a hemostatic corner stitch (Fig. 6). Suture-ligate any bleeding vessel that is seen. Then remove the sponges, irrigate the cavity, and diathermize or suture any remaining bleeding sites. If there is a large vessel bleeding deep in the prostatic cavity and it can't be seen, insert a strong suture into the inner aspect of the capsule and pull the capsule inside out. The bleeding source can then be seen and suture-ligated.

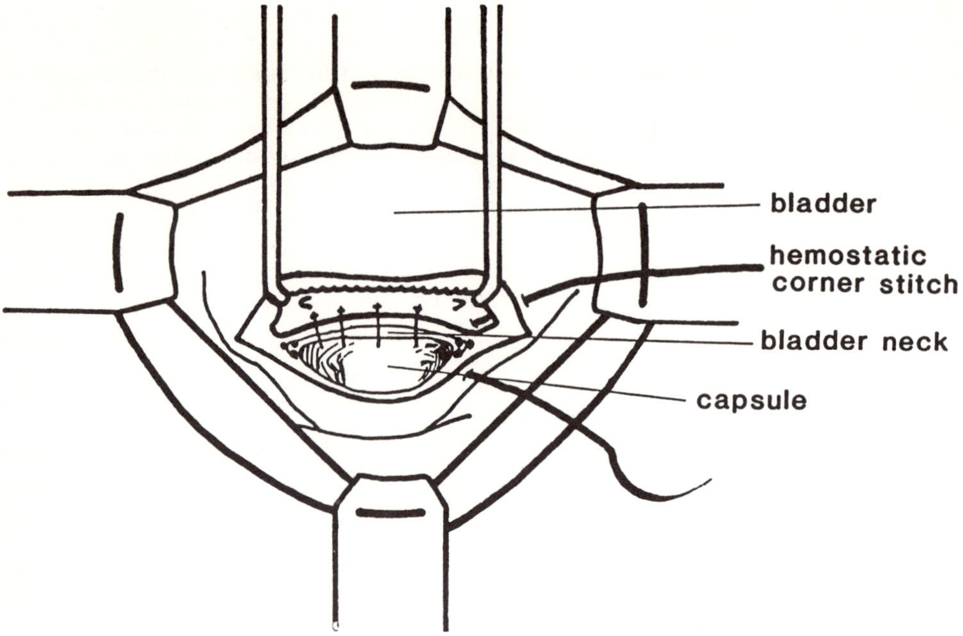

Figure 6: *Open surgery to control post-prostatectomy hemorrhage. The bladder and prostate are exposed through a retropubic approach. The capsule of the prostate is opened transversely.*

Despite these maneuvers, bleeding may continue. If so, open the bladder, pass a two-way 22 Fr. hemostatic Foley catheter through the urethra into the bladder, and then pack the prostatatic fossa firmly with a vaginal roll. Leave the end of the roll long so it can be brought out suprapubically. Alternatively, Penrose drains may be used as packing. Inflate the Foley balloon with 40 ml of saline and pull it down firmly onto the packing. If bleeding is controlled, close the bladder with interrupted sutures, place a retropubic drain, and suture the end of the vaginal roll to the skin. Place traction on the catheter using a 2-pound waterbag for 24 hours, and place the catheter to straight drainage. Broad-spectrum antibiotics are administered. If the bleeding is controlled, remove the packs after 72 hours. During the removal, repeatedly soak the packs with sterile saline to make the removal as untraumatic as possible. The balloon of the Foley catheter is deflated and the catheter pushed up into the bladder. Once the packs are out, again inflate the balloon and gently pull it down against the bladder neck.

Bladder neck sutures and prostatic fossa sutures have been used during open prostatectomy to reduce postoperative bleeding.[48-51] Hryntschak's method is claimed to offer reliable control of postoperative hemorrhage.[48,52] Unfortunately, this leads to a high incidence of urethral stricture. The procedure was modified so that the prostatic fossa is compressed with a figure-of-8 no. 2 plain catgut suture, which was then fixed to a 22 Fr. Couvelaire catheter.[49] In a controlled clinical trial, Hahne and Van der Linden compared vesical neck closure (using this modification) to use of hemostatic balloon catheters[53] and found no difference between the two with respect to blood loss or duration of hospital stay. However, in this study, patients treated with vesical neck closure experienced catheters falling out prematurely and an increased incidence of incontinence at 1-year follow-up. Malament described a removable the purse-string suture of the bladder neck,[50] but this has not gained widespread acceptance. The difficulty is that these sutures are placed at the time of open prostatectomy, when we cannot determine which patients will bleed severely postoperatively and who might benefit from the technique. Since the incidence of severe bleeding is low and the sutures may cause bladder neck stenosis, we do not use them, and prefer meticulous attention to hemostasis at the time of prostatectomy and the use of other methods afterwards if needed.

When hemorrhage and blood clots persist in blocking the urethral catheter, using a suprapubic catheter for drainage is preferable. A large bore tube is inserted into the bladder during a suprapubic cystostomy. This permits easier evacuation of clots and avoids the complications associated with prolonged indwelling urethral catheters, including urethritis, epididymitis, stricture, and fistula.

On occasions when hemorrhage is severe, even the largest caliber suprapubic catheters may become obstructed, so that bladder overdistension and detrusor spasm occur leading to sepsis, increased hemorrhage, pain, debility, and possible death. Lapides[54] concluded that in this situation, the lethal aspect of the uncontrolled bleeding was not due to the blood loss but from the increased intravesical pressure and bladder overdistension. Thus he advocated directing treatments toward providing low pressure drainage of the bladder with easy egress of clots. He described approaching the bladder by a Pfannenstiel incision, retracting the recti, and making a 10 cm transverse incision through the anterior bladder wall. All wounds were left open and dressings were applied around the area to catch the drainage. No drains were used and no tight bandages were applied. Clots that formed did not cause obstruction, pain, or septicemia. The wounds closed spontaneously shortly after the hemorrhage ceased.

Ligation of the internal iliac arteries has been performed, but as in severe bleeding from the bladder, it is usually unsuccessful due to extensive collateral circulation.

H. Arteriographic Embolization

Arteriographic embolization for post-prostatectomy hemorrhage has been reported by Perieras et al.[55] They reported a patient who had cirrhosis, which elevated PTT, and developed severe bleeding that failed to respond to vast volumes of fresh frozen plasma, EACA, fulguration of bleeding points, and packing of the prostatic fossa. Pelvic arteriography showed bleeding from right-sided vesical arterial branches. The right internal iliac artery was catheterized and embolized with 1 ml of Gelfoam. The bleeding from the prostate stopped immediately and did not recur (see Chapter 7 for further discussion of embolization). We advise using arterial embolization if the bleeding is life-threatening, if the patient is unfit for further surgery, or if all other methods have failed.

V. Disorders of Hemostasis Causing Post-Prostatectomy Hemorrhage

Prostatectomy is especially hazardous in patients with impaired hemostasis. Even minor surgical procedures in such patients without adequate hematologic control may provoke significant hemorrhage and delayed healing.

The hemostasis defects may be of the primary hemostatic platelet plug, the coagulation mechanism, fibrinolysis, or the blood vessel constriction, each of which are discussed in previous chapters. There is often specific treatment for these disorders which has to be used in addition to the general treatment measures already discussed.

While Lapides[54] treated four patients with persistent post-prostatectomy hemorrhage due to disordered hemostasis, and advised that the bleeding will stop after 6–7 weeks when re-epithelialization of the denuded prostatic fossa occurs, there are other approaches available. First, the nature of the disorder and the severity of the deficiency must be established. Owen et al.[56] reviewed 1,416 patients who underwent surgery between 1956 and 1961 and were investigated for blood coagulation function. Of the patients investigated because of unexpected hemorrhage and who were found to have definite coagulation defects, only 17 of 34 had a personal or family history of bleeding. Therapeutic requirements for successful surgery in patients with coagulation disorders have been defined by Biggs.[57] Adequate laboratory facilities and sufficient supplies of the appropriate therapeutic material should be available during and after the operation.

Kernoff[58] treated five patients with hemophilia or Christmas disease who underwent prostatectomy and reviewed another seven cases from the literature. After accurate diagnosis of the type and severity of the coagulation disorder, the prostatectomy was performed with prior replacement of the appropriate factor in concentrated form. Therapy was controlled by specific assays. Minimum levels of factor VIII or IX in the first postoperative week were not less than 25%. (The present practice is to aim for minimum levels of 35–40%.) Thereafter the replacement dosages were gradually reduced. The postoperative period of the five patients was complicated by hematuria, and in two patients by clot obstruction. Increasing the dosage of factor VIII or IX was not a reliable way of stopping the hematuria. On the other hand, insufficient replacement therapy in the cases reviewed in the literature resulted in severe bleeding complications.[58] EACA can be used in addition to traditional factor replacement. EACA was used in addition to factor replacement in 20 patients with hemophilia and other bleeding disorders.[23] It was a valuable supplement in those where there was local fibrinolysis. Steiger et al.[59] and Barkhan[60] reported a good hemostatic effect of EACA in the treatment of hematuria in hemophiliac patients.

In liver disease, primary fibrinolysis can be problematic.[61,62] In hematologic diseases such as acute nonlymphoblastic leukemia and polycythemia vera, fibrinolytic bleeding has been described.[63,64] Again, it can be controlled using EACA.[23]

Blood Vessel Constriction as Part of Coagulation.

Contraction of the blood vessels is necessary for hemostasis. Without vessel contraction, full axial force of the blood flow would dislodge the developing plug. Contraction of the vessels is produced by local vasoconstrictors and by muscular contraction of the prostatic fossa following prostatectomy. This mechanism can be affected by various rare bleeding disorders, for example Ehlers-Danlos syndrome, or much more commonly when the prostatic fossa is prevented from contracting by residual prostatic tissue or by blood clot.Residual prostatic tissue often remains in patients with prostate cancer since it is customary to resect a good voiding channel rather than attempt a complete resection. Post-prostatectomy hemorrhage tends to be greater in patients with prostatic neoplasm than BPH because of increased local fibrinolysis and because the residual malignant tissue prevents contraction of the fossa. Furthermore, blood clot commonly prevents fossa contraction. Treatment is largely preventative by insuring that the gland is well resected and that hemostasis is meticulously complete. Blood clot needs to be removed by simple irrigation through a Foley catheter, and if this fails, by endoscopic removal.

VI. Summary

Marked bleeding from the prostate fossa is not uncommon after enucleative or transurethral prostatectomy. Postoperative bleeding interferes with bladder drainage leading to sepsis, increased hemorrhage, intractable pain, debility, and death. The hemorrhage-related MR is 0.3% following TUR prostate and between 0.5–2.4% after open prostatectomy. Preventive measures to avoid postoperative bleeding and prompt recognition and aggressive treatment if it occurs are essential to minimize the morbidity and mortality. Preventive measures include preoperative assessment of the hemostatic mehanism, meticulous hemostasis at surgery and, during TUR, avoidance of inadequate resection especially at the apex of the prostate.

Many drugs have been used to reduce post-prostatectomy hemorrhage with very little success. EACA substantially reduces postoperative bleeding but has little effect on bleeding during surgery. Dicynene reportedly reduces blood loss during and after TUR for BPH, but it is not required for most patients since the blood loss of TUR is small and it has not been used for patients with severe post-prostatectomy bleeding.

Significant post-prostatectomy hemorrhage should be recognized if clots obstruct the bladder drainage or if continuous bladder irrigation is unable to keep the urine a rose color. Treatment is started immediately with replacement of blood and evacuation of all the blood clots. Simply syringing is used, and if this fails, endoscopic clot removal is required. Under anesthesia all the clots are removed through a resectoscope sheath. The resectoscope loop is used to disrupt the clots and they are removed by a combination of repeated syringe irrigation and loop extraction. Any bleeding point can then be identified and meticulously coagulated. After this we like to insert a 22 Fr. three-way hemostatic Foley catheter into the bladder, start continuous bladder irrigation, and give EACA. The catheter balloon is inflated in the bladder using 30 cc of saline and is snugged down against the bladder neck. If there is appreciable bleeding, the balloon is further inflated with an additional 10 or 20 ml of saline. If bleeding persists, the catheter is placed on traction; the best method is to fasten a cord to the catheter, run the cord over a pulley at the end of the bed, and attach a 1-pound waterbag weight. The traction should be removed after 3–4 hours and the situation re-evaluated. If necessary, the traction can be reapplied and maintained for up to 24 hours. Continuous bladder irrigation is started with saline running in briskly for 20 minutes; the rate is then adjusted so as to keep the outflow pink. The catheter drainage tube is led over the rail at the side of the bed to distend the bladder and allow the irrigant to enter the bladder. We administer EACA in the irrigant using a solution of 4 grams of EACA in 1 liter of saline. EACA can be administered orally or intravenously if preferred. If bleeding persists and clot retention occurs, we repeat the cystoscopy, clot evacuation and fulguration of bleeding point, again followed by catheter traction, continuous bladder irrigation, and EACA.

Should bleeding continue, the bladder can be irrigated for 1 hour using a 1 in 10,000 solution of silver nitrate. Arteriographic embolization has been used but we do not have personal experience of this technique. However, we would advise reserving embolization for situations where the bleeding is life-threatening, especially if the patient is unfit for further surgery and when other efforts have failed.

If the previous measures fail, open surgery is necessary. Through a suprapubic approach, the capsule of the prostate is opened as in a retropubic prostatectomy. The fossa is packed to stop venous bleeding. Hemostatic corner stitches are inserted and any bleeding arteries are identified and suture-ligated. The packs are removed and the venous bleeding points are coagulated with the diathermy or are sutured. If bleeding continues, a Foley catheter is introduced through the urethra into the bladder, the bladder is opened, and the prostatic fossa is firmly packed with a vaginal roll. The balloon of the catheter is inflated and the catheter is pulled down firmly on top of the packing. The catheter is placed on traction for 24 hours using a 2-pound waterbag weight. The end of the vaginal roll is brought out suprapubically and antibiotics are given. The pack is gently removed after 72 hours. If bleeding recurs, it may be necessary to repack the fossa. We do not like to use Hyrntschak-type bladder neck or prostate sutures after routine open prostatectomy since they are unnecessary for most patients and may cause bladder neck stenosis. Likewise, we prefer packing of the prostatic fossa and catheter traction rather than Hyrntschak sutures if open surgery is needed to control post-prostatectomy hemorrhage. When blood clots persistently block the urethral catheter, it is preferable to use a large-caliber suprapubic catheter instead. This allows easier removal of the clots and avoids the complications of a prolonged indwelling urethral catheter. If, despite all the aforementioned techniques, the bleeding continues to be severe so that even the suprapubic catheters blocks with clots, we advocate resorting to Lapides' procedure of making a wide cystotomy and leaving all the wounds open. Blood is transfused to keep pace with the bleeding. Loose dressings are applied to catch the drainage. Clots form without causing obstruction, pain, or septicemia. The wounds close spontaneously as soon as the bleeding ceases. Ligation of the internal iliac arteries may be performed, but it is usually unsuccessful.

Prostatectomy is especially hazardous in patients with disordered hemostasis. The disorder may be of the primary hemostatic plug, the coagulation mechanism, fibrinolysis, or the blood vessel constriction. There is often specific treatment for these disorders that has to be used in addition to the general measures and these are summarized in Table I of Chapter 10. In these patients bleeding may persist for 6–7 weeks after the operation until the denuded prostatic fossa re-epithelializes.

REFERENCES

1. Singh M. Tresidder GC, Blandy JP. The evaluation of transurethral resection for benign enlargement of the prostate. *Br J Urol.* 45:93–102, 1973.
2. Bergman RT, Turner R, Barnes RW, Hadley HL. Comparative analysis of 1,000 consecutive cases of transurethral prostatic resection. *J Urol.* 74:533–545, 1955.
3. Wines RD, Lane V, O'Flynn JD. Post-prostatectomy bleeding: Active management by early endoscopic haemostasis and packing in a series of 3,219 prostatectomies. *Aust NZ J Surg.* 43:274–277, 1973.
4. Perrin P, Barnes R, Hadley H, Bergman RT. Forty years of transurethral prostatic resections. *J Urol.* 116:757–758, 1976.
5. Lund BL, Dingsor E. Benign obstructive prostatic enlargement. *Scand J Urol Nephrol.* 10:33–38, 1976.
6. Salvaris M. Retropubic prostatectomy: An evaluation of 1200 operations. *Med J Aust.* 47:370–376, 1960.
7. Slade N, Andrews GL, Tovey GH, Wilson F. Blood loss in prostatic surgery. *Br J Urol.* 36:399–405, 1964.
8. Madsen RE, Madsen PO. Influence of anesthesia form on blood loss in transurethral prostatectomy. *Anesth Anal* (Cleveland). 46:330–332, 1967.
9. Madsen, PO, Kaveggia L, Atassi SA. The effect of estrogens (premarin) and regional hypothermia on blood loss during transurethral prostatectomy. *J Urol* 92:314–316, 1964.
10. Robson CJ, Sales JL. The effect of local hypothermia on blood loss during transurethral resection of the prostate. *J Urol* 95:393–395, 1966.
11. Bruce AW, Zorab J, Still B. Blood loss in prostatic surgery. *Br J Urol.* 32:422–426, 1960.
12. Frank RM, Lloyd FA. A clinical study of the effectiveness of adrenosem in transurethral resection. *J Urol.* 82:243–246, 1959.
13. Weisenthal CL, Meade RC, Owenby J, Irwin RI. An investigation of kutapressin as a hemostatic agent in transurethral surgery of the prostate. *J Urol.* 86:346–349, 1961.
14. Madsen PO, Strauch AE, Barquin OP, Malek GH. The lack of hemostatic effect of polyestradiol phosphate and carbazochrome salicylate in transurethral prostatectomy. *J Urol.* 99:786–787, 1968.
15. Pearson BS. The effect of trasylol and amino caproic acid in post-prostatectomy haemorrhage. *Br J Urol.* 41:602, 1969.
16. Symes JM, Hardy DG, Sutherns K, Blandy JP. Factors reducing the rate of infection after trans-urethral surgery. *Br J Urol.* 44:582–586, 1972.
17. Negus D, Pinto DJ, Brown N. Platelet adhesiveness in postoperative deep-vein thrombosis. *Lancet.* 1:220–224, 1969.
18. Foley FEB. A hemostatic bag catheter: A one piece latex rubber structure for control of bleeding and constant drainage following prostatic resection. *J Urol.* 38:134–139, 1937.
19. Weyrauch HM. In: *Surgery of the Prostate.* Philadelphia, W.B. Saunders Co., 1959.
20. Salvaris M. In: *Operative Urology.* J. Blandy, Oxford, Blackwell Scientific Publications, 149, 1978.
21. Andersson L. Antifibrinolytic treatment with epsilon-aminocaproic acid in connection with prostatectomy. *Acta Chir Scand.* 127:552–564, 1964.
22. McNicol GP, Fletcher AP, Alkjaersig N, Sherry S. The use of epsilon-aminocaproic acid, a potent inhibitor of fibrinolytic activity, in the management of postoperative hematuria. *J Urol.* 86:829–837, 1961.
23. Nilsson IM, Andersson L, Björkman SE. Epsilon-aminocaproic acid (EACA) as a therapeutic agent based on 5 years' clinical experience. *Acta Med Scand.* (Suppl) 448:1–46, 1966.

24. Gormsen J, Haxholdt BF. The heparin tolerance test and thromb-embolic incidence in surgery. *Acta Chir Scand.* 120:121–136, 1961.
25. Bergin JJ. The complications of therapy with epsilon-aminocaproic acid. *Med Clin N Am.* 50:1669–1678, 1966.
26. Naeye RL. Thrombotic state after a hemorrhagic diathesis, a possible complication of therapy with epsilon-aminocaproic acid. *Blood.* 19:694–701, 1962.
27. Vinnecombe J, Shuttleworth KE. Aminocaproic acid in the control of haemorrhage after prostatectomy: A controlled trial. *Lancet.* 1:230–232, 1966.
28. Gordon-Smith IC, Hickman JA, El Masri SH. The effect of the fibrinolytic inhibitor epsilon aminocaproic acid on the incidence of deep-vein thrombosis after prostatectomy. *Br J Surg.* 59:522–524, 1972.
29. Black WD, Hatch FE, Acchiardo S. Aminocaproic acid in prolonged hematuria of patients with sicklemia. *Arch Intern Med.* 136:678–681, 1976.
30. Borgstrom S. Investigation on the effect of dicumarol and early ambulation in the prevention of postoperative thrombo-embolism in a surgical material strongly disposed to thrombosis. *Acta Chir Scand.* (Suppl) 150:32, 1950.
31. Mayo ME, Halil T, Browse NL. The incidence of deep-vein thrombosis after prostatectomy. *Br J Urol.* 43:738–742, 1971.
32. Andersson J. Combined prophylaxis of haemorrhage and thrombosis after prostatectomy. *Acta Chir Scand.* 130:393–398, 1965.
33. Gormsen J, Andersen A, Gammelgaard A. Prostatectomy during anticoagulant therapy. *Acta Chir Scand.* 120:380–387, 1961.
34. Gollub S. In discussion, Deysine M, Cliffton EE. Mechanism of action of epsilon-aminocaproic acid in the control of hemorrhage. *Ann NY Acad Sci.* 115:291–301, 1964.
35. Andersson L. Fibrinolysis in patients with prostatic cancer. *Acta Chir Scand.* 126: 172–180, 1963.
36. Griffin JD, Ellman L. Epsilon-aminocaproic acid (EACA). *Semin Thromb Hemostas.* 5:27–40, 1978.
37. Parton LI. Treatment of post-prostatectomy haemorrhage. Hyryntshak prostatectomy –520 Cases. *Br J Urol.* 41:600–601, 1969.
38. Crile GW. *Blood Pressure in Surgery: Experimental and Clinical Research.* Philadelphia, J.B. Lippincott Co., 1903, pp. 288–291.
39. Gardner WJ, Storer J. The use of the G-suit in control of intra-abdominal bleeding. *Surg Gynecol Obstet.* 123:792-798, 1966.
40. Paris PM. Antishock garments (Letter). *N Engl J Med.* 305:960, 1981.
41. Pelligra R, Sandberg EC. Control of intractable abdominal bleeding by external counterpressure. *JAMA.* 241:708–713, 1979.
42. Batalden DJ, Wichstrom PH, Ruiz E, Gustilo RB. Value of the G-suit in patients with severe pelvic fracture. *Arch Surg.* 109:326-328, 1974.
43. Burdick JF, Warshaw AL, Abbott WM. External counterpressure to control postoperative intra-abdominal hemorrhage. *Am J Surg.* 129:369–373, 1975.
44. McCullough DL, McLaughlin AP, Warshawsky AB. The gravity suit: A useful device in complicated urologic hemorrhage. *Urology.* 6:468–470, 1975.
45. Cangiano JL, Kest L. Use of a G-suit for uncontrollable bleeding after percutaneous renal biopsy. *J Urol.* 107:360–361, 1972.
46. Shenasky JH, Gillenwater JY. The renal hemodynamic and functional effects of external counterpressure. *Surg Gynecol Obstet.* 134:253–258, 1972.
47. Espinosa MH, Updegrove JH. Clinical experience with the G-suit. *Arch Surg.* 101: 36–69, 1970.
48. Hryntschak T. Suprapubic prostatectomy with primary closure of the bladder by an original method. Springfield, Illinois, Charles C. Thomas, Publisher, 1955.
49. Beck AD, Gaudin HJ. The Hryntschak prostatectomy. III. A modified technique of closing the vesical neck and prostatic cavity. *J Urol.* 104:739–744, 1970.
50. Malament M. Maximal hemostasis in suprapubic prostatectomy. *Surg Gynecol Obstet.* 120:1307–1312, 1965.

51. Nicoll GA, Riffle GA II, Andersen FO. Suprapubic prostatectomy. The removal of purse string: A continuing comparative analysis of 300 consecutive cases. *J Urol.* 120: 702–704, 1978.
52. Beck AD, Gaudin HJ. The Hryntschak prostatectomy. I. A review of 1,345 cases. *J Urol.* 103:637–640, 1970.
53. Hahne B, Van der Linden W. Vesical neck closure versus balloon catheter in suprapubic prostatectomy: A controlled clinical trial. *J Urol.* 120:699–701, 1978.
54. Lapides J. Principles of treatment of persistent post-prostatectomy hemorrhage. *J Urol.* 106:913–914, 1971.
55. Pereiras RV, Jr., Meier WL, Katz ER, Viamonte M, Jr. Arteriographic embolization treatment for post-prostatectomy hemorrhage. *Urology.* 9:705–707, 1977.
56. Owen CA, Thompson JH, Bowie EJ. Evaluation of bleeding tendencies in surgical patients. *Med Clin N Am.* 46:935–946, 1962.
57. Biggs R, Matthews J. The plasma concentration of factor VIII in the treatment of hemophilia. In: *Treatment of Haemophilia and Other Coagulation Disorders.* Biggs R, and Macfarlane RG, Eds. Chapter VI. Oxford, Blackwell Scientific Publications, 1966.
58. Kernoff PB. Prostatectomy in haemophilia and Christmas disease. *J Urol.* 44:51–57, 1972.
59. Steiger B, White JG, Krivit W. Epsilon-aminocaproic acid for hematuria in hemophilia. *Lancet.* 82:421–424, 1962.
60. Barkham P. Haematuria in a haemophiliac treated with epsilon-aminocaproic acid. *Lancet.* 82:421–424, 1962.
61. Fletcher AP, Biederman O, Moore D, Alkjaersig N, Sherry S. Altered fibrinolytic mechanisms in hepatic cirrhosis and its potential clinical significance. *Trans Assoc Am Physicians.* 76:280–288, 1963.
62. Astrup T, Rasmussen J, Amery A, Poulsen HE. Fibrinolytic activity of cirrhotic liver. *Nature.* 185:619–620, 1960.
63. Nilsson IM, Sjoerdsma A, Waldenstrom J. Antifibrinolytic activity and metabolism of 6-aminocaproic acid in man. *Lancet.* 1:1322–1326, 1960.
64. Bjorkman SE, Laurell CB, Nilsson IM. Serum proteins and fibrinolysis in polycythemia vera. *Scan J Clin Lab Invest.* 8:304–308, 1956.

Chapter 12

The Role of Chemotherapy in the Management of Hematuria Due to Neoplasms of the Urinary Tract

Mark S. Huberman, M.D.

I. Introduction

Urinary tract malignancies are a frequent cause of urologic bleeding. In renal cell carcinoma, approximately 60% of patients present with hematuria, with the classic triad of pain, hematuria, and flank mass occurring much less frequently[1] (Fig. 1). In the less common carcinoma of the renal pelvis, hematuria is a finding at presentation in 80–90% of patients.[1] Hematuria is also the most common initial symptom with carcinoma of the ureter occurring in about 74% of cases.[1] Additionally, hematuria is the most frequent presenting manifestation of bladder cancer, occurring in approximately 70–80% of patients.[1] Prostatic carcinoma, as well as nonurologic malignancies with local extension into the urinary tract such as rectal and cervical carcinomas, may also cause urologic bleeding.

A. Systemic Therapies

1. Selection of Drugs

The efficacy of systemic therapy using either hormonal or cytotoxic chemotherapy in urologic cancer and its role in the management of neoplastic urinary tract bleeding vary depending on the primary tumor. Table I summarizes the current systemic therapies available for primary urologic tract malignancies. A

From Bern MM (ed.): *Urinary Tract Bleeding: Diagnosis and Control by Medical, Radiologic, and Surgical Techniques*. Mount Kisco, NY, Futura Publishing Co., Inc., 1985.

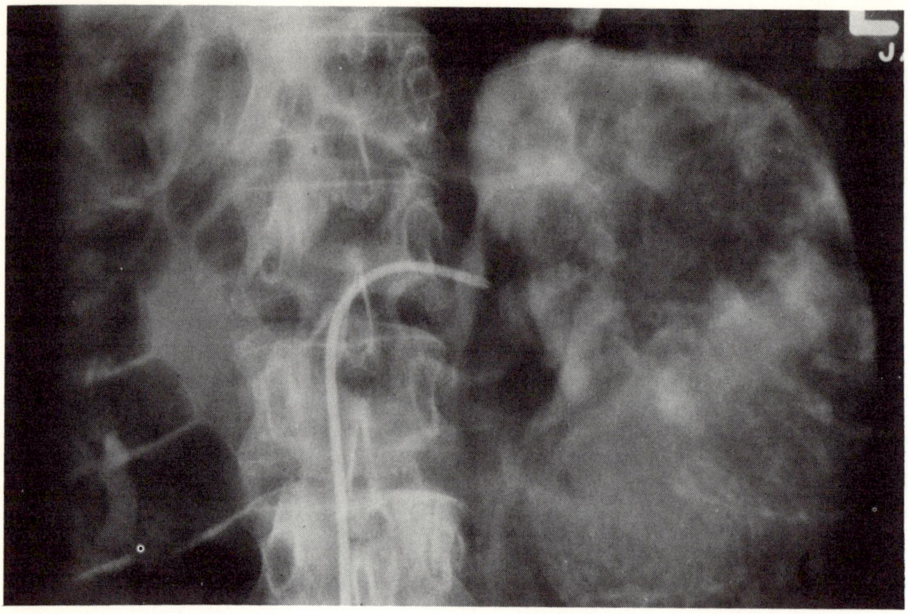

Figure 1: *Renal artery angiogram demonstrating a hypernephroma.* (From the Learning File *of the Center for Devices and Radiological Health, FDA, case GU603.)*

Table I
Systemic Therapy in Advanced Urologic Malignancy

Tumor Type	Chemotherapy	Hormone Therapy
Renal cell carcinoma	Vinblastine Response rate is low and treatment remains experimental	Early encouraging reports not substantiated
Transitional cell carcinoma of the renal pelvis	Cis-platinum Role is to be defined	None
Bladder cancer	Cis-platinum and other single agents appear equivalent to combinations	None
Prostate cancer	Several effective single agents No advantage to combinations presently. Role of simultaneous cytotoxic and hormone therapy to be defined.	Estrogens or Orchiectomy as primary treatment
Testicular cancer	Cis-platinum, Vinblastine, and Bleomycin High cure rate.	None

full discussion of systemic therapy by each tumor type will follow. The decision of whether to use systemic chemotherapy at all, and which therapy, should be based on the extent of the disease, knowledge of prior therapy and its efficacy, and the overall medical condition of the patient. These decisions are best made with the help of a medical oncologist and ideally, after communications between urology, radiation therapy, and medical oncology. The discussions in this chapter should serve as an introduction and guide to the questions involved in these often very complex clinical problems.

2. *Responses*

With the exception of testicular carcinoma, none of the primary urinary tract malignancies of adulthood is curable with present types of systemic drug therapies. Thus, the realistic goals of chemotherapy when used for diseases other than testicular carcinoma are palliation of symptoms and prolongation of survival.

The results of most chemotherapy trials are reported in terms of response rate, which is the percentage of patients whose tumor undergoes a pre-defined reduction in size following treatment. Most, but not all, studies describe partial and complete responses. A partial remission is a greater than 50% decrease in the sum of the perpendicular diameters of measurable tumor masses. A complete response is when all clinical and radiographic evidence of tumor disappears. Response rates reported in any single article in the literature may be based on other definitions. Thus, responders in one study may not be considered responders in another study, and great care must be taken when making comparisons. These differences in the reporting techniques are not altogether unreasonable. As an example, prostate cancer is by it biologic nature difficult to evaluate, i.e. measurable tumor masses do not often exist and it is difficult to evaluate objectively changes in osteoblastic metastases. Thus, alternative parameters are used.

For most urologic malignancy, with the exception of testicular cancer, complete responses are infrequent using currently available chemotherapy and/or hormonal treatments. Responses usually occur within 6–8 weeks of the initiation of treatment with either cytotoxic or hormonal therapy. Generally, partial responses are associated with symptomatic improvement and prolongation of survival when responding patients are compared to nonresponding patients. Unfortunately, the duration of these responses tends to be short, generally measured in months with the exception of testicular or hormonally sensitive prostatic carcinoma.

3. *Pharmacology of Chemotherapy Agents*

The pharmacology of anticancer drugs must also be considered in making decisions regarding therapy of urologic malignancies. Several cytotoxic drugs are eliminated by the renal route. Cis-platinum (Platinol®) and methotrexate are excreted in the urine. Both drugs are potentially nephrotoxic in patients with renal insufficiency due to any cause, particularly in the obstructive uropathies. Doses of these drugs must be decreased or alternative drugs selected in the presence of renal insufficiency. Newer drugs such as VP16-213 (Etoposide®) may also need dose reduction due to renal failure. Patients with bladder atony or outlet obstruction with long retention time in the bladder may be at risk for cyclophosphamide-induced cystitis.

B. Localized Therapies

Local therapies have the advantage of increasing the concentration of drugs (or radiation) delivered to the tumor, while reducing the systemic toxicities. In recent years, options for local treatment have increased to include regional infusion and embolization, in addition to the local radiation and instillation therapies (see Chapters 8, 13, and 14).

1. *Instillation Therapy*

The most extensive experience with chemotherapeutic agents in urologic malignancies has been in the treatment of superficial noninvasive bladder cancer. These can be treated with a variety of local modalities. Of those with superficial disease, between 50% and 70% will form new tumors, with about 30% progressing in grade or stage.[2–5]

Several drugs such as Thio-TEPA, mitomycin-C (Mutamycin®), bleomycin (Blenoxane®), and more recently doxorubicin (Adriamycin®) have been instilled directly into the bladder. (Chapter 13 discusses the details of intravesical therapy).

2. *Infusion Therapy*

Arterial infusion therapy has the advantage of delivering high concentrations of drug to the tumor while sparing the patient systemic side effects from intravenous therapy.[6] This approach takes advantage of the steep dose-response curves[7] and allows an increase of five to 30 times the concentration of drug delivered to the tumor,[8] the latter obtained if the artery is occluded proximally. A variety of situations affect the success of this approach including (1) sensitivity of the tumor to the drug, (2) tolerance of arterial endothelium to the drug, (3) success of selective catheter placement, (4) patient's changing position, (5) hemodynamics within the vessel catheterized, (6) effects of pulsatile flow, and (7) shunting away from the tumor, among others.[6,9]

3. *Embolization Therapy*

Embolization creates ischemia in the tumor. The degree of the vascular occlusion depends upon (1) the proximity of the occlusion to the tumor, (2) the abundance of collateral vessels, and (3) the material used to occlude the vessel. The latter materials used include Gelfoam®, polyvinyl alcohol foam particles, stainless steel coils, autologous clot or tissue, starch spheres, and jelling or sclerosing agents.[6] This embolization technique can be coupled with intra-arterial infusion of chemotherapy. The participation of an interventional radiologist is required for these approaches (see Chapter 8).

II. Tumor Types

A. Renal Cell Carcinoma (Adenocarcinoma or Hypernephroma)

At the time of diagnosis of renal carcinoma (Fig. 2a, b), about 25–50% of patients will already have stage IV or metastatic disease.[6,11] In addition, a significant number of resected patients will eventually develop metastases. This makes systemic therapy a necessary course in a great many patients. Yet, carcinoma of the kidney continues to be one of the most chemotherapy-resistant types of cancer. No cytotoxic agent has been reported that consistently effects a higher response rate than vinblastine (Velban®). Hrushesky and Murphy reported a 25% response rate in 135 patients with renal cell carcinoma treated with vinblastine.[12] However, some of their "responses" did not actually fit the usual criteria for partial response. Combination therapy, which includes vinblastine, often produces a somewhat lower response rate.[13] While vinblastine is possibly a useful agent, the realistic likelihood of response is no more than 10–15%. Thus, there is presently no standard chemotherapeutic approach for this disease. Chemotherapy remains basically investigational, with definite need for improvement.

In hamsters, diethylstilbesterol can induce renal cell carcinoma.[14] In these same animals, testosterone or progesterone inhibited tumor growth. Extensive investigation of progestational agents in human renal adenocarcinoma was begun. Although there were reported initial response rates of 15–17%, more recent studies involving over 400 patients with stricter response criteria showed response rates less than 5%.[1,13] Thus, there is no convincing evidence that hormonal management of human renal cell carcinoma has any significant bene-

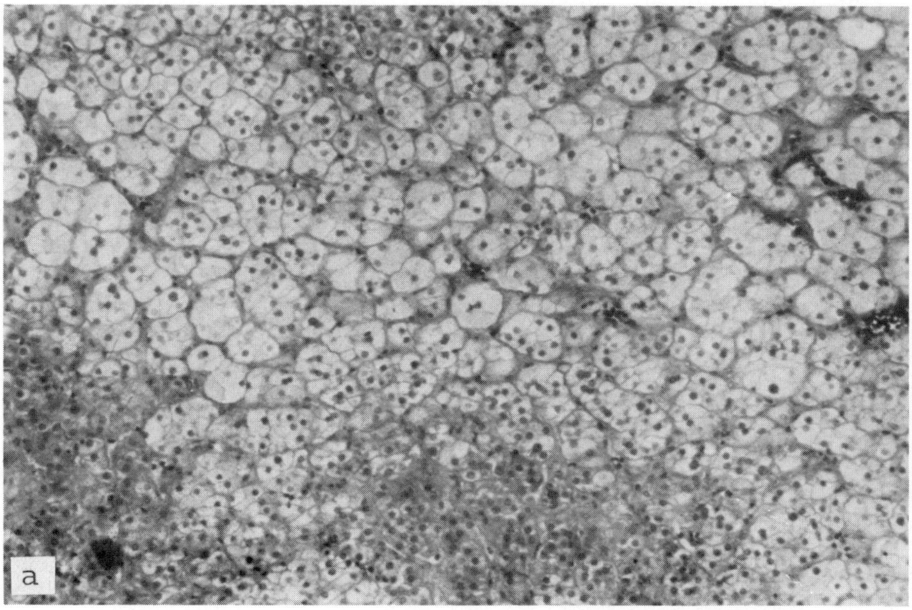

Figure 2: *Photomicrographs of renal cell carcinoma.* **a.** *Clear cell type.*

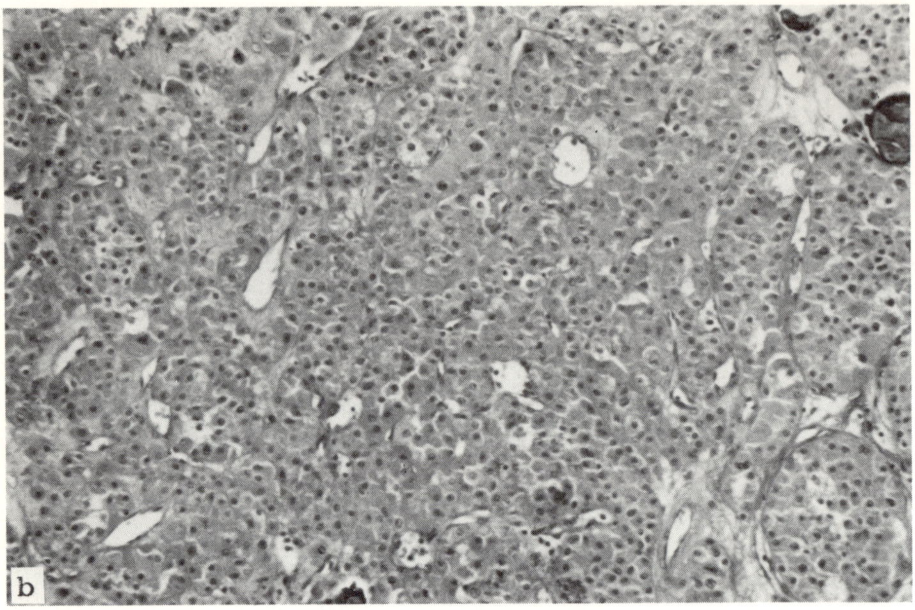

Figure 2: **b.** *Dark cell type.*

fit. Therefore, patients with urologic bleeding from hypernephroma (Fig. 2) are unlikely to be helped by any current systemic therapy and local modalities of treatment should be applied.

Transitional cell carcinoma of the renal pelvis is less common than classic renal cell carcinoma, and chemotherapy has had a rather limited evaluation (Fig. 3). However, early experience suggests that cis-platinum (Platinol®) may be an active agent in this disease as it is with the more common transitional cell carcinoma of the urinary bladder.

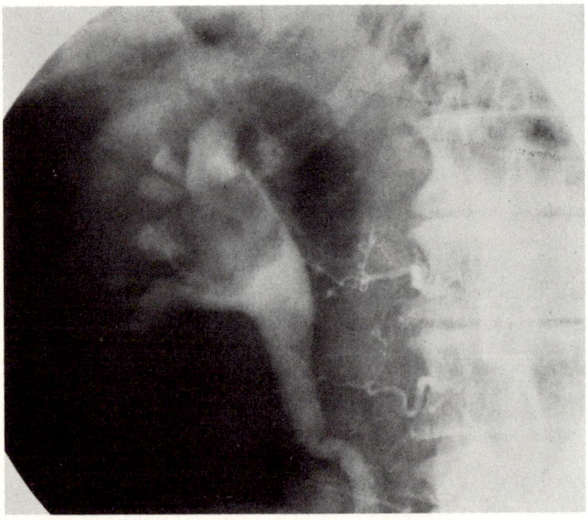

Figure 3: *Excretory phase following renal artery angiogram demonstrating a transitional cell carcinoma of the renal pelvis. (From the Learning File of the Center for Devices and Radiological Health, FDA, case GU704.)*

Wallace et al. have recently reviewed the treatment of renal carcinomas using infusion and/or emboli therapy and their complications.[6] Transcatheter arterial embolization for the disease was first proposed by Lalli et al. in 1969.[15] A variety of materials, including radioactive gold, have been used as discussed above.[15,16] In several series, embolization has been combined with other therapies such as hormones and nephrectomy, making the role of the embolization difficult to interpret.[17–19] There is no clear evidence of survival advantage for these types of treatments. However, embolic therapy can control bleeding and other symptoms referable to the tumor.[6]

Arterial embolization has also been useful as an adjunct to surgical biopsy or excision and for prosthetic fixation of bones damaged by metastatic renal carcinoma. Preoperative arterial embolization appears to have significantly reduced the surgical blood loss from these hypervascular lesions.[20,21]

B. Ureteral Neoplasms

Chemotherapy remains an area for investigation in treatment of carcinoma of the ureter (Fig. 4). This is primarily due to the limited experience available with drug therapy in this rare tumor. As the majority of ureteral cancers are transitional cell in origin, it is likely that the role of chemotherapy is similar to that of transitional cell carcinoma of the bladder.[1]

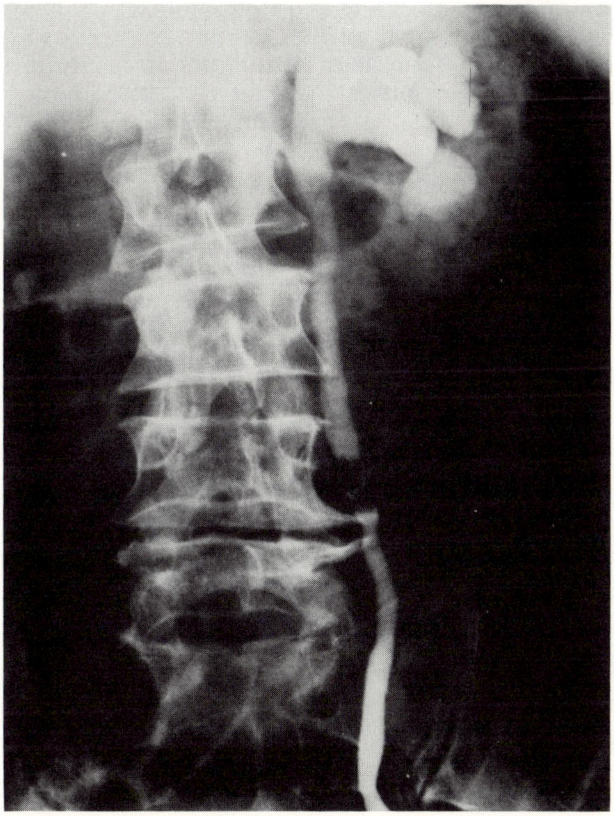

Figure 4: *Excretory phase of intravenous pylegram demonstrating a carcinoma of the ureter. (From the Learning File of the Center for Devices and Radiological Health, FDA, case GU703.)*

C. Bladder Cancer

1. *Systemic Therapy*

Hematuria occurs in 70–80% of patients with bladder cancer (Fig. 5). It is often total and without pain. The magnitude of hematuria is not related to the stage or grade of the tumor; it may even be sporadic.[2] Additional urinary tract symptoms may appear including frequency, urgency, decreased urinary flow, or pain—symptoms not dissimilar from those of infection. Therapy for this neoplasm is based on clinical staging systems (see Table II). These clinical staging systems are not as accurate as the pathological staging systems.[24,25] Transitional cell carcinoma causes 85% of these tumors, with the remainder due to squamous cell and adenocarcinomas[2] (Figs. 6, 7). These latter forms are rarely superficial at presentation and have a poorer prognosis.

There have been a number of active cancer chemotherapeutic agents in bladder cancer that, when used alone, can lead to remission rates varying from 10% to 40%.[26] Yet chemotherapy has only a palliative role in advanced bladder cancer. Most of the responses are partial, with only a small percentage of complete remissions. In addition, responses are usually of short duration in the several-month range. The drugs with single-agent activity against bladder cancer include: cis-platinum, methotrexate, doxorubicin, cyclophosphamide, vinca alkaloids, mitomycin-C, and 5-fluorouracil (5-FU). Cis-platinum has the highest single-agent activity for transitional cell carcinoma.[27] It is possible that metastatic sites respond better than local and regional sites.[25]

Methotrexate induces remission in 29% of cases, with an undefined optimal dose schedule.[28] Doxorubicin induces responses in about 21% of patients.[29]

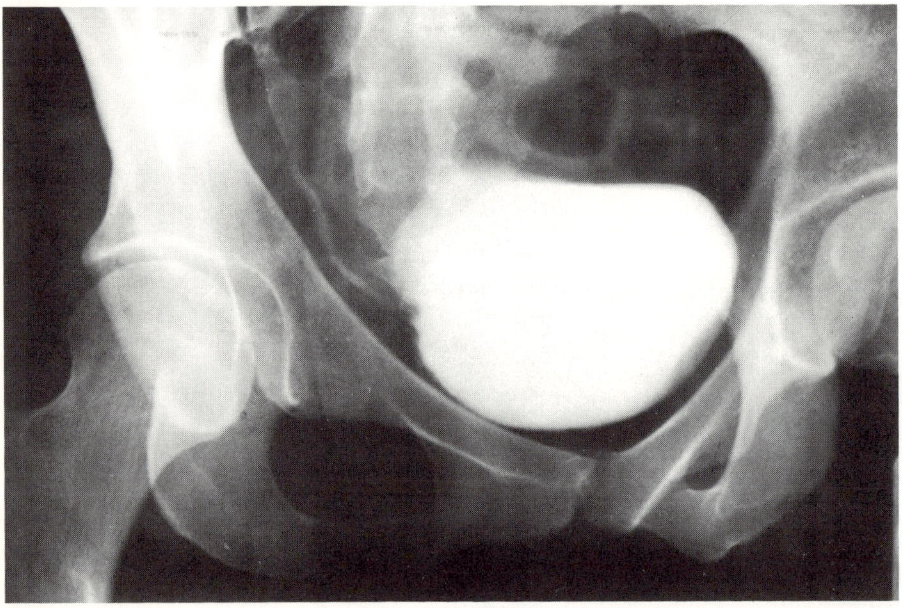

Figure 5: *Transitional cell carcinoma of the bladder.*

Table II
Clinical Staging of Bladder Carcinoma

	Sites Of Disease	Stage[22]	TNM System[23]
Superficial	Carcinoma in situ	0*	T_{iS}*
	To bladder mucosa only	0	T_a
	To lamina propria only	A	T_1
	To muscle: < ½ of muscle depth	B_1	T_2
Deep	> ½ of muscle depth	B_2	T_{3A}
	To perivesical fat	C	T_{3B}
	To adjacent organ	D	T_4
	To pelvic lymph nodes	D_1	N_{1-3}
	To extrapelvic lymph nodes or distant organ	D_2	N_4M_1

*Carcinoma in situ can be found in bladder (Tish), ureter (Tisu), prostatic urethra (Tis pr u), or prostatic ducts (Tispd).

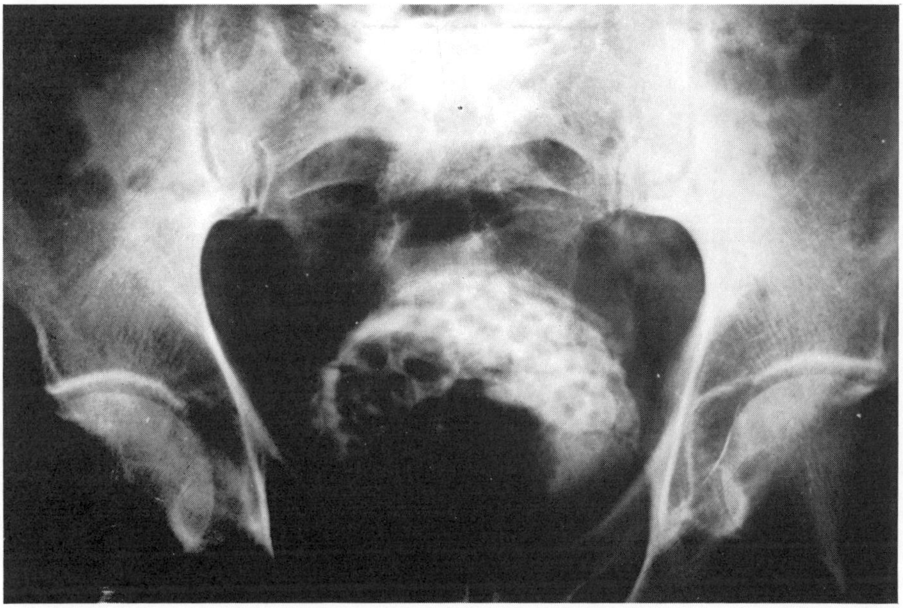

Figure 6: *Adenocarcinoma of the bladder.*

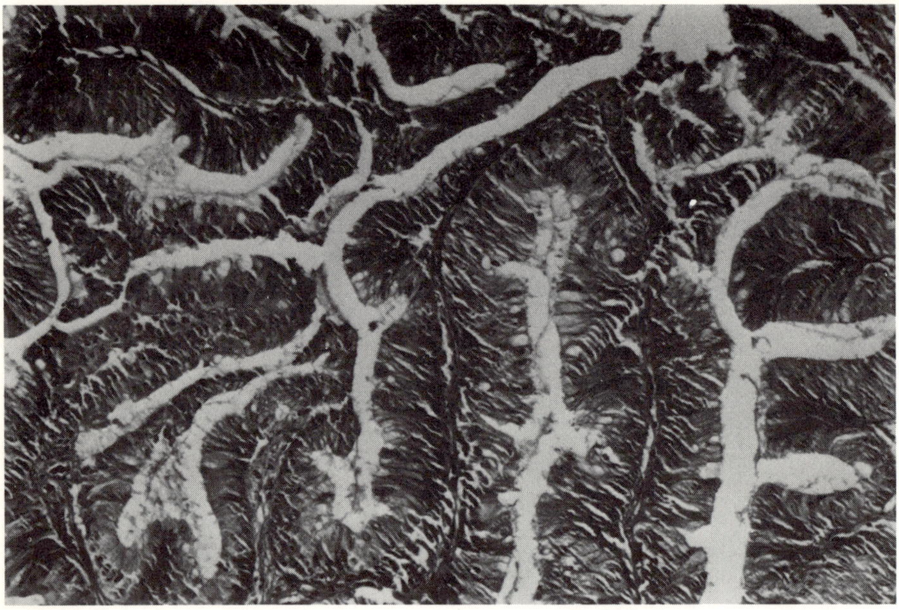

Figure 7: *Photomicrograph of adenocarcinoma of the bladder (100×).*

Vincristine and vinblastine lead to 10–18% response rates, respectively.[27] These responses are all of short duration and are negatively biased by prior therapy.

The role of combination chemotherapy in advanced bladder cancer is still being defined. Early reports of combining two to three active agents, usually including cyclophosphamide, doxorubicin, and platinum, gave response rates that vary from 26% to 90%. The majority of these trials were not randomized. Randomized trials have not yet shown an advantage for combination chemotherapy in bladder cancer over single agent treatment.[1,26,30–32] Studies that compared platinum to a combination of cyclophosphamide, doxorubicin, and platinum showed no significant advantage. The combination therapy did have more side effects.[26,31] Additionally, another study that compared platinum to cyclophosphamide plus platinum showed no advantage to the combination.[32] Several other combination trials are discussed by Yagoda[25] in greater detail expanding this analysis to involve other combinations.

Therefore, based on current data, meaningful palliation of advanced bladder cancer can be achieved at best in about 20–30% of patients with the most active single agent being cis-platinum. Responses usually occur within several weeks and generally last 3 to 6 months, though significantly longer remission durations have been noted. Ongoing studies to identify new active drugs and improve the combination therapies are being conducted. In addition, the National Bladder Cancer Group is conducting a study using platinum as adjuvant therapy in patients completing pre-op radiation therapy and radical cystectomy. Clearly, it is necessary to develop more efficacious programs in this difficult-to-manage disease.

2. *Transcatheter Intra-arterial Infusion of Chemotherapy For Bladder Cancer*

Intra-arterial chemotherapy for bladder cancer was first reported by Byron in 1961.[33] Subsequently, 5-FU and then mitomycin were infused.[34,35] Recently, Wallace and his group from M. D. Anderson Hospital have reported on the use of bilateral internal iliac artery infusion of chemotherapeutic agents in patients with advanced bladder cancer.[6,36] In their reports they described patients with symptomatic pelvic disease, which was either isolated or was part of more widely spread metastatic disease. All patients had pelvic pain or hematuria. Cis-platinum was infused over 24 hours with protection of the renal function by hydration and mannitol diuresis. This program was repeated every 4 weeks for a total of three courses. Forty percent of the patients achieved a complete response and 20% achieved a partial response. Significantly, pelvic pain was controlled in 12 of 15 patients, and hematuria was controlled in eight out of 10 patients. Ten of these patients had failed prior systemic chemotherapy, and three were receiving concomitant systemic therapy with cyclophosphamide and doxorubicin. An additional two patients who did not respond to cis-platinum infusion did respond to a combination of 5-FU infusion through the iliac arteries and systemic doxorubicin plus mitomycin-C.

In another study, 29 patients received intra-arterial 5-FU while receiving systemic doxorubicin and mitomycin-C.[37,38] Of these, 58% had complete responses, including 12 of 20 with transitional cell carcinoma and four of four with adenocarcinoma. There was a survival advantage for the responders. Another group of patients was treated with intra-arterial cis-platinum along with systemic cyclophosphamide and doxorubicin.[39] Complete remissions were observed in 39% of the patients, again with a survival advantage for complete responders.

These combination approaches make the evaluation of the role of infusion therapy when used alone more difficult. Comparative trials are now appropriate. In addition, there were two cases of transient acute tubular necrosis and one lower extremity embolus that did resolve spontaneously. Transient peripheral neuropathy also occurred. Pulmonary complications occurred in three patients. Leukopenia with fever was common. Nevertheless, the ability to control bleeding in 80% of patients is quite impressive. Wallace et al. report that while in their experience systemic chemotherapy effects a high response rate particularly with pulmonary metastases, there is less ability to control pelvic and retroperitoneal disease with systemic therapy. Thus, the role of infusional therapy in the management of urinary tract malignancy is exciting, but must for now remain investigational.

D. Prostate Cancer (Fig. 8)

There has been an extensive experience with hormonal manipulation as systemic therapy for advanced prostate cancer. The role for cytotoxic chemotherapy in this disease is still being defined. Hormone therapy, usually orchiectomy or oral diethylstilbesterol (DES), when used as primary therapy is associated with palliation in 50–80% of patients with advanced prostate cancer.[1,40] Urologic bleeding caused by prostate cancer is often well managed by hormonal

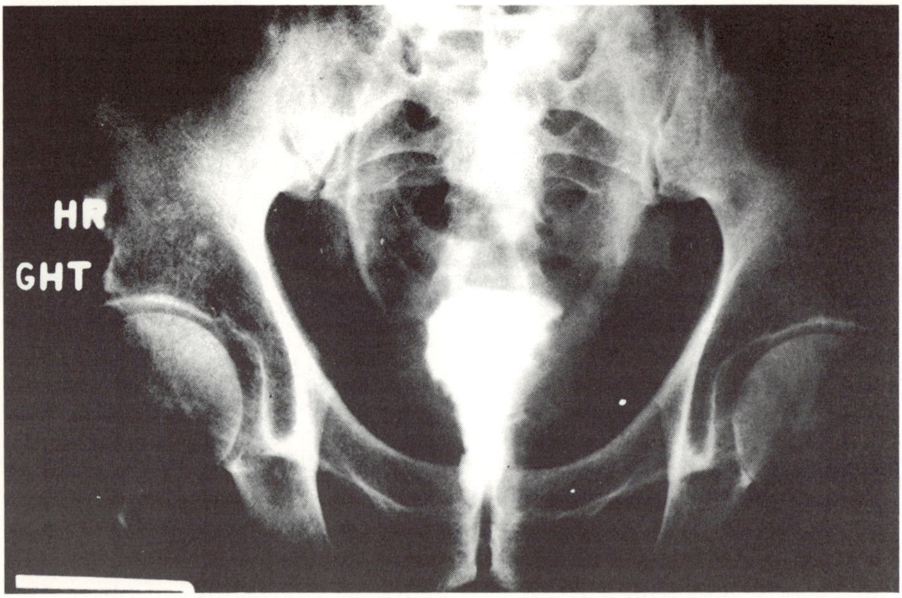

Figure 8: *Prostatic carcinoma involving the bladder. (From the* Learning File *of the Center for Devices and Radiological Health, FDA, case GU719.)*

manipulation in patients who have not failed prior hormone therapy. It is, however, recognized that hormonal therapy has limited impact on survival in these patients.[1,41]

The choice of which hormonal therapy to choose is based primarily on patient acceptance and potential toxicity. DES at 5.0 mg per day is associated with a significant risk of death from cardiovascular and/or thromboembolic disease.[41] This risk is considerably lower at a dose of 1.0 mg per day DES. The risk of cardiovascular mortality of a DES dose of 3.0 mg per day has not been systematically evaluated. Orchiectomy, on the other hand, has not been associated with any excess risk of cardiovascular mortality. Also, orchiectomy is not associated with painful gynecomastia, as is seen in patients receiving DES. (The DES-associated gynecomastia can be prevented by pre-treatment low-dose radiation to the breasts.) Recently the gonadotropin-releasing hormone analogue, leuprolide, was shown to have similar efficacy to DES for the initial hormonal management of metastatic prostate cancer.[59] Leuprolide was associated with less gynecomastia, nausea and vomiting, and thromboembolic phenomena than DES.

Secondary hormonal maneuvers in prostate cancer are generally much less successful, with fewer objective responses. The reported response rate is less than 20% of patients treated.[1,41] These secondary hormonal therapies include (1) orchiectomy after DES, (2) DES after orchiectomy, (3) higher-dose estrogen, diethylstilbesterol diphosphate (Stilphostrol®) (4) anti-androgen therapy such as cyproterone acetate, (5) surgical or medical adrenalectomy with aminoglutethemide, (6) hypophysectomy, (7) progestational therapy, or (8) anti-estrogen therapy with Tamoxifen.

The role of cytotoxic chemotherapy in advanced prostate cancer needs to be further defined. Clinical investigations in this situation are hampered by some biological factors seen in patients with this disease. Frequently, this disease occurs in elderly men who have significant underlying medical problems. There is difficulty in evaluating objective response in most patients with prostate cancer since osteoblastic bone involvement is difficult to quantitate. Frequently, these patients do not have disease that can be easily measured, such as soft tissue masses or pulmonary nodules. Many standard chemotherapeutic agents have not been systematically tested in prostate cancer. Still, there are a number of single agents that are associated with response rates ranging from 15% to 46%.[1,42,43]

Many of these drug evaluations included the concept of "disease stabilization" in the criteria for judging response. When response criteria includes "disease stabilization," the single agents with activity against prostatic carcinoma include 5-fluorouracil, cyclophosphamide, doxorubicin, cis-platinum, dacarbazine (DTIC®), lomustine (CCNU®), nitrogen mustard, streptozotocin, vincristine (Oncovin®), hydroxyurea, estramustine (Emcyt®), and prednimustine. The last two drugs are interesting newly synthetized agents that combine a nitrogen mustard moiety with estradiol or prednisone. The rationale behind the development of estramustine is that the estrogen-sensitive cells will selectively take up the drug that will carry the nitrogen mustard directly to the cell.

The difficulty in evaluating the role of combinations of chemotherapy in prostate cancer is similar to that in bladder cancer. There are reports of higher response rates using combinations of two or three of the active drugs. However, in five published randomized studies that compared single-agent therapy to multi-agent therapy in metastatic prostate cancer, no advantage was shown for the combinations.[44–48]

The simultaneous use of cytotoxic drugs and hormone therapy is now being tested, but presently it is too early to reach conclusions. Information is available that compares cytotoxic therapy to second- or third-line hormone therapy. Studies from the National Prostate Cancer Project have suggested that although objective responses to cytotoxic chemotherapy in prostate cancer are low, palliation and possibly survival are better with drug therapy than with secondary or tertiary hormonal manipulations in the patients who have failed their primary hormonal therapy.[49]

Clearly, more work is to be done. All of the standard drugs and any new drugs need to be well tested in prostatic cancer. Criteria for response in these drug studies need to be standardized and further refined. Patients failing primary hormonal therapy should be strongly considered for chemotherapy trials in view of the poor results with use of secondary hormonal therapy.

E. Carcinoma of the Urethra

Carcinoma of the urethra is a very rare disease. Hematuria is a common presenting complaint of primary disease. Local management is appropriate for localized disease. At this time, there is very limited experience with chemotherapy in this disease, and this precludes further meaningful discussion. Basically, the decisions to use therapy are based on clinical need and the cell type involved.

F. Testicular Cancer

Testicular carcinoma is rarely associated with urinary tract hemorrhage. However, it is included in this discussion as an example of the genitourinary tract tumor that is highly amenable to cure with systemic chemotherapy. Using combinations of Velban,® platinum, and bleomycin, several different investigators have reported complete response rates and long-term, disease-free survival in 60–75% of patients with advanced testicular carcinoma.[50] Thus, this disease appears curable with combination chemotherapy in the majority of patients.

G. Secondary Tumors or Nonurologic Tumors

There are a number of nonurologic malignancies that may involve the urinary tract and cause bleeding. These generally arise in other pelvic or abdominal organs and invade the urinary tract secondarily. Surgery or radiotherapy may have a role for localized problems especially if there is no evidence of metastatic disease. Chemotherapy, however, may ultimately be required. The role of chemotherapy for these tumors is outlined in Table III. The more common secondary tumors including colorectal and cervical carcinoma tend to be rather resistant to chemotherapy although occasional palliation may be achieved by cytotoxic therapy. More sensitive tumors such as carcinoma of the ovary or Hodgkins' and non-Hodgkin's lymphoma are often more responsive to combination chemotherapy. This modality should be considered especially if the particular patient has not received previous chemotherapy. Rarely, myeloma or Waldenstrom's macroglobulinemia involve the urinary tract system and lead to bleeding. Prostatic involvement is probably more common in this uncommon event. These tumors are similarly quite responsive to chemotherapy. Finally, sarcomas originating in the pelvis or retroperitoneum or primary sarcomas of the urinary tract are intermediately sensitive to chemotherapy, particularly Adriamycin-containing regimens.

Persistant, local disease from these sources can often be very problematic for the patient causing pain, bleeding, discharge, and fistuli. In selected circumstances arterial infusion has been used, but with generally poor results. Since 1952, infusion of a number of drugs including nitrogen mustard, methotrexate, 5-FU, FUDR, bleomycin, mitomycin, and the vinca alkaloids have been used in carcinoma of the cervix and vagina.[51–57] More recently, the group at M. D.

Table III
Systemic Therapy in Nonurologic Tumors Involving Urinary Tract

Tumor Type	Chemotherapy
Ovarian cancer	High response (50–70%) to primary combination therapy
Lymphoma (Hodgkin's and non-Hodgkin's)	Combination chemotherapy very effective
Colorectal cancer	Low response rates (15–20%)
Cervical cancer	Low response rates (20–30%)
Sarcoma	30–40% response rate to doxorubicin alone or in combination

Anderson Hospital have reported their experience with Cis-platinum by iliac artery infusion in nine patients with low-grade persistent or recurrent cervical cancer.[58] In this small series, a response rate of 33% was observed. However, it is unclear whether similar results might not have been achieved with systemic chemotherapy.

III. Conclusion

The control of advanced urothelial cancers, or cancers derived from adjacent tissues, persists as a major problem—testicular cancer not withstanding. More clinical experimentation is needed using various combinations of surgery, radiation, and chemotherapy given by infusion or systemically. Hematuria, which is often a first symptom and which frequently persists as a clinical problem, can respond to these various modalities when they are selected judiciously by experts in the field.

References

1. Paulson DF, Perez CA, Anderson T. In: *Genito-urinary malignancies: Principles and Practice of Oncology*. DeVita VT, Hellman S, Rosenberg SA, Eds. Philadelphia, J.B. Lippincott Co. pp. 732–785, 1982.
2. Fisher HAG. Diagnosis and management of superficial bladder cancer. *Clin Cancer Briefs*. 6:3–12, 1984.
3. Lerman IL, Hutter RUP, Whitmore WF, Jr. Papilloma of the urinary bladder. *Cancer* 25:333–342, 1970.
4. Williams JL, Hammond JC, Saunders N. T_1 bladder tumors. *Br J Urol*. 49:663–668, 1977.
5. Heney N, Ahmed S, Flanagan MJ, Frable W, Corder MP, Hafermann MD, Hawkins IR, for National Bladder Collaborative Group. Superficial bladder cancer: Progression and recurrence. *J Urol*. 130:1083–1086, 1978.
6. Wallace S, Charnsangavej C, Carrasco H, Bechtel W. Infusion–embolism. *Cancer*. 54:2751–2765, 1984.
7. Frei E, III. Effect of dose and schedule on response. In: *Cancer Medicine*. Holland JF, Frei E, III, Eds. Philadelphia, Lea and Febiger, 1973, pp. 717–730.
8. Anderson JH, Gianturco C, Wallace S. Experimental transcatheter intra-arterial infusion-occlusion chemotherapy. *Invest Radiol*. 16:496–500, 1981.
9. Kaplan WD, D'Orsi CJ, Ensminger WD, Smith EH, Levin DC. Intra-arterial radionuclide infusion: A new technique to access chemotherapy infusion patterns. *Cancer Treat Rep*. 62:699–703, 1978.
10. Kato T, Nemoto R, Mori H, Takahashi M, Tamakowa Y, Harada M. Arterial Chemoembolization with microencapsulated anticancer drug. *JAMA*. 245:1123–1124, 1981.
11. Johnson DE, Samuels ML. Chemotherapy for metastatic renal carcinoma. In: *Chemotherapy: Fundamental Concepts and Recent Advances*. Proceedings, University of Texas Cancer Center. M.D. Anderson Hospital and Tumor Institute, 19th Annual Clinical Conference in Cancer. Chicago, Year Book Medical Publishers, 1975, pp. 493–503.
12. Hrushesky WJ, Murphy GP. Current Status of the therapy of advanced renal carcinoma. *J Surg Oncol*. 9:277–288, 1977.
13. Bodey GP. Current States of Chemotherapy in Metastatic Renal Carcinoma. In: *Cancer of the Genito-urinary Tract*. Johnson DE, Samuels ML, Eds. New York, Raven Press, pp. 67–72, 1979.

14. Bloom HJG. Hormone treatment of renal tumors—Experimental and clinical observations. In: *Tumors of the Kidney and Ureter*. Riches EW, Ed. Baltimore, Williams and Wilkins Co., pp. 311–320, 1964.
15. Lalli AF, Peterson N, Bookstein JJ, Roentgen-guided infarction of kidney and lung: A potential therapeutic technique. *Radiology*. 93:434–435, 1969.
16. Lang EK. Superselective arterial catherization as vehicle for delivering radioactive infarct particles to tumors. *Radiology*. 98:391–399, 1971.
17. Swanson DA, Johnson DE, von Eschenbach AC, Chiung VP, Wallace S. Angioinfarction plus nephrectomy for metastatic renal cell carcinoma: An update. *J Urol*. 130:449–452, 1983.
18. Dekernion J. Treatment of advanced renal cell carcinoma: Traditional methods and innovative approaches. *J Urol*. 130:2–7, 1983.
19. Tykka H, Oravisto KJ, Lehtonen T, Sarna S. Active specific immunotherapy of advanced renal cell carcinoma. *Eur. Urol*. 4:250–258, 1978.
20. Carpenter PR, Ewing JA, Cook AJ, Kuster AH, Tallberg T. Angiographic assessment and control of potential operative hemorrhage with pathologic fractures secondary to metastasis. *Clin Orthop*. 123:6–8, 1977.
21. Bowers TA, Murray JA, Charnsangavej C, Soo C-S, Chuang VP, Wallace S. Bone metastasis from renal carcinoma. *J Bone Joint Surg*. 64-A:749–754, 1982.
22. Jewett–Strong–Marshall Staging System.
23. International Union Against Cancer. *Tumor–Node–Metastasis staging system*. 3rd edition, 1978.
24. Whitmore WF, Jr. Management of bladder cancer. *Curr Prob Cancer*. 4:1–48, 1979.
25. Yagoda A. Chemotherapy for advanced urothelial Tract Cancer. *Clin Cancer Briefs*. 6:13–24, 1984.
26. Yagoda A. Phase II trials in bladder cancer at Memorial Sloan-Kettering Cancer Center, 1975–1978. In Johnson DE, Samuels ML, Eds. In: *Cancer of the Genitourinary Tract*. New York, Raven Press, 1979, pp. 107–119.
27. Yagoda A. Progress in chemotherapy for cancers of the urothelium. *Urology*. (Suppl 4) 23:118–123, 1984.
28. Richie JP, Shipley WU, Yagoda A. Bladder cancer. In: *Cancer: Principles and Practice in Oncology* 2nd Edition. De Vita VT, Hellman S, Rosenberg SA, Eds. Philadelphia, J.B. Lippincott Co., 1984.
29. Yagoda A. Chemotherapy for advanced urothelial cancer. *Semin Urol*. 1:60–74, 1983.
30. Samuels ML, Logothetis C, Trindade A, Johnson DE: Cytoxan Adriamycin and Cisplatinum (CISCA) in metastatic bladder cancer. Proc. *AACR*. 21:137, 1980.
31. Khandekar JD, Elson PJ, Dewys WD, et al: Comparative activity and toxicity of Cis-diammine dichloroplatinum (DDP) vs cyclophosphamide (CTX), Adriamycin (ADR), and DDP(CAD) in disseminated transitional cell carcinomas of the urinary tract. (DRCUT). *Proc ASCO*. 22:461, 1981.
32. Einstein A, Soloway M, Corder M, et al: Diamminedichloroplatinum (DDP) vs DDP plus cyclophosphamide for metastatic bladder cancer. *Proc ASCO*. 22:461, 1981.
33. Byron RL, Perez FM, Yonemoto RH, Bierman HR, Gildenhorn HL, Kelley KH. Left brachial arterial catherization for chemotherapy in advanced intra-abdominal malignant neoplasms. *Surg Gynecol Obstet*. 112:689–696, 1961.
34. Nevens JE, Hoffman AA. Use of arterial infusion of 5-fluorouracil either alone or in combination with super voltage radiation as a treatment for carcinoma of the prostate and bladder. *Am J Surg*. 130:544–549, 1975.
35. Ogata J, Migita N, Nakamura T. Treatment of carcinoma of the bladder by infusion of the anticancer agent (mitomycin C) via the interrenal iliac artery. *J Urol*. 110: 667–670, 1973.
36. Wallace S, Chuang VP, Samuels M, Johnson D. Transcatheter intra-arterial infusion of chemotherapy in advanced bladder cancer. *Cancer*. 49:640–645, 1982.
37. Logothetis CJ, Samuels ML, Wallace S, Chuang V, Trindade A, Grant C, Haynie TP, III,

Johnson DE. Management of pelvic complications of malignant urothelial tumors with combined intra-arterial and IV chemotherapy. *Cancer Treat Rep.* 66:1501–1507, 1982.
38. Logothetis CJ, Samuels ML. Intra-arterial chemotherapy for malignant urothelial tumors. *Cancer Bull.* 36:47–52, 1984.
39. Logothetis CJ, Samuels ML, Selig DE, Wallace S, Johnson DE. Combined intravenous and intra-arterial cytoxan, adriamycin, and cis-platinum (Cisca) in the management of select patients with invasive urothelial tumors. *Cancer Treat Rep.* 69:33–38, 1985.
40. Paulson DF: The role of endocrine therapy in the management of prostatic cancer. In: *Genito-urinary Cancer.* Skinner DG, and de Kornion JB Eds. Philadelphia, W.B. Saunders, 1978, p. 388.
41. Byar DP: The Veterans' Administration Cooperative Urological Research Group's studies of cancer of the prostate. *Cancer.* 32:1126–1130, 1973.
42. Murphy GP (Ed.) *Prostatic Cancer.* Littleton, MA, PSG Publishing Co., 1979.
43. Torti FM, Carter SK. The chemotherapy of prostatic adenocarcinoma. *Ann Int Med.* 92:681–689, 1980.
44. Chlebowski RT, Hestorff R, Sardoff L, Weiner J, Bateman JR. Cyclophosphamide (NSC 26271) versus the combination of adriamycin (NSC 123127), 5-fluorouracil (NSC 19893) and cyclophosphamide in the treatment of metastatic prostatic cancer: A randomized trial. *Cancer.* 42:2546–2552, 1978.
45. Smalley RV. A phase II evaluation of three-drug combination of cyclophosphamide, doxorubicin, and 5-fluorouracil in patients with advanced bladder carcinoma or stage 4 metastatic carcinoma. *J Urol.* 125:191–195, 1981.
46. Soloway MS. Comparison of estramustine phosphate and vincristine alone or in combination for patients with advanced hormone refractory carcinoma of the prostate. *J Urol.* 125:664–667, 1981.
47. Muss HB, Howard V, Richards F, White D, Jackson DV, Cooper R, Stuart JJ, Resnick MI, Brodkin R, Spurr CL. Cyclophosphamide versus cyclophosphamide, methrotrexate, and 5-fluorouracil in advanced prostatic cancer: A randomized trial. *Cancer.* 47:1949–1953, 1981.
48. Murphy GP, Gibbons RP, Johnson DE, Prout GR, Schmidt JD, Soloway MS, Loening SA, Chu TM, Gaeta JF, Saroff J, Watsman Z, Slack N, Scott WW. The use of estramustine and prednimustine versus prednimustine alone in advanced metastatic prostate who have received prior irradiation. *J Urol.* 121:763–765, 1979.
49. Murphy GP. Chemotherapeutic treatment of a national randomized trial basis by the National Prostatic Cancer Project. In: *Cancer of the Genito-urinary Tract.* Johnson DE, and Samuels ML, Eds. New York, Raven Press, pp. 249–260, 1979.
50. Einhorn LH. Testicular cancer as a model for a curable neoplasm: The Richard and Hinda Rosenthal Foundation Award Lecture. *Cancer Res.* 41:3275–3280, 1981.
51. Cromer JK, Bateman JC, Berry GN. Kannelly J, Klopp CT, Platt LI. Use of intra-arterial nitrogen mustard therapy in the treatment of cervical and vaginal cancer. *Am J Obstet Gynecol.* 63:538–548, 1952.
52. Krakoff IH, Sullivan RD. Intra-arterial nitrogen mustard in the treatment of pelvic cancer. *Ann Intern Med.* 48:839–850, 1958.
53. Sullivan RD, Wood AM, Clifford P, Duff JK, Trussel R, Nary DK, Burchenal JH. Continuous intra-arterial methotrexate with simultaneous intermittent intramuscular citrovorum factor therapy in carcinoma of the cervix. *Cancer Chemother Rep.* 8:1–6, 1960.
54. Hulka JF, Bisel HF. Combined intra-arterial chemotherapy and radiation treatment for advanced cervical carcinoma. *Am J Obstet Gynecol.* 91:486–490, 1965.
55. Morrow CP, Disaia PJ, Mangan CF. Continuous pelvic arterial infusion with bleomycin for squamous carcinoma of the cervix recurrent after radiation therapy. *Cancer Treat Rep.* 61:1403–1405, 1977.
56. Lipshitz G, Railsback LD, Buschsbaum HJ. Intra-arterial pelvic infusion chemotherapy in advanced gynecologic cancer. *Obstet Gynecol.* 52:476–479, 1978.

57. Swenerton KD, Evers JA, White GW, Boyes DA. Intermittent pelvic infusion with vincristine, bleomycin, and mitomycin-C for advanced recurrent carcinoma of the cervix. *Cancer Treat Rep.* 63:1379–1381, 1979.
58. Carlson JA, Jr., Freedman RS, Wallace S, Chuang VP, Wharton JT, Rutledge FN. Intra-arterial cis-platinum in the management of squamous cell carcinsoma of the uterine cervix. *Gynecol Oncol.* 12:92–98, 1981.
59. Garnick MB, for the Leuprolide Study Group. Leuprolide versus diethylstilbesterol for metastatic prostate cancer. *N Engl J Med* 311:1281–1286, 1984.

Chapter 13

Instillation Chemotherapy for Bladder Tumors

Robert E. Desautels, M.D.

I. Introduction

Urinary bladder neoplasms are frequently associated with hematuria, and since these make up 2–3% of all visceral neoplasms, hematuria due to bladder neoplasm is fairly common. Bladder neoplasms are the most common neoplasms of the urinary tract, including the kidney.[1] Their spectrum extends from benign papillomas to aggressive carcinomas (Figs. 1 and 2). About 70% of these bladder cancers are superficial at the time of presentation. Even benign-appearing papillomas tend to "progress" toward more aggressive disease once they recur (Fig. 3 and 4). Of the superficial tumors, 50–70% will form new masses after primary treatment, and 30% of these progress in grade or stage.[2-4] Moreover, it may be difficult to distinguish benign papillomas from well-differentiated papillary carcinomas. Other benign tumors capable of causing hematuria include fibromas, myxomas, leiomyomas, neurofibromas, angiomas, granular cell myoblastomas, and others.[1] The primary malignancies include bladder carcinoma (including transitional cell (85%), squamous cell (10%), and adenocarcinomas (5%)) and sarcomas. At least 80% of bladders removed for invasive carcinoma show multifocal areas of carcinoma *in situ*.

Management decisions should be based on the clinical stage (see Table I) and, when appropriate, should involve instillation therapy surgery, radiotherapy, or systemic chemotherapy.[5] Instillation of topical agents (intravesical therapy) has been used for more than 20 years in attempt to eliminate, control, and protect against recurrence of low-grade and low-stage tumors occurring in the urinary bladder. Survival is generally good using this approach for superficial T_a or T_1 lesions (see Table II of Chapter 12). Unfortunately, following primary therapy there is a high incidence of recurrence of bladder tumors,

From Bern MM (ed.): *Urinary Tract Bleeding: Diagnosis and Control by Medical, Radiologic, and Surgical Techniques*. Mount Kisco, NY, Futura Publishing Co., Inc., 1985.

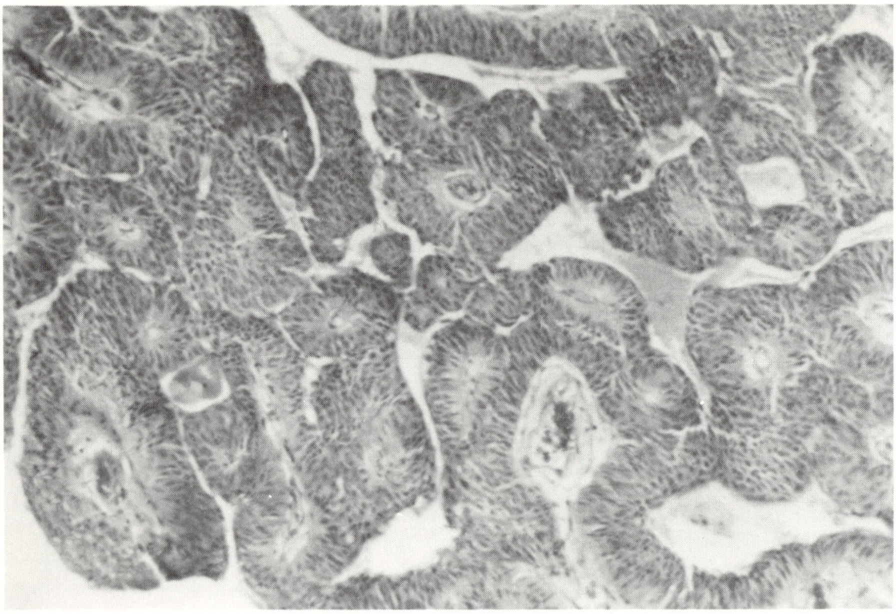

Figure 1: *Photomicrographs demonstrating a transitional cell papilloma, low grade. (100×).*

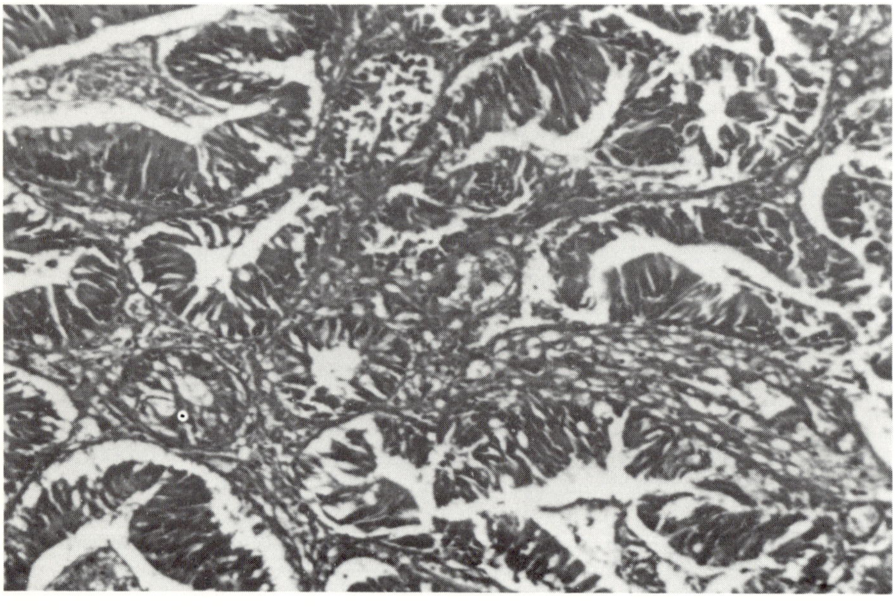

Figure 2: *Photomicrograph demonstrating adenocarcinoma of bladder (250×).*

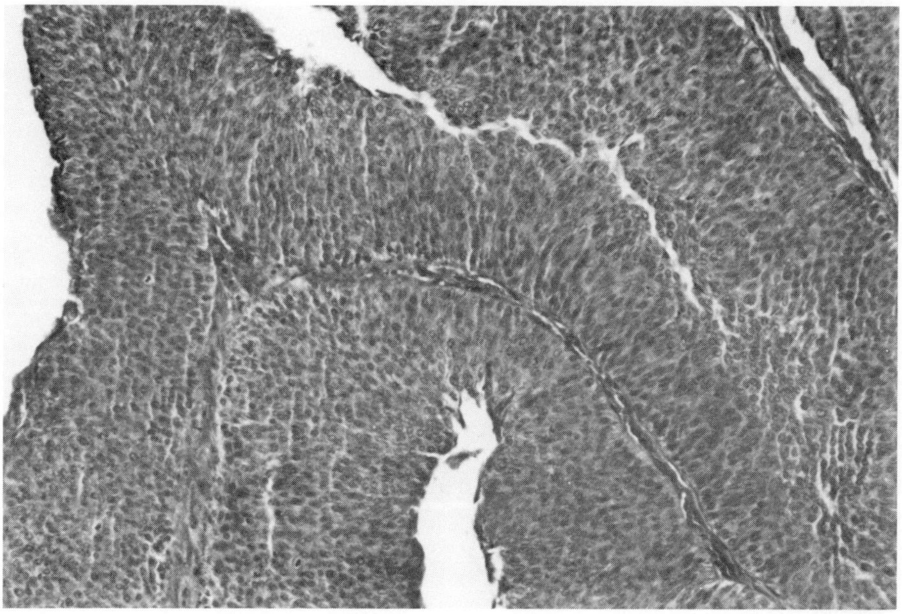

Figure 3: *Photomicrograph demonstrating low grade transitional cell carcinoma (100×).*

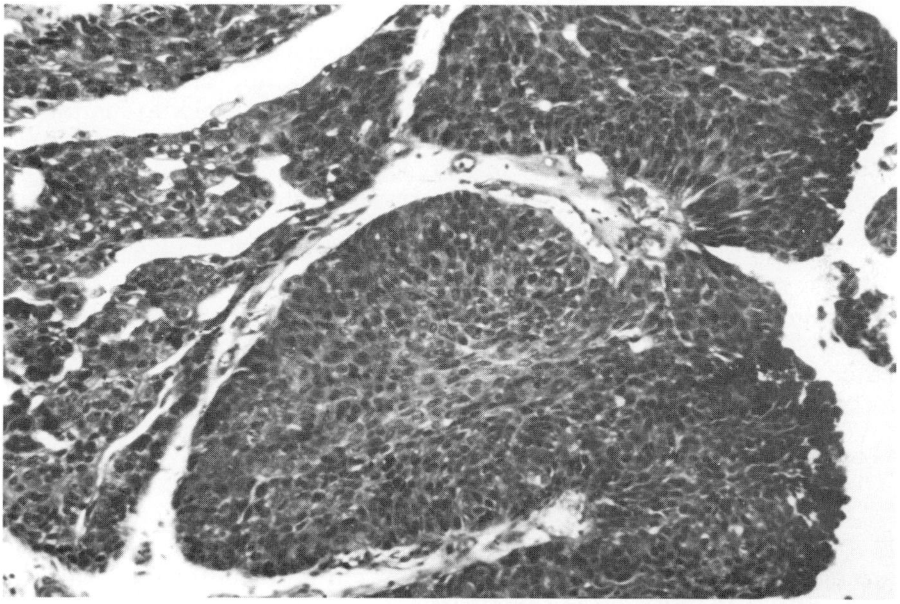

Figure 4: *Photomicrograph demonstrating high grade transitional cell carcinoma comparing this figure to Figure 3, the change in the grade at the time of recurrence can be appreciated.*

Table I
Grade and Stage of Bladder Cancers

Use of Topical Chemotherapy	Grade	Stage	Characteristic
yes	Papilloma or Grade I	0, T_{is} and T_a	No invasion beyond mucosa
		A or T_1	Carcinoma *in situ* Invasion to lamina propria only
maybe	Grade II	B_1 or T_2	Invasion to less than ½ of muscle depth
usually no	Grades III or IV	B_2, T_{3A} and higher	Invasion to greater than ½ of muscle depth and beyond

ranging from 50% to 70%, mostly occurring within 6–12 months of primary therapy.[2,3,6,7]

A. Staging

1. *Modalities Used for Staging*

The use of topical chemotherapy requires that the tumor(s) be limited to the luminal surface of the bladder. Any tumor penetrating beyond the superficial luminal layer will be inadequately treated by the technique. Thus, staging of the tumor to determine the boundaries of the disease is very important when planning instillation therapy. For this effort, the cytoscopic appearance and resection through the cytoscope of the bladder tumor provides helpful information about the invasive characteristics of the tumor or tumors. Papillary tumors with narrow stalks are usually noninvasive and are low grade, whereas papillary tumors with a broad base are more likely to be invasive and a higher grade. Sessile tumors tend to be invasive and are high grade. Deformity of the bladder wall adjacent to the tumor and neovascularity are indications of invasiveness.

Biopsy specimens of the tumor including tissue taken from the tumor base and from underlying bladder wall provide histologic aid in determining stage. Random biopsies of bladder wall in areas apparently free of tumor indicate whether carcinoma *in situ* or potential precursor lesions exist such as atypia, hyperplasia, or dysplasia.

A bimanual rectoabdominal palpitation of the bladder with the patient under anesthesia can yield further evidence of tumor penetration. If a mass, thickening, induration, or fixation of the bladder is appreciated, there will be more extensive disease. A soft, movable bladder is a favorable sign.

CT scan of the bladder and ultrasound often yield valuable information about regional extensions. These modalities can indicate the extent of tumor involvement of the bladder mucosal surface and wall, as well as indicate the possible presence of disease outside the bladder and in lymph nodes. In cases of muscle infiltrate, chest x-ray and bone scans can help rule out distant metastasis.

Stage Assignment: Two staging systems are used: The Jewett-Strong-Marshall system, and the TNM (Tumor-Node-Metastasis) system (see Table II of

Chapter 12). These two systems differentiate the superficial from the deeper lesions. Unfortunately, even when using the best skills, they are applied only with about 80% accuracy, making the understaging of superficial lesions rather common.[8] Staging errors are greatest for the deeper penetration lesions.[5,8] For example, tumors thought to have superficial muscle invasion (T_2 or B_1) have a high likelihood of being understaged (Figs. 5–7).

TABLE II
Parameters for Follow-up of Patients Under Treatment

Local	Urinalysis and cytology for (hematuria and evidence of tumor cells).
	Cystoscopy, every 2–3 months.
	Biopsies of bladder every 3–4 months or sooner as indicated.
	CT scan to be used selectively if there is a question of possible extension.
Systemic	CBC and platelet count before administration of thiotepa.
	Examine for palmar rash when using with mitomycin-C;
	Fever, malaise, pulmonary symptoms when using BCG.

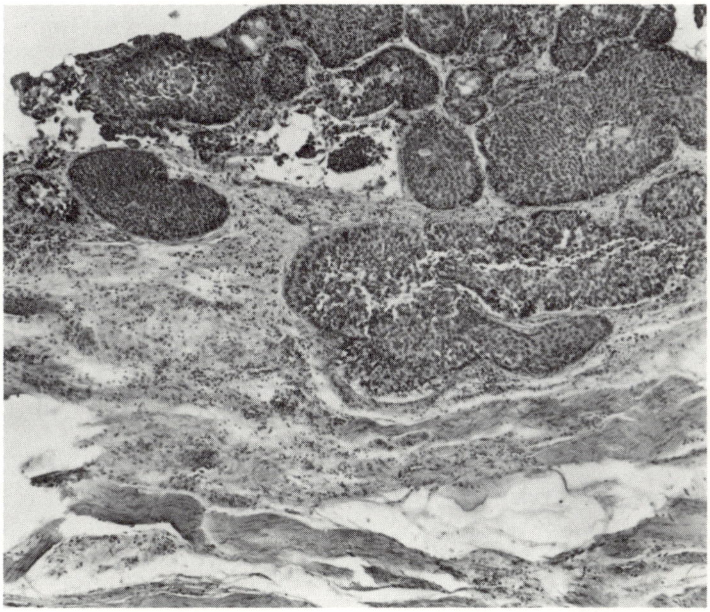

Figure 5: *Photomicrograph demonstrating superficial invasion of transitional cell carcinoma of the bladder (40×).*

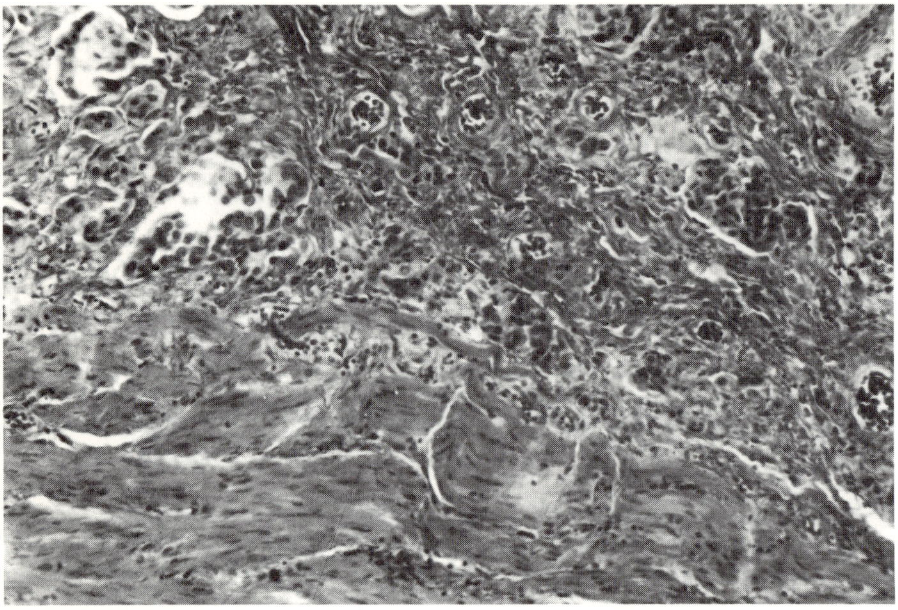

Figure 6: *Photomicrograph demonstrating invasion of muscle (less than one-half of muscle thickness) by transitional cell carcinoma of the bladder (100×).*

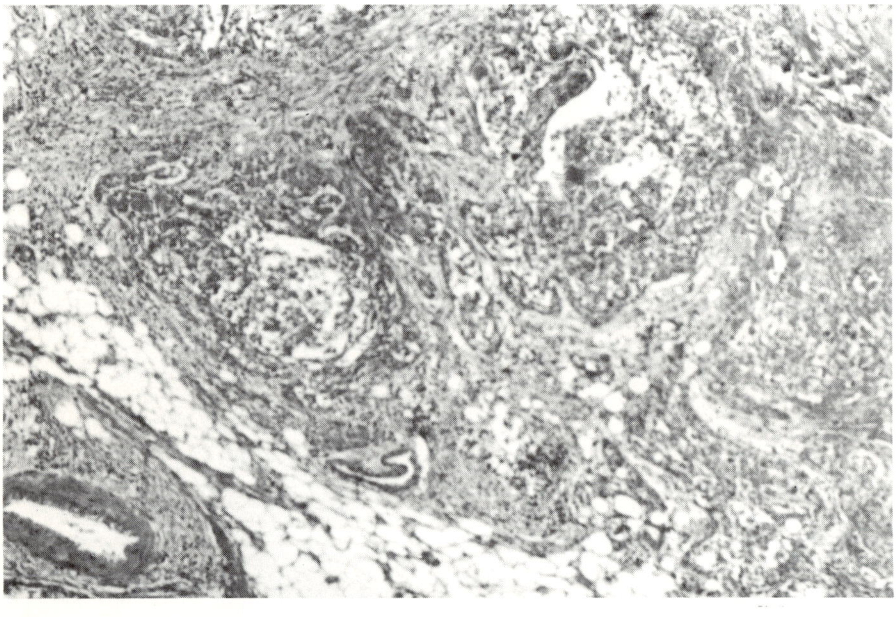

Figure 7: *Photomicrograph demonstrating invasion through the muscle to the serosa of the bladder by transitional cell carcinoma of the bladder (40×).*

B. Tumor Grade

The grade of the tumor will also influence the accuracy of the staging, and the subsequent clinical success.[4] The higher grades of tumor (grade II and above) and carcinoma *in situ* can spread beyond the bladder before there is evidence by surface examination of significant invasion (see Table I). Carcinoma *in situ* is in fact an inexact term, representing a specific stage, but a variety of grades of tumor, often with high malignant potential[9] (Fig. 8a,b). It may appear as a local or diffuse process, alone or concomitantly with papillary lesions. Its natural history is not predictable.[5,9] Despite its name, carcinoma *in situ* may exist at sites beyond the bladder. Thus, small tumors must be respected for their possibly lethal behavior; the larger the number of tumors or larger the mass of the tumor, the poorer the result.[10-12]

II. Case Selection and Case Exclusion

The maximal tumor control with the least damage to the patient is the goal of treating bladder cancer. This requires careful avoidance of understaging the tumor.[13] Surgery and radiotherapy can be applied singularly or in combination, with varying results. The combined opinions of the surgeons and the radiotherapists are indispensable.

By careful case selection, many patients can be saved from bladder resections. Intravesical chemotherapy is applied to treat superficial residual tumors after local surgical control with transurethral resections and as prophylaxis against new tumor formation. The majority of patients selected for topical chemotherapy are those with frequent recurrences of low-grade and low-stage

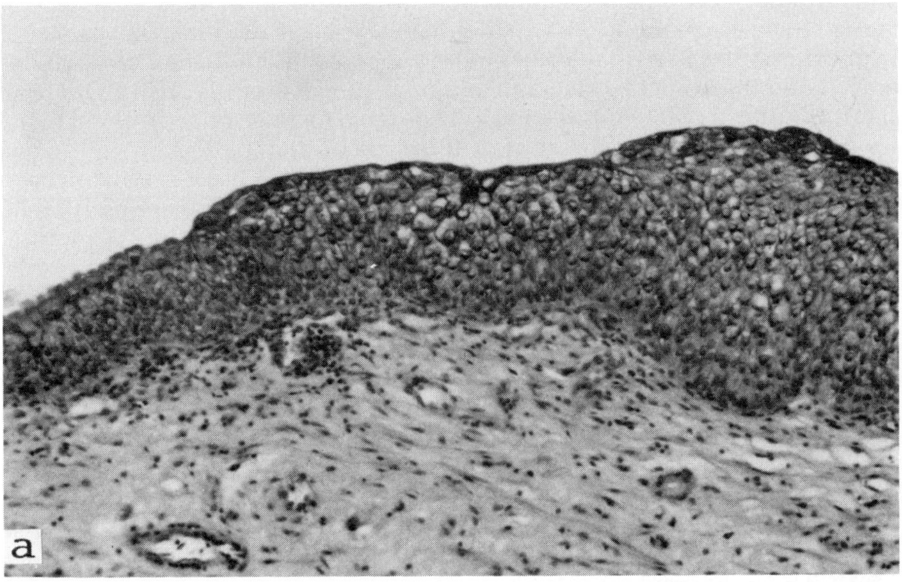

Figure 8: a,b. *Photomicrographs demonstrating the carcinoma* in situ (**a:** *100×).*

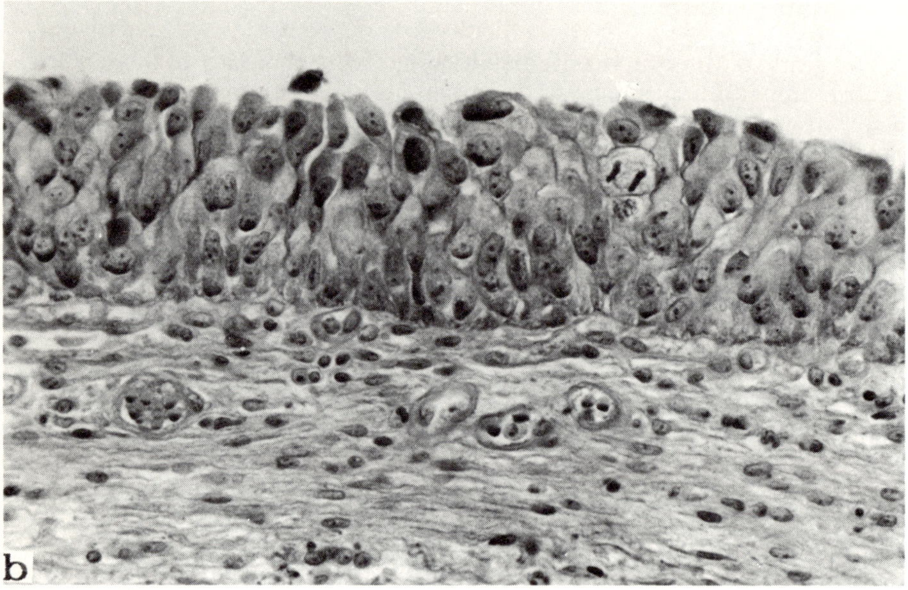

Figure 8.b.: *(250×).*

tumors (see Table I). Individuals with higher grade tumors that are small and have low stage may still benefit from this form of treatment; here, however, the therapy must be carried out with great care and with respect for the potential of deeper penetration.

Aside from some adverse reactions to intravesical therapy, the major clinical problem is to decide whether or not continued therapy is appropriate. Although there are patients with high-grade, low-stage disease, as is particularly true for carcinomas *in situ*, whose tumors appear to be eradicated, they are in the minority, and they must be selected and monitored carefully. Failure to rapidly gain initial control of the tumor should be a signal to move on to surgical therapy. It has been apparent from the start of this type of therapy that certain patients respond well while others fail to respond and have subsequent extension beyond the bladder if appropriate additional therapy is not provided in a timely fashion. Generally, unless complete and rapid response occurs within 3 months of therapy, the treatments should be abandoned.

One reason that radical surgery has presented such bad survival results appears to be that it was often applied too late following unrecognized failure of other more common measures. A favorable surgical outcome can be anticipated when appropriate primary therapy is employed for an appropriate length of time. Thus, while a complete initial response following instillation therapy argues well for its future, a partial response is associated with increased mortality. In some of the studies, there has been a mortality rate of about one out of three patients whose disease has extended while therapy continued. As example of the value of careful monitors, 15 of 45 patients treated with intravesical thiotepa for prophylactic effect who were found to have no tumor at the end of 12 months had positive urine cytologies.[14] These patients require other therapy.

TABLE III
Effects of Topical Chemotherapy

Local	Destruction of tumor cells with preservation of normal mucosa. Biopsies show degeneration and vacuolization of superficial cells.
Systemic	Absorption through bladder with possible bone marrow depression—occurs with thiotepa and rarely with epodyl. Rash—palmar surface of hands and genitalia following mitomycin C. General effects of BCG infection.

The follow-up observations required vary to some extent with the agent being used (see Table II). In general, cystoscopy should be performed every 2 to 3 months and biopsies of the bladder are taken routinely every 3 to 4 months or specifically as indicated for suspicious areas. Urinalysis and urinary cytology also may be useful. A complete blood count and platelet count is done prior to each treatment, especially with thiotepa.

III. Drugs Available

A. General Pharmacology

The ideal agents used for topical intravesical chemotherapy should cause damage to tumor cells with minimal effect on the surrounding normal mucosa. There should be no systemic toxicity. Biopsy specimens following therapy should show degeneration and vacuolization of superficial tumor cells, and in the case of BCG therapy, local inflammatory reactions.

Systemic absorption of the agent through the bladder mucosa is a serious pharmacologic consideration. Absorption is by passive diffusion. Rates of absorption appear to be related to molecule size and lipid solubility. It has been shown that a molecular weight of 200 is the critical limit beyond which absorption is unlikely to take place.[15]

Jones and Swinney in 1961 and Veenema et al. in 1962 demonstrated that thiotepa (Triethylenethiophosphoramide), an alkylating agent, when instilled into the bladder destroyed low-stage tumors in some individuals.[16,17] Subsequently it was shown that selected tumors can be destroyed in a third or more of the individuals receiving instillation therapy. Thiotepa has a molecular weight of 189 and up to one-third of it is absorbed following instillation into the bladder.

Consequently, thiotepa can create potentially serious systemic problems by excessive absorption via the bladder mucosa. Serious bone marrow suppression must be avoided by limiting the dose and the exposure time. Additional agents since then have been added to the therapeutic options. These newer agents are poorly absorbed, with tumoricidal activity but without causing significant injury to normal bladder tissue.[15] Epodyl, on the other hand, has a molecular weight of 262 and mitomycin C has a molecular weight of 334. They are absorbed poorly. Rarely epodyl has been associated with bone marrow depression. Doxorubicin, mitomycin C, and BCG have not presented such problems.

B. Drug Selection

Drug selection depends mainly on the experience of the operator with a given drug or drugs and their expected toxicities, since all of the commonly used agents have approximately the same degree of success.[18] Thiotepa has had the largest clinical trials, starting in 1961. It generally will be tolerated with mild secondary dysuria or hematuria, but must be monitored for its effect upon the bone marrow. Mitomycin C and Adriamycin are perhaps safer since they have little or no systemic absorption. They may be tried when there has been failure after thiotepa or if there was excessive marrow suppression.[19,20] 5-Flourouracil has limited efficacy and is rarely used in this fashion. Epodyl, also an alkylating agent, has had most use in Europe.

Bacillus Calmette-Guérin (BCG) acts through immune hypersensitivity plus local inflammation and may work when the other agents fail. BCG has been shown to reduce the number of new tumors when used for prophylaxis.[21-24] It has been successfully used for carcinoma *in situ*.[9] It can cause transient hematuria, dysuria, frequency, fever, arthralgia, plus nausea and vomiting. High doses can cause a tuberculosis-like syndrome needing treatment.

C. Use of Intravesical Agents (See Table 4)

1. *Thiotepa*

The alkylating agent, thiotepa, is the most commonly used and most readily absorbed agent. A number of cases of pancytopenia occasionally causing death have been reported. Thus dose limitation is important. Reduction of the instilled dose from 90 mg in 100 cc distilled H_2O to 30 mg in 30 cc distilled water for 2 hours has resulted in a significant reduction of bone marrow depression caused by absorption of the drug.[14,16] A course is comprised of four weekly instillations followed by cystoscopy 1 month later. If there is no response after three courses, the treatment should be terminated. Forty-five percent of patients can show a complete response. Prophylaxis against recurrence is given every 4 weeks for 2 years if the response has been complete. Cytoscopy is performed every 3 months together with cytology and bladder biopsies.[25,26]

2. *Epodyl*

The alkylating agent, epodyl, a di-epoxide of myleran, has been used in England and appears to have about the same rate of tumor control as thiotepa but without the problems of absorption and bone marrow depression.[27-29] One hundred milligrams in 100 cc of distilled H_2O is instilled weekly for 12 weeks. If partial or complete remission occurs, therapy is repeated every month for 1 year, then every other month for the second year, and then every third month thereafter. With this therapy, two out of three patients responded completely. Un-

TABLE IV
Drugs Available

Trade Name	*Generic Name*	*Action*
Thiotepa	Triethylenethiophosphoramide	Alkylating agent
Epodyl	Triethylene glycol diglyceridyl ether	Alkylating agent
Adriamycin	Doxorubicin	Antibiotic, interference in DNA synthesis
Mutamycin	Mitomycin-C	Antibiotic, alkylating agent
BCG	Bacillus Calmette-Guérin	Immunologic effect

fortunately, again the majority of patients with partial and no response died of progressive disease, including 27% of patients with noninvasive disease.[27-29]

3. *Doxorubicin hydrochloride*

Doxorubicin hydrochloride, an antitumor antibiotic isolated from cultures of *Streptomyces peucetius*, var. *caesius*, has had moderately extensive trials using 50 mg in 100–150 cc of normal saline instilled into the bladder for one-half hour. Therapy is given monthly with repeat cytoscopic examinations every 3 months. No evidence of absorption through the bladder mucosa has been found in blood samples taken at the time of therapy. Complete responses from 3–21 months have been described in up to 62% of patients.[20,26,30-32]

4. *Mitomycin C*

Mitomycin C, an alkylating agent and antibiotic, produces interstrand and intrastrand deoxyribonucleic acid across links causing inhibition of deoxyribonucleic acid synthesis. It is instilled into the bladder in a dose of 30–40 mg in 30–40 ml of distilled H_2O for 2 hours. Therapy is continued weekly for 8 weeks and cytoscopy is performed after 12 weeks. Most patients with complete response are continued on therapy at monthly intervals with cytoscopic evaluation at 3-month intervals. Sixty-nine percent of patients have had complete response and 17.5% of patients have had a partial response.[33,34] No evidence of systemic toxicity has been seen and serum samples taken during therapy fail to show evidence of drug absorption.[35]

5. *BCG*

Use of *Bacillus Calmette-Guérin* (BCG) in the therapy of melanoma led to its trials treating superficial noninvasive bladder tumors. A study in mice using a strain of bladder cancer cells demonstrated 90% complete regression of tumor when given BCG at time of cell injection and 50% when given BCG 10 days beforehand.[36] Therapy is usually given with 120 mg of the bacillus in 50 ml of saline instilled for 2 hours at weekly intervals for 6 weeks, starting 10 days after the cystoscopy and biopsy of the bladder tumors. In early studies, 5 mg of BCG was also injected intradermally with each intravesical treatment.[21] Cytoscopy was repeated 4–6 weeks after cessation of therapy and then at 3- to 6-month intervals. A 59% complete response rate was found on follow-up, averaging 19 months long. Tumor grade appeared to be an important determinant in that the higher grade tumors were significantly less likely to respond to the treatment.[22,37,38] It does not appear necessary to give intradermal therapy simultaneously with the intravesical therapy.

Delayed hypersensitivity reaction with BCG can be induced in the bladder of immunized hosts.[39] These reactions can be produced by intracavitary administration of the agent in the presence of a disrupted vesical epithelium or systemic administration. The therapy does not appear effective in advanced tumors. As outlined above, side effects of fever, malaise, occasional nausea, and pulmonary infection may occur. Routine isoniazide has not been necessary. The use of larger doses (6×10^9 organisms) for longer periods of time appears to produce an even greater effect with no recurrences found in a group of patients treated prophylactically after removal of tumor.[22] However, in this group there was a high incidence (28%) of systemic side effects, including fever, malaise, and in a few patients pulmonary disease requiring antituberculous therapy.

IV. Final Comments

Most patients with bladder carcinoma appear to present when the disease is curable, even if cure requires cystectomy. Obviously, however, not all patients require cystectomy and may be well managed by less dramatic therapy, such as instillation chemotherapy. Case selection is critical. Of all individuals with bladder tumors, less than 10% will require cystectomy. When a patient dies of bladder cancer under these circumstances, an error in planning has probably occurred.

There is no evidence that a combination of radiation and chemotherapy provides an additional benefit to treatment of these lesions. Likewise, combinations of drugs or the routine sequential use of intravesical drugs do not significantly improve the results. The goal of local therapy is to cure the disease, while causing minimal side effects. If the patient subsequently dies of the tumor, intravesical chemotherapy, obviously, should not have been used initially in the individual. It is therefore important to select only those patients for topical chemotherapy whose disease is unlikely to become invasive. By limiting therapy to only those patients who show a complete response within 3 months of beginning therapy, this goal can be met to a large degree. Recurrence of tumor following an initial complete response does not necessarily indicate a failure since the recurrence may still respond completely and promptly. However, following such an event, even greater surveillance should be applied. It is essential that rigid limits be placed on this type of therapy because with each of the drugs studied there has been a significant mortality by carcinoma in those patients who show partial or no response.

New modalities for local therapy hold some promise. Laser therapy, photoradiation therapy using hematoporphyrin as a cell sensitizer, plus prevention of recurrence with agents such as pyridoxine are experimental modalities that need

TABLE V
Treatment Plans for Instillation Therapy

Drug	Dosage	Frequency of Therapy and Follow-up	Duration of Therapy	Response Rates
Thiotepa	30 mg/30 ml distilled H_2O given for 2 hours	Weekly for 4 weeks followed by cystoscopy 1 month after each course	Three 4-week courses then every 3 months for 2 years if free of disease	Up to 47% complete
Epodyl	100 mg/100 ml of normal saline given for 2 hours	Same	Same	Up to 66% complete
Adriamycin	50–80 mg/100 ml of normal saline given for 2 hours	Monthly for 4 months followed by cystoscopy every 3–4 months	One 4-month course, then every 3 months for 2 years if free of disease	Up to 61% complete
Mitomycin C	30 mg/30 ml distilled H_2O given for 2 hours	Weekly for 8 weeks, followed by cystoscopy at 12 weeks, and every 3 months thereafter	One 8-week course, then monthly for 2 years if free of disease	Up to 69% complete
BCG	120 mg BCG/50 ml of normal saline for 2 hours with 5 mg BCG intradermally	Weekly for 6 weeks, followed by cystoscopy at 3 months, and every 3 months thereafter	6-week course	59% complete
	or			
	6×10^9 T organisms/60 ml of normal saline given for 2 hours with no intradermal injection	Weekly for 6 weeks followed by cystoscopy every 3 months	6-week course, then every 2 weeks for 3 months, then monthly until a total of 24 months	Marked prophylactic effect up to 100%

further development. If interest in these approaches is sustained, comparative studies with the heretofore standard therapies will be needed using studies that are well controlled and stratified for grade of tumor and stage.

References

1. Robbins SL. The lower urinary tract. In: *Pathology*. Philadelphia, W.B. Saunders Company, 3:1060–1066, 1967.
2. Lerman RI, Hutter RV, Whitmore WF, Jr. Papilloma of the urinary bladder. *Cancer*. 25:333–342, 1970.
3. Williams JL, Hammonds JC, Saunders N. T_1 bladder tumors. *Br J Urol*. 49:663–668, 1977.
4. Henry N, Ahmed S, Flanagan MJ, Frable W, Corder MP, Hafermann MD, Hawkins IR. Superficial bladder cancer: Progression and recurrence. *J Urol*. 130:1083–1086, 1983.
5. Fisher HAG. Diagnosis and management of superficial bladder cancer. *Clin Cancer Briefs*. 6:3–12, 1984.

6. Pyrah LN, Raper FP, Thomas GM. Report of a follow-up of papillary tumors of the bladder. *Br J Urol.* 36:14–25, 1964.
7. Nichols JA, Marshall VF. Treatment of histologically benign papilloma of the urinary bladder by local excision and fulguration. *Cancer.* 9:566–567, 1956.
8. Whitmore WF, Jr. Management of bladder cancer. *Curr Prob Cancer.* 4:1–48, 1979.
9. Herr HW. Carcinoma in situ of the bladder. *Semin Urol.* 1:15–22, 1983.
10. Cooper PH, Wasiman J, Johnson WH, Skinner DG. Severe atypia of transitional epithelium and carcinoma of the urinary bladder. *Cancer.* 31:1055–1060, 1973.
11. Soto EA, Friedell GH, Tiltman AJ. Bladder cancer as seen in giant histologic sections. *Cancer.* 39:447–455, 1977.
12. Soloway MS, Murphy W, Rao MK, Cox C. Serial multiple-site biopsies in patients with bladder cancer. *J Urol.* 120:57–59, 1978.
13. Soloway MS. Rationale for intensive intravesical chemotherapy for superficial bladder cancer. *J Urol.* 123:461–466, 1980.
14. Koontz WW, Jr, Prout GR, Jr, Smith W, Frable W, Minnis JE. The use of intravesical thiotepa in the management of non-invasive carcinoma of the bladder. *J Urol.* 125: 307–312, 1981.
15. Maluf NSR. Further studies on absorption through human bladder. *J Urol.* 73: 830–835, 1955.
16. Jones HC, Swinney J. Thiotepa in the treatment of tumour of the bladder. *Lancet.* 2:615–618, 1961.
17. Veenema RJ, Dean AL, Jr , Roberts M, Gingerhut B, Chowhury BK, Tarassoly H. Bladder carcinoma treated by direct instillation of Thiotepa. *J Urol.* 88:60–63, 1962.
18. Abbassian A, Wallace DM. Intracavitary chemotherapy of diffuse noninfiltrating papillary carcinoma of the bladder. *J Urol.* 96:461–465, 1966.
19. Prout GR, Griffin PP, Nocks BN, de'Furia MD, Dali JJ. Intravesical therapy of low stage bladder carcinoma with mitomycin C: Comparison of results in untreated and previously treated patients. *J Urol.* 127:1096–1098, 1982.
20. Edsmyr F, Berlin T, Boman J, Duchek M, Esposti PL, Gustafsson H, Wijkstrom H, Collste LG. Intravesical therapy with Adriamycin in patients with superficial bladder tumors. *Eur Urol.* 6:132–136, 1980.
21. Morales A, Ottenhof P, Emerson L. Treatment of residual, noninfiltrating bladder cancer with bacillus Calmete-Guérin. *J Urol.* 125:649–651, 1981.
22. Brosman SA. Experience with bacillus Calmette-Guérin in patients with superficial bladder cancer. *J Urol.* 128:27–30, 1982.
23. Morales A, Eidinger D, Bruce AW. Intracavitary bacillus Calmette-Guérin in the treatment of superficial bladder tumor. *J Urol.* 116:180–183, 1976.
24. Camacho F, Pinsky CM, Kerr D, Whitmore W, Oettgen H. Treatment of superficial bladder cancer with intravesical BCG. *Proc ASCO.* 21:359, 1980.
25. Burnand KG, Boyd PJ, Mayo ME, Shuttleworth KED, Lloyd-Davies RW. Single dose intravesical thiotepa as an anjuvant to cystodiathermy in the treatment of transitional cell bladder carcinoma. *Br J Urol.* 48:55–59, 1976.
26. Horn Y, Eidelman A, Walach N, Ilian M. Intravesical chemotherapy in a controlled trial with thiotepa versus doxorubicin hydrochloride. *J Urol.* 125:652–654, 1981.
27. Riddle PR, Wallace DM. Intracavitary chemotherapy for multiple noninvasive bladder tumour. *Br J Urol.* 43:181–184, 1971.
28. Riddle PR. The management of superficial bladder tumors with intravesical epodyl. *Br J Urol.* 45:84–87, 1973.
29. Riddle PR, Khan O, Fitzpatrick JM, Oliver RT. Prognostic factors influencing survival of patients receiving intravesical epodyl. *J Urol.* 127:430–432, 1982.
30. Banks MD, Pontes JE, Izbicki RM, Pierce JM, Jr. Topical instillation of doxorubicin hydrochloride in the treatment of recurring superficial transitional cell carcinoma of the bladder. *J Urol.* 118:757–760, 1977.
31. Jacobi GH, Durth K-H. Studies on the intravesical action of topically administered G^3 H-doxorubicin hydrochloride in men: Plasma uptake an tumor penetration. *J Urol.* 124: 34–37, 1980.

32. Yu H, Glashan R, Robinson MR, Richards B, Fryszman A, Daponte D, Cooper EH. Changes in the urine protein profile following intravesical doxorubicin. *J Urol.* 128:272–275, 1982.
33. Defuria MD, Bracken RB, Johnson DE, Soloway MS, Merrin CE, Morgan LR, Miller HC, Crooke ST. Phase I-II Study of mitomycin C topical therapy for low-grade, low-stage transitional cell carcinoma of the bladder: An interim report. *Cancer Treat Rep.* 64:225–230, 1980.
34. Soloway MS, Murphy WM, DeFuria MD, Crooke S, Finebaum P. The effect of mitomycin C on superficial bladder cancer. *J Urol.* 125:646–648, 1981.
35. Nissenkorn I, Herrod H, Soloway MS. Side effects associated with intravesical mitomycin C. *J Urol.* 126:596–597, 1981.
36. Pang ASD, Morales A. Immunoprophylaxis of a murine bladder cancer with high dose BCG immunizations. *J Urol.* 127:1006–1009, 1982.
37. Lamm DL, Thor DE, Harris SC, Reyna JA, Stogdill VD, Radwid HM. Bacillus Calmette-Guérin immunotherapy of superficial bladder cancer. *J Urol.* 124:38–40, 1980.
38. Lamm DL, Thor DE, Winters WD, Stogdill VD, Radwin HM. BCG immunotherapy of bladder cancer: Inhibition of tumor recurrence and associated immune responses. *Cancer.* 48:82–88, 1981.
39. Coe JE, Feldman JD. Extracutaneous delayed hypersensitivity, particularly in the guinea-pig bladder. *Immunology.* 10:127-136, 1966.

Chapter 14

Radiotherapy in the Treatment of Hematuria

Miljenko V. Pilepich, M.D.

I. Radiotherapy in the Treatment of Hematuria Secondary to Benign Processes

Radiotherapy for hematuria caused by non-neoplastic disease is generally based on the anticipated "sclerosing" effect of irradiation on blood vessels. It is well known that radiation causes tissue fibrosis and obliteration of blood vessels (Figs. 2–4) to a degree closely correlated with the total dose of irradiation and the pattern of fractionation. The same total dose will produce considerably more fibrosis-sclerosis if larger individual fractions are utilized. If conventional 200-rad-per-day fractionation is used, fibrosis will usually be clinically evident following doses exceeding 5,000 rad. Fibrosis and blood vessel sclerosis are among the so-called "late" effects of radiotherapy and require at least several months to develop.

It is very difficult to evaluate objectively the use of radiotherapy as a "sclerosing" agent in the treatment of hematuria produced by benign conditions such as arterial or venous malformations of the genitourinary tract, since most of the information on this subject is anecdotal. In 1961, Mathes and Mayer[1] reported on the use of irradiation in patients with essential "hematuria thought to be secondary to vascular abnormalities." The treatment consisted of 1,500 rad to the affected kidney. Bleeding stopped in six of eight cases.

In an extensive review of the use of ionizing radiation in the treatment of benign disease published in 1977 by the United States Department of Health, Education, and Welfare,[2] only a few reports of the use of irradiation for benign diseases of the genitourinary tract are identified. These include a report on the use of irradiation in hemangioma of the bladder[3] and several reports[4–9] on the treatment of bladder papillomas using a variety of doses and techniques (intra-

From Bern MM (ed.): *Urinary Tract Bleeding: Diagnosis and Control by Medical, Radiologic, and Surgical Techniques*. Mount Kisco, NY, Futura Publishing Co., Inc., 1985.

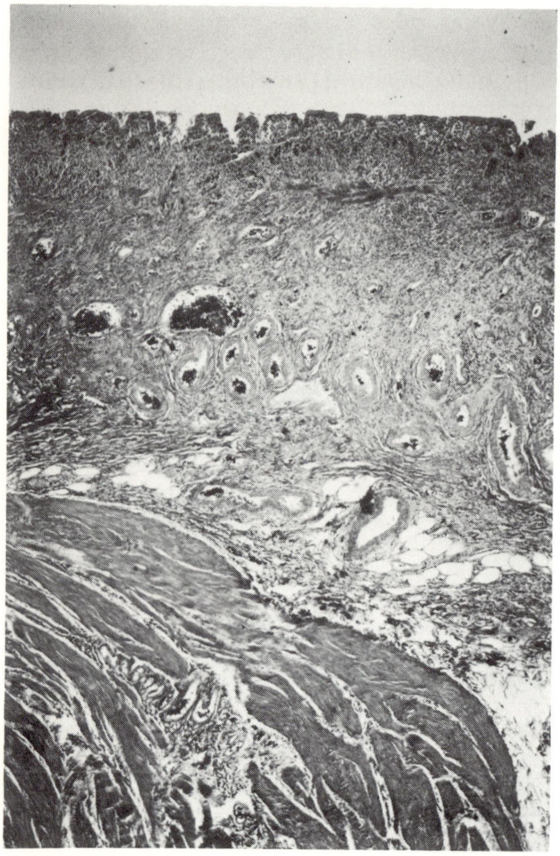

Figure 1: *Photomicrograph demonstrating acute radiation-induced cystitis (250×).*

cavitary application of isotopes, interstitial implants, and external beam radiotherapy). Although favorable and prolonged responses have been observed, the reported results are difficult to interpret because the studies involved no control or "alternate therapy" groups. The irradiation techniques employed in these studies were frequently suboptimal by today's standards and were quite likely to produce normal tissue injuries and hematuria secondary to treatment itself. Recurrent hematuria in many cases might have been related to irradiation rather than the underlying disease.

Acute radiation-induced cystitis may appear shortly following a course of irradiation as a so-called "hemorrhagic radiation cystitits." (Fig. 1). This type of bleeding, usually with dysuria, frequency, and nocturia, is related to acute injury of the affected epithelial (mucosal) surface. It is rare with properly fractionated external beam radiotherapy, but is more likely to occur with massive doses (more than 3,000 rad), especially if delivered by intracavitary isotopes. By cystoscopy, the mucosa is seen to be hyperemic with occasional petechiae. This disease is usually self-limited and can be treated symptomatically and with treatment breaks from the radiotherapy.[10]

More commonly, post-irradiation hematuria is related to late, permanent damage to the blood vessels in the mucosa of the urinary tract. This damage is manifested by telangiectasia and fragility of the mucosa and may result in recurrent chronic bleeding occurring several months to many years after completion of therapy. This type of bleeding may recur for many years. The frequency of post-irratiation hematuria will depend on the dose-fractionation pattern of irradiation and can be expected in approximately 5–10% of patients with pelvic malignancies irradiated with curative intent.[11–15] Larger doses and larger individual fractions can be expected to produce more normal tissue and blood vessel damage and a higher incidence of post-irradiation bleeding. Cytoscopy reveals hypertrophied dilated vessels with erythema, edema, or bleeding. Telangectasia may appear on the otherwise pale atrophic epithelium.[10] By light microscopy, there will be interstitial fibrosis, endarteritis obliterans, fibrosis of the muscularis, and vascular sclerosis (Figs. 2–4).

II. Radiotherapy in the Treatment of Hematuria Secondary to Malignant Tumors

The effectiveness of radiotherapy in relieving bleeding from a malignant tumor is, in principle, related to the radioresponsiveness and radiosensitivity of the tumor. The terms "radiosensitivity" and "radioresponsiveness" are often used interchangeably in the daily clinical parlance. More specifically, however,

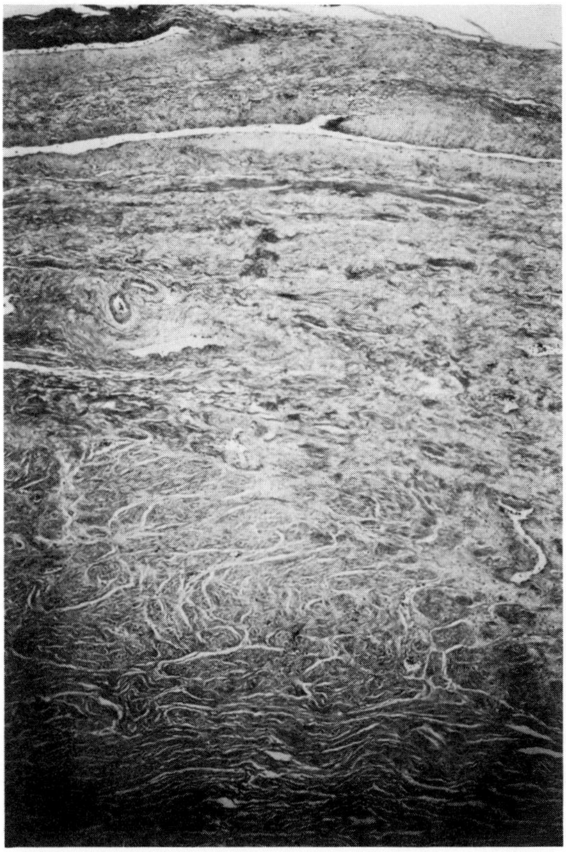

Figure 2: *Photomicrograph demonstrating chronic radiation-induced cystitis (250×).*

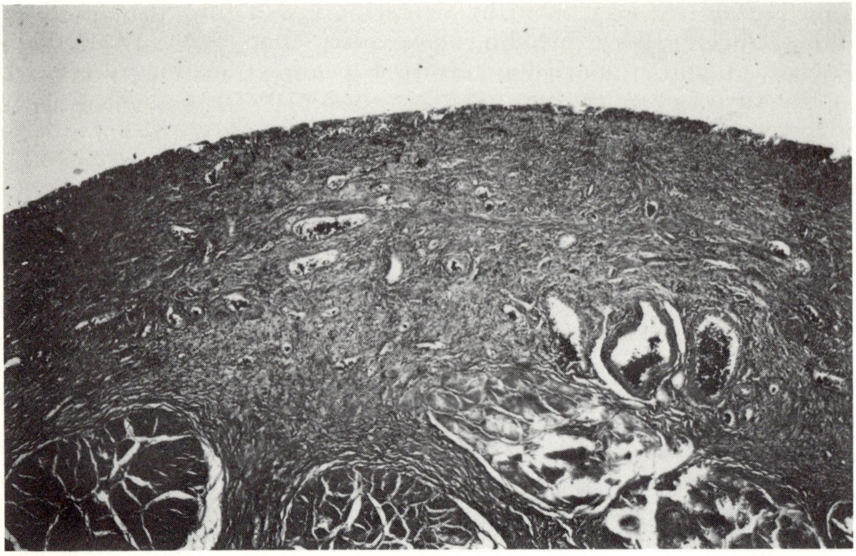

Figure 3: *Photomicrograph demonstrating chronic active radiation-induced cystitis (250×).*

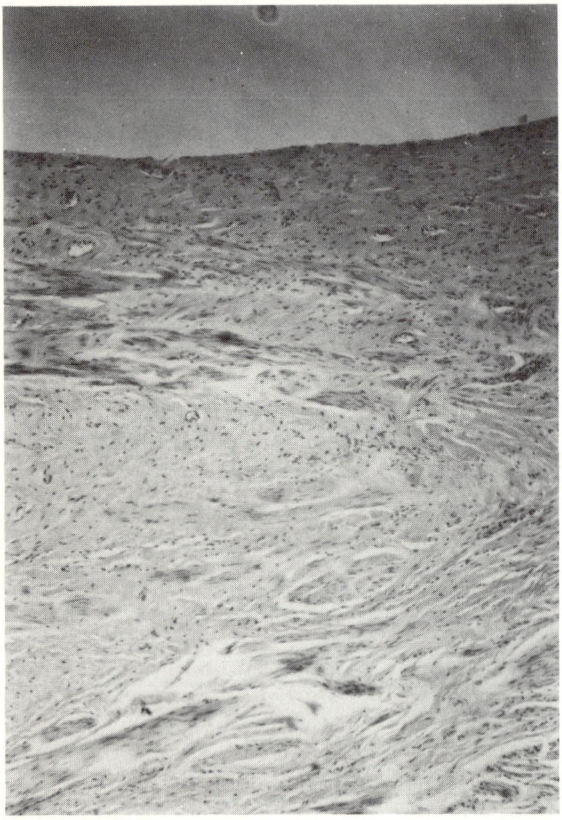

Figure 4: *Photomicrographs demonstrating chronic radiation-induced fibrosis of the bladder (250×).*

the term "radiosensitivity" refers to the inherent susceptibility of tumor cells to radiation-induced cell kill. "Radioresponsiveness" is a clinical term that refers to the observed rate of tumor regression. In this context, a radioresponsive tumor is one that shrinks rapidly following exposure to radiation. Since the rate of tumor regression following a course of radiotherapy depends not only on the radiosensitivity of the tumor cells but also on the tumor cell kinetics and the properties of the tumor stroma, some otherwise "radiosensitive" tumors that are also highly radiocurable may be poorly responsive in the sense that the tumor may take many months or even several years to regress completely. Carcinoma of the prosate is a prime example of a tumor with this type of response; these cells demonstrate radiosensitivty similar to that of other epithelial tumors, but clinically the tumor may take 2 years or even longer before it resolves completely.

The degree to which irratiation relieves bleeding from a tumor varies widely, depending on tumor type and mode of radiation delivery. Improvement may be noted before there is complete, or even partial, tumor response and bleeding may cease within a few days, several weeks, or a number of months.

When asked to provide palliation for patients with hematuria secondary to malignancies of the genitourinary tract, the radiation oncologist must be aware of the clinical situation in its entirety, plans for further therapeutic manipulation, prognosis, and predicted survival. It is essential to identify potentially curable patients and treat them as such. Delivery of short-course, inadequate-dose, or inappropriately fractionated radiotherapy aimed simply at relief of hematuria may prevent further radiotherapy with curative intent in the future. Similarly, radiotherapy, unless given at an appropriate time and in an appropriate form, may compromise subsequent surgical intervention. Even when the goal is purely palliation, an accurate assessment of the patient's general condition, relevant medical problems, tumor extent, and predicted clinical course and survival are essential in choosing the optimal treatment format. In a patient with widely disseminated disease and brief predicted survival, one would not embark on a protracted high-dose course of radiotherapy that would consume a major portion of their remaining life span. A similar course, however, could be highly appropriate for a patient with long predicted survival for whom radiation therapy may mean years of hematuria-free life.

Such radiotherapeutic parameters as field, dose, and fractionation will depend upon the type of tumor, tumor site and extent, and the predicted clinical course. The treatment may range from a single fraction of 1,000 rad to full 7- to 8-week course approaching 7,000 rad. Due to simplicity and ease of administration, external beam irradiation is used almost exclusively. In exceptional circumstances (e.g., advanced tumors of the urethra or bleeding produced by gynecological tumors invading the bladder), intracavitary and interstitial brachytherapy may be employed.

A. Renal Cell Carcinoma

Nephrectomy is the mainstay of treatment in renal cell carcinoma and is sometimes advocated even in the presence of metastatic disease. Hematuria is a frequent presenting symptom and may remain a serious therapeutic problem in patients who do not undergo resection (nephrectomy).

The response of renal cell carcinoma to irradiation varies considerably from patient to patient.[16] While some tumors respond within a few weeks to modest doses (e.g., 3,000 rad), most require considerably higher doses. Because tumor responsiveness is unpredictable and often limited and because a patient may live a number of years with locally advanced or even metastatic disease, irradiation to substantial doses approaching the normal tissue tolerance for the area is usually indicated. A dose to the renal bed of about 4,000–5,000 rad in 4 to 5 weeks appears appropriate.

B. Carcinoma of the Renal Pelvis and Ureter

Although little information is available on the radiotherapy of these tumors, it appears that the transitional and squamous cell carcinomas of these sites show a degree of response to radiotherapy similar to that of carcinoma of the bladder.[17]

C. Carcinoma of the Bladder

Radiotherapy is frequently utilized for palliation in advanced carcinoma of the bladder and appears equally effective in transitional and squamous cell tumors. Responses can be striking. Green and George found a correlation between the total doses of radiotherapy and (1) the percentage of patients with hematuria showing a response, and (2) the duration of responses.[18] They observed a permanent relief of hematuria in 2 of 12 patients receiving less than 4,000 rad and 10 of 23 receiving more than 4,000 rad.

Chan et al.[19] reported on the use of single-dose, whole-pelvis, megavoltage irradiation repeated two to three times at 3- to 4-week intervals. Bleeding ceased promptly in all patients. This approach is attractive for practical reasons (expediency) but should be used with caution in patients with extended predicted survival since large-fraction irradiation can harm normal tissues.

D. Carcinoma of the Prostate

Hematuria in patients with carcinoma of the prostate is usually associated with extension of the prostate tumor into the bladder neck and the base of the bladder. Even if permanent control-cure is not an aim, radiotherapy to high doses ranging between 6,000 and 7,000 rad in 7 to 8 weeks might be justified, since a substantial proportion of patients survive for long periods of time. While evaluating the response, one must remember the slow progression rate following irradiation. Abatement of heamturia may require several weeks or even several months.

F. Secondary Malignancies

A number of malignant tumors may invade the genitourinary tract either through direct extension (carcinoma of the cervix, rectum, ovary) or hematogenously. Lymphomas and leukemias involve the genitourinary tract in a significant percentage of patients in whom radiotherapy, in modest doses, provides highly effective means for the relief of hematuria.[20–22]

The basic principle of individual treatment tailoring is as valid in patients with hematuria due to secondary malignancies as in those with primary malignancies of the genitourinary tract. Radiotherapeutic parameters (dose, field, fractionation) should be dictated by the extent of tumor, plans for further management, and predicted course.

References

1. Mathes GL, Mayer RF. Cobalt radiation for essential hematuria. *JAMA*. 177:10–13, 1961.
2. *A Review of the Use of Ionizing Radiation for the Treatment of Benign Diseases*. Vol. 1. U.S. Department of Health, Education, and Welfare, 1977.
3. Liang DS. Hemangioma of the bladder. *J Urol*. 79:956–960, 1958.
4. Dickson RJ, Lang EK. Treatment of papillomata of the bladder with radioactive colloidal gold (Au^{198}). *Am J Roentgenol Radium Ther Nucl Med*. 83:116–122, 1960.
5. Durrant DR, Laing H. Treatment of multiple superficial papillary tumor of the bladder by intracavity yttrium-90. *J Urol*. 113:480–482, 1975.
6. Einhorn J, Hultberg S, Nilson AE. Treatment of papillomatosis of the bladder with radioactive arsenic ^{76}As. *Acta Radiol. (Ther)* (Stockholm) 2:1–16, 1964.
7. Ellis F, Oliver R. Treatment of papilloma of bladder with radioactive colloidal gold Au^{198}. *Br Med J*. 1:136–139, 1955.
8. Thompson N. Bladder papilloma: An analysis of 75 cases. *Br J Surg*. 47:419–424, 1960.
9. Wallace DM. Intracavitary radiation for multiple non-filtering bladder tumours. *Br J Urol*. 43:177–180, 1971.
10. Goldberg ID, Bloomer WD. Urinary tract toxic effects of cancer therapy. *J Urol*. 132:1–6, 1984.
11. Ram MD. Visceral complications of supervoltage radiotherapy for carcinoma of the bladder. *Br J Surg*. 57:409–412, 1970.
12. Villasanta U. Complications of radiotherapy for carcinoma of the uterine cervix. *Am J Obstet Gynecol*. 114:717–726, 1972.
13. Pilepich MV, Perez CA, Walz BJ, Zivnuska FR. Complications of definitive radiotherapy for carcinoma of the prostate. *Int J Radiat Oncol Biol Phys*. 7:1341–1348, 1981.
14. Kottmeier HL. Complications following radiation therapy in carcinoma of the cervix and their treatment. *Am J Obstet Gynecol*. 88:854–866, 1964.
15. Strockbrine MF, Hancock JE, Fletcher GH. Complications in 831 patients with squamous cell carcinoma of the intact uterine cervix treated with 3000 rad or more whole pelvis irradiation. *Am J Roentgenol*. 108:293–304, 1970.
16. Bratherton DG. Tumours of the kidneys and suprarenals. III. The place of radiotherapy in the treatment of hypernephroma. *Br J Radiol*. 37:141–146, 1964.
17. Brady LW, Gislason GJ, Faust DS, Kazem I, Antoniades J, Davis JA. Radiation therapy: A valuable adjunct in the management of carcinoma of the ureter. *JAMA*. 206:2871–2874, 1968.
18. Green N, George FW. Radiotherapy of advanced localized bladder cancer. *J Urol*. 122:750–751, 1979.
19. Chan RC, Bracken RB, Johnson DE. Single-dose whole-pelvis megavoltage irradiation for palliative control of hematuria or ureteral obstruction. *J Urol*. 122:750–751, 1979.
20. Grooms AM, Morgan SK, Turner WR. Hematuria and leukemic bladder infiltration. *JAMA*. 223:193–194, 1973.
21. Sufrin G, Keogh B, Moore RH, Murphy GP. Secondary involvement of the bladder in malignant lymphoma. *J Urol*. 118:251–253, 1977.
22. Weimar G, Culp DA, Loening S, Narayana A. Urogenital involvement by malignant lymphomas. *J Urol*. 125:230–231, 1981.

Chapter 15

Bleeding in Renal Transplant Patients

Peter N. Madras, M.D.,

and

Anthony P. Monaco, M.D.

I. Coagulation Problems of Renal Transplantation

The variety and amount of surgery associated with transplantation are undergoing rapid growth. The hematologic complications of this specialty include not only coagulation problems, but also those associated with immunosuppression and neoplasia. While coagulation problems are seen in liver, pancreas, heart, and kidney recipients, this chapter focuses on the coagulation problems associated with surgical therapy in the patient with end-stage renal failure. These hemorrhagic problems include those seen in operations used for preparation for transplantation, for access procedures, for immunosuppression, and for the transplant and its complications. The surgeon must adhere to the principles of hemostasis as applied in all surgery, but with even greater attention to details.

The number and variety of surgical procedures employed in patients with end-stage renal disease is growing. These operations relate to:

- Vascular and peritoneal access
- Surgical preparation for transplantation
- Transplantation
- Immunosuppression.

A tabulation of these procedures is presented for the reader's perspective.

Vascular and Peritoneal Access Operations

- Prosthetic percutaneous shunts (Scribner)
- Radial-cephalic fistulas

From Bern MM (ed.): *Urinary Tract Bleeding: Diagnosis and Control by Medical, Radiologic, and Surgical Techniques.* Mount Kisco, NY, Futura Publishing Co., Inc., 1985.

- Brachial fistulas
- Prosthetic indwelling shunts
  - Bovine
  - Expanded polytetrafluoroethylene
  - Umbilical vein grafts
- Saphenous vein shunts
- Subclavian catheters (Uldall)
- Femoral vein catheters
- Chronic indwelling shunts (Tenchkoff)
- Acute peritoneal access
  - Chronic-Tenchkoff
  - Temporary or acute catheters

Operations Relating to Immunosuppression

- Splenectomy
- Thoracic duct drainage
- Bone marrow infusion

Examples of Preparative or Delayed Surgery for Transplantation

- Cholecystectomy
- Ulcer Surgery
- Appendectomy
- Uni- or bilateral nephrectomy
- Parathyroidectomy

Operations Related to the Transplant

- Renal transplantation
- Transplant nephrectomy
- Transplant exploration
- Renal vascular hypertension
- Ureteral strictures and leaks
- Renal biopsy

Bleeding associated with renal transplantation may be arbitrarily divided into three separate categories: (1) bleeding associated with uremia and dialysis; (2) bleeding associated with surgical procedures; and (3) bleeding associated with immunosuppression.

A. Bleeding Associated With Uremia and Dialysis

The uremic state predisposes to bleeding in a variety of ways (see Chapters 1 and 2). Approximately 20% of all patients with renal failure are thrombocytopenic, but with platelet counts that rarely fall below 50,000.[1,2] Abnormal platelet function rather than actual number may be the more important determinant of their bleeding tendency. The bleeding time appears to correlate reasonably well with the clinical tendency to hemorrhage.[1,3] Screening any uremic patient prior to surgery is mandatory. The usefulness of the screening tests is slightly limited by the fact that they will be abnormal secondary to the uremia in many of the patients. However, their usefulness includes their provocation of specific therapies in order to optimize hemostasis when the tests are markedly abnormal.

Coupled with the thrombocytopathy and thrombocytopenia of uremia, dialysis membranes themselves induce profound changes in platelets.[4] The dialysis membranes cause sequestration and degranulation of platelets and activation of the complement system.[5–8] Heparin used in hemodialysis can "spill over" into the patient's circulation, further enhancing the hemorrhagic tendency. Special means to minimize this effect are discussed in Chapter 16 by Yoburn and Bern.

B. Bleeding Associated With Surgical Procedures

There is no doubt that the uremic patient tends to lose more blood at operation than the nonuremic counterpart. Particular surgical care should be applied to minimize this loss, using the best principles of hemostasis applied in all operations. Certain maneuvers in the uremic patient are particularly treacherous. As an example, undermining, often necessary to create space for the vascular access devices, would ordinarily be of little concern in patients without uremic coagulopathy. Vessels contract and thrombose poorly. Lymphatic vessels share in some of these faults. The surgeon is soon aware that there is significantly more blood and lymphatic fluid loss from the uremic patient.

1. Bleeding Associated With Vascular Access Surgery

The problem of a hematoma in the surgical field is not unusual in the uremic patient. However, as most access surgery is performed on small vessels in a superficial operative field, bleeding is seen uncommonly from the anastomosis itself. In the preparation of radial artery-to-cephalic vein fistula (Ciminio-Brescia fistula), relatively little dissection is required. Placement of other permanent indwelling access devices, including autogenous saphenous vein, requires more surgery to elevate skin flaps or tunneling. In the uremic patient, both of these procedures can be hazardous. Not only is platelet function, clot retraction, and vessel spasm abnormal, but the patient must often undergo hemodialysis and anticoagulation in the immediate postoperative period, thus compounding the possibility of bleeding.

Such bleeding is multifactorial in origin, and prevention of bleeding is based on the recognition of the important principles. Preoperative dialysis or other therapies can reverse some of the bleeding tendencies.[9] Tunneling and undermining are hazardous but necessary maneuvers, since direct visualization of the entire length of the vascular bed is not available. Tension on skin and subcutaneous tissues must be minimized and compulsive attention given to hemostasis before skin incisions are closed.

Bleeding from the anastomosis occurs more frequently when using certain vascular prostheses, notably the expanded polytetrafluouroethylene devices. This annoying bleeding presents from the actual needle holes in the graft used for suturing. It will usually stop with patiently applied pressure, but the amount of time sacrificed to this bleeding may be great. Minimization of this bleeding depends on the use of the finest possible tapered needle swagged to a monofilamentous material. We usually use 6-0 or 7-0 polypropylene. The use of mineral oil on this suture material helps prevent the polypropylene from "sawing" through the expanded polytetrafluoroethylene graft, and results in smaller needle holes and less bleeding.

Another type of hemorrhage is seen almost exclusively with use of the expanded polytetrafluoroethylene graft. This bleeding manifests itself as a brisk hemorrhage or an expanding hematoma at the skin incision line at one end of the graft. It frequently follows the first or second use of the graft, and is usually interpreted by the dialysis nurse or physician as a disruption of the anastomosis. Understanding this form of hemorrhage requires knowledge of the nature of the expanded polytetrafluoroethylene graft. The expanded polytetrafluoroethylene access prosthesis is a matrix of 20 to 30 micron pores, which allows tissue ingrowth. Occasionally serum will ultrafilter through these pores, creating seroma surrounding the graft and preventing desired ingrowth. The graft then rests in the seroma, surrounded by a connective tissue capsule. When the dialysis needle is removed, the bleeding occurs into this seroma. The blood then follows a low resistance path to the end of the prosthesis. If the skin incision is weak, the blood will present externally; if the incision is healed, an expanding hematoma will develop at the end of the graft, often quite remote from the puncture site. The medical attendant usually will apply pressure to the area of the hematoma or hemorrhage rather than to the true site of the bleeding. While pressure to the previous puncture site will yield secure hemostasis, the source of the bleeding is frequently not recognized until the hematoma has become large enough to require surgical drainage.

Bleeding from any prosthesis may occur from simple overuse after the graft has been repeatedly punctured in the same region. Not only is the wall of the prosthesis weakened by this practice, but the patient's skin and subcutaneous tissue in the area are attenuated scars. The latter appears to occur more often in diabetic patients. Eventually, the region can erode and alarming hemorrhage may occur. This hemorrhage is easily controlled by simple pressure directly over the bleeding point until the area is oversewn surgically. Final surgical correction of this situation requires replacement of the prosthesis. Attempts to replace the attenuated length of graft with a new segment and to apply a skin flap have met with only temporary success. Prevention of this problem is usually possible by having an awareness of some technical factors. First, as in all vascular surgery, the synthetic prosthesis should be used only after having considered all other alternatives. Autogenous vein should be considered as the prosthesis of choice. Second, the depth of the tunnel must leave a thin layer of subcutaneous tissue between the prosthesis and the skin, especially in diabetic patients. More superficial placement of the prosthesis has two detrimental effects: (1) it leaves a region of skin without adequate nutrition, and (2) it provides the dialysis nurse with a very easy target for access, allowing the most vulnerable areas of skin to undergo the most frequent needle punctures.

In the diabetic patient with uremia, there is another cause of late hemorrhage related to the use of the vascular prosthesis. The incisions used for their graft implantation seem to be more susceptible to breakdown after prolonged use even after uneventful healing. Usually the breakdown occurs at the proximal or distal anastomosis. When this occurs, the prosthesis may be visible in the base of what is now a skin ulcer. Once exposed, the graft should be considered infected. If the exposed area is remote from the anastomosis and no drainage or cellulitis is evident, the situation is not urgent. Although attempts to salvage such a prosthesis have been successful occasionally, this is not our experience. Failure then presents as hemorrhage, necessitating emergency intervention, or metastatic infections.

If confronted with such an exposed graft, cultures are obtained from the incision, the graft, and the blood. The patient is then placed on antibiotics covering for *Staphylococcus* and *Streptococcus* while awaiting the results of those cultures. During this period the wound is covered with betadine dressings and the patient is observed in the hospital.

Under appropriate antibiotic coverage the prosthesis is removed. The surgeon is then confronted with the decision either to leave a remnant of the prosthesis near the anastomosis to serve as an arterial patch (and thus preserve the arterial lumen) or to remove all the foreign material and risk compromising the lumen. The former course is advised only if the anastomosis itself is not exposed. If the surgeon elects this procedure, the patient must be observed frequently and the surgeon must be prepared to remove remaining foreign material to control either infection or hemorrhage.

A recent variant of the subclavian catheter, as modified by Uldall, is now a popular prosthesis for acute dialysis.[10] A number of sources of hemorrhage exist associated with the use of this device. During its insertion, the subclavian artery or the vein might be injured, either by the needle or due to the stiff catheter itself. Perforations of the superior vena cava, apparently after the catheters have functioned normally, have been described. This is due presumably to an erosion of the vessel by the catheter. This complication has been implicated in the death of a patient. Because of this risk and because of the occurrence of infection of device following its protracted use, it has become our practice to implant the single-cuffed Tenchkoff catheter in the external jugular vein, threading it into the superior vena cava when longer but yet still temporary vascular access is required. Mechanical disconnection of the distal end fitting is possible, particularly when the patient is out of the hospital, causing alarming blood loss. This can hardly happen to responsible individuals, but with increasing acceptance of this device, it could happen by human error or neglect.

While bovine grafts are not commonly implanted today, many are still in use for vascular access. This prosthesis has a limited lifetime, similar to its duration when used as a vascular bypass in the femoro-popliteal position. It is therefore probable that bovine grafts will be seen by the access surgeon for a number of years ahead. Thus the questions about managing these failed bovine grafts arise. Removal of this graft is a difficult operation. It is not possible to remove it with a small incision, delivering the graft with traction. The prosthesis adheres strongly to surrounding tissues and must be dissected away, leaving behind a raw and bleeding surface. It has been our practice to leave the bed of a bovine graft open to granulate if there is any concern for hemostasis or infection following the removal of this device.

2. *Bleeding Associated With Renal Transplantation*

The clinical presentation of hemorrhage in the transplant recipient is variable and, at times, may be unrecognized or difficult to diagnose. Possible causes and presentation of post-transplant bleeding as well as investigation and the appropriate therapy will be discussed.

a. Causes of Early Hemorrhage After Renal Transplantation: Intraoperative blood loss during renal transplantation is usually not sufficient to warrant transfusion. In spite of this, our policy is to administer one unit of blood, usually starting early in the operation. In addition to increasing the hematocrit, this unit serves to increase the intravascular volume.

Prior to application of the vascular clamps, the patient is given sufficient heparin to increase clotting time to infinity. This, coupled with the uremic state, will cause diffuse but slight bleeding. This bleeding usually stops soon after the incision is closed, but still requires adequate drainage of the operative field. Reversal of the heparin dose with protamine is not always necessary.

Although kidney transplantation is a largely vascular operation, bleeding at the anastomosis is rare, as it is usually rectified by the surgeon at the time of operation. The other causes of bleeding are more subtle, requiring an understanding of the pathophysiology and the surgery of renal transplantation.

Bleeding from the pelvis of the donated kidney is a major pitfall for the transplant surgeon. In retrieving a kidney for donation, either living-related or cadaver, surgical trauma to small vessels in the pelvis of the kidney often occurs. Under conventional circumstances, these vessels would retract, thrombose, and not bleed. However, other problems exist for the transplanted kidney. The donor is heparinized, adding to the hemorrhage tendency in the donated organ. The donated kidney is then perfused with cold solution, which contains vasodilators and anticoagulants. During perfusion or cold storage, the potential bleeding sites are undetectable. However, when the kidney is reimplanted and arterial flow resumes, open vessels in the renal pelvis may bleed. The bleeding may be delayed occasionally until after the incision is closed.

Two other potential sources of bleeding appear in the operative field. The cut ends of the cord or round ligament and the epigastric vessels may bleed. The epigastric artery and vein are routinely sacrificed and doubly ligated to prevent bleeding.

A kidney undergoing hyperacute or acute rejection may become swollen and rupture, presenting as bleeding into the operative field. This is unusual today with improved tissue typing. Nevertheless, an acute rejection may occur at any time after the transplant and can carry with it the possibility of rupture of the kidney.

All of the above sources create clinically similar and often indistinguishable clinical situations. Detection of blood loss in the immediate post-transplant period may be difficult except when the bleeding presents through surgical drains. However, the presence of drains does not ensure that the blood loss will be detectable externally. The absence of overt blood loss is not evidence that the patient is not bleeding.

Normally on the first postoperative day, the transplant recipient complains only of localized incisional pain. Accumulation of blood in the space surrounding the transplanted kidney manifests by inordinate discomfort in the operative region, often with back pain or flank pain. The patient appears distressed and ill. Pressure over the bladder may cause urgency despite a functioning indwelling urinary catheter. The patients may complain of tenesmus. If enemas are given, they are often retained due to ileus secondary to the hematoma, and invarably add to the patient's discomfort. Pressure on the retroperitoneum by the infiltrating fluid may lead to nausea and vomiting, distension and ileus.

Examination of the patient discloses a tense, tender incision. Hematoma could be confused with the mere bulk of the transplanted kidney, especially if the wound is dry with surgical drains in place. The patient will be pale, but hypotension, tachycardia, and thirst are later signs of bleeding. Falling urine output is unreliable in the transplant recipient. Ecchymosis in the region of the incision is a late and nonspecific sign, possibly only reflecting the blood that found its way through the tissue plains during the surgical procedure.

The diagnosis of a fluid collection around a transplanted kidney is best made by the ultrasound scan. Computerized scans may distinguish blood from urine or lymph, but this distinction is not often the issue at hand. Angiography usually is not needed, since the question to be decided in the early post-transplant course is whether or not to re-explore the patient. If a large volume of fluid is found, whether of blood or urine density, exploration is indicated.

When re-exploring the recent transplant, the surgeon should suspect the renal pelvis as the most likely source of bleeding, followed by the epigastric vessels or the divided cord or round ligaments. Failure to locate bleeding in these areas will lead to further inspection of the cut muscle layers, the bladder, the ureteral tunnel, and finally, the anastomosis. If a specific bleeding site is found in any of these structures, it is usually easily controlled.

It is not uncommon that no distinct bleeding is found on exploration of the transplanted kidney. After evacuation of clots, the entire field may reveal no hint of the source of blood loss. In this situation, it is reasonable to suppose that the bleeding vessel was in the renal pelvis and that it stopped spontaneously after sufficient tamponade resulted from the hematoma. The incision is closed and drains are left in place. In the usual case, bleeding will not recur. The improvement in the clinical state of the patient following evacuation of the retroperitoneal hematoma justifies having performed the exploration even when no primary bleeding site is identified.

b. Hematuria: Bleeding in the early post-transplant period may also present as hematuria. Hematuria in modest amounts is almost invariable for about 48 hours after a transplant. However, if heavy, this bleeding may lead to significant problems. It may become a source of urinary tract obstruction by blocking the urinary catheter and it may make it difficult to accurately record the urinary output.

The source of bleeding in the lower urinary tract following transplantation may be the bladder mucosa, the cut end of the implanted ureter or the ureteral artery, and the kidney itself. Ureteral obstruction either from bleeding in the kidney, which can clot in the ureter, or from bleeding in the submucosal tunnel, which occludes the ureter by extralumenal pressure, must be considered as causes of acute oliguria in the early post-transplant period. It is our practice not to perform a mucosal approximation as part of the ureteroneocystostomy, thus allowing free access for blood in the submucosal tunnel to the bladder. This type of bleeding is usually limited, and replacement isn't required, but it may lead to obstruction of the bladder outlet, with bladder distension. If bladder obstruction does occur, especially in the neuropathic bladder, there can be further hemorrhage and further lower urinary tract obstruction. Meticulous irrigation of the Foley catheter and changing the catheter as often as necessary are essential in managing these patients.

Occasionally, and more commonly in diabetic patients with neurogenic bladder dysfunction, enough clotted blood may accumulate in the bladder so that patency will not be re-established even with irrigation or catheter change. Assessment of the amount of clot in the bladder can be obtained by ultrasonic scans and the results may be startling. When the bladder is distended with clots, further mucosal bleeding can occur. By emptying the bladder, the detrusor muscle contracts, helping to stop further bleeding. In rare cases surgical exploration of the bladder is needed to remove the clot. Supra-pubic drainage is necessary.

c. Vascular Defects: Arterial or venous thrombosis of the transplanted vessels may present as urinary tract hemorrhage and oliguria (see below). In the early postoperative period, this is often attributed to acute tubular necrosis or rejection. If the patient still has his own kidneys, the urine output will be an unreliable sign of thrombosis. Thus, it is essential to obtain a perfusion scan and an echo on all oliguric patients in the immediate postoperative period, especially if their output suddenly decreases after a period of normal flow.

d. Late Causes of Renal Transplant Hemorrhage: Once the patient acquires stable function in the transplanted kidneys, bleeding from the kidney is rare. Healing obliterates the potential retroperitoneal plane in 4–6 weeks, so there is little chance for a large, occult blood loss into that area. Thus, the most likely route of escape for blood at this time is via the urinary tract, presenting as hematuria, either gross or microscopic. The causes of late hemorrhage are acute or chronic rejection, trauma to the kidney, and venous arterial thrombosis. All of these may, but usually do not, lead to swelling of the kidney, which in turn could cause rupture of the kidney.

Diagnosis of the causes of late hemorrhage is usually not difficult. Trauma is ascertained by history and physical examination. Acute rejection can occur in the patient who has neglected to take the prescribed immunosuppressive drugs. Besides hematuria, there is pain and tenderness over the transplant. Bleeding from the transplanted kidney may present as sudden anuria due to ureteral obstruction, which may or may not be painful. The kidney may become enlarged, but in the early period after obstruction, enlargement of the kidney may not have had time to develop. Infection or embolization to the kidney could also lead to this outcome. Diagnosis of this problem is helped by ultrasonic examination.

When considering the causes of late hematuria, one must not overlook the patient's native kidneys. Kidneys with polycystic disease are well known to bleed after transplantation. Infection, calculi, tumors, lower urinary tract pathology, and lesions of the patient's own kidneys all may present as urinary tract bleeding. Interestingly, tumors of the native kidneys do not often appear.

The bladder can accumulate massive amounts of clotted blood, occasionally without the obvious clinical signs. These clots can become an extremely troublesome cause of lower urinary tract obstruction. When the clots cannot be removed by cystoscopy, re-exploration of the bladder may be necessary. The diabetic recipients with neuropathic bladders may have painless bladder distension due to outlet obstruction; the diagnosis of oliguria necessitating hemodialysis may be considered, having overlooked the true cause of the problem. A resultant danger of this type of hemorrhage is massive distension of the vesicle wall, leading to high pressures within the detrusor muscle, with strangulation of the distal end of the ureter and possible stricture or disruption.

The management of this type of postoperative hematuria lies in assuring patency of the urinary catheter, through frequent irrigations and catheter changes when necessary. Replacement of blood loss is rarely needed. It has been our experience that the blood loss from hematuria is usually slight, though it may persist for weeks following cadaveric transplantation, even in the face of normal or improving renal function.

e. Bleeding Associated With Transplant Nephrectomy: Hemorrhage is the major potential hazard of transplant nephrectomy. As the causes of hemorrhage are multifactorial, avoidance of this complication is dependent on recognition of the causes.

Transplant nephrectomy is performed for specific indications other than rejection. If a rejected kidney is asymptomatic, there is no reason to remove it. The usual indications for this operation are: (1) uncontrollable infection in the transplant; (2) fulminant rejection with consumptive coagulopathy; (3) infarction with or without hemorrhage from the kidney; (4) preparation for another renal transplantation, particularly if the patient has had bilateral transplants in the past, and (5) systemic illness attributable to the presence of the transplanted organ, characterized by fever, malaise, arthropathy, and other signs and symptoms similar to serum sickness.

In many of these situations, coagulopathy should be anticipated. If the patient is having a severe rejection, then it is likely that some consumption of coagulation factors and platelets is occurring. In this situation, it is usually possible to control the rejection with high dose steroids for 1 or 2 days while the patient is prepared for the transplant nephrectomy. This preparation consists, in part, of enlisting the aid of the hematologist for management of the possible coagulation defects.

Correction of the coagulopathy is essential prior to transplant nephrectomy since this operation requires dissection of large planes of adherent tissues between the kidney and the surrounding soft tissues of the host, which precludes a bloodless dissection. Thus the hemostatic mechanisms of the patient are essential to stop the blood loss.

The technique of this procedure centers on the prevention of blood loss. It is generally agreed that the capsule of the kidney may be left in place in a subcapsular dissection. This approach is satisfactory if the kidney is completely thrombosed and will not bleed. Dissection of the hilum of the kidney is best performed from an intracapsular plane in order to minimize the risk of trauma to the iliac artery and vein. The renal vessels are then ligated, leaving a stump of transplanted vessel to be used as a patch on the hosts' iliac vessels. These stumps will thrombose without significant risk of hemorrhage.

Following removal of the transplant, the entire field is drained and loosely closed. It is anticipated that significant oozing will occur, often requiring blood replacement. It is sometimes necessary to re-explore the incision in order to evacuate a hematoma. Rarely, however, will a discreet bleeding site be found. Once again, prior to re-exploration, it is essential to rule out coagulopathy.

Bleeding from vascular anastomoses is a rare occurrence. While venous anastomosis rarely can be a source of late hemorrhage, we have not experienced such a problem. The tissue pressure surrounding a transplant is close to venous pressure so that tamponade occurs quickly.

Arterial bleeding from the anastomoses is also not common but, when present, it is usually secondary to infection. The patient is febrile and complains of tenderness in the incision, which often radiates to the back and the ipsilateral hip. Superficial layers of the incision may not reflect the deeper infection. There may be deteriorating renal function. The differential diagnosis usually includes rejection, urinary tract infection, and deep wound infection.

If the infection goes unrecognized, the arterial closure following the transplant nephrectomy may become infected. Typically, it will not disrupt or cause massive hemorrhage immediately. The initial bleeding will be in small amounts (analogous to the aorto-duodenal fistula that may present as occult blood loss in the stool). The early anastomotic bleeding may be asymptomatic or may only exacerbate an already painful incision. Ultrasonic or CT scanning will recognize the existence of fluid in the nephrectomy field. Gas bubbles seen on the CT scan would yield the diagnosis of infection requiring exploration.

At exploration, the mixture of blood and pus is evacuated and large drains are left in the operative field. At this point, it is probably not possible to determine whether the arterial anastomosis is infected. The correct management is to ensure adequate drainage of the surgical field and to give appropriate antibiotics. If the arterial anastomosis is infected, it remains in danger of disruption at any time, though probably it would not occur during the initial drainage procedure. The likelihood of eradicating the anastomotic infection is not great, even though it is theoretically possible since there is no prosthetic material in the field. The ultimate fate of the infected transplant arterial anastomosis can be massive hemorrhage presenting as frank bleeding into the incision. This requires immediate surgical control of the common or external iliac artery and removal of the graft.

The surgeon then may be confronted with the management of the infected host artery. In the earlier days of renal transplantation, the internal iliac artery was used to supply the graft. This artery can be ligated with minimal risk to the host. Recently, the external iliac artery has become the host vessel of choice for implanting the donor renal artery. Owens reported that six patients who bled from an infected iliac anastomosis underwent ligation of the external iliac artery without developing distal ischemic symptoms. In contrast to the benign course after ligation of the external iliac artery, those patients in whom an attempt was made to repair the artery all re-bled. Four of the 11 patients died due to hemorrhage.[11] If this vessel is ligated, there is about a 50% chance that the patient will lose the leg unless an arterial reconstruction is performed. However, any bypass would require prosthetic material and this would have to circumvent an already infected field. Thus, the surgeon is justifiably reluctant to ligate the external iliac artery.

The alternative to ligation of the vessel is to suture the external iliac arteriotomy and hope that it will heal with approriate antibiotics. Over 70% of these lesions will not heal and disruption will occur in 1–3 weeks. If disruption does occur after the transplant nephrectomy, the surgeon probably has no choice but to ligate the common or external iliac artery and to hope for limb survival. An extra-anatomic bypass could then be performed with greater safety since the original infection would have been treated for some time.

It is probable that more than half of the infected arteriotomies heal with appropriate antibiotics. The arterial infections must be considered as endarteritis and treated as such. This would include 3–6 weeks of intravenous antibiotics and debridement of the infected areas if there is evidence of persistent localized infection.

Although anastomotic infections are serious complications, it is important to realize that they are distinctly rare. On our transplant service, over 300 transplants have been performed over the past 15 years and we have encountered this complication only twice. The first case involved the internal iliac artery and was managed easily by ligation. The second patient is currently hospitalized and was managed with antibiotics after removal of the renal graft. A second transplant was performed without obvious sequelae related to the previously infected iliac artery.

C. Bleeding Associated With Immunosuppression

There are three general categories of hemostatic problems associated with immunosuppression: those associated with steriods, with bone marrow suppression, and with sepsis. The aspects of these problems specific to transplantation will be reviewed.

Ulcers due to the effect of uremia upon the gastrointestinal tract are usually secondary to underdialysis and are not part of the syndrome now under consideration. They will respond to better dialysis and will not recur if the patient can be given normal renal function. Acid-peptic disease will be exacerbated by the use of steriods. The general rule is to treat this disease when recognized before proceeding with a transplant. Duodenal ulcers are now manageable with conventional medical treatment. Before the introduction of cimetidine, patients with duodenal ulcers often would undergo therapeutic surgery. Since the advent of cimetidine, it is possible to transplant patients with a history of previous duodenal ulcers with less risk. Before transplant surgery, endoscopy and radiographic examinations must confirm that the ulcer is inactive. If the patient has a history of active bleeding from the ulcer or had a previous perforation, it is still wise to perform definitive surgery in preparation for transplantation. It is more difficult to offer guidelines for the patient who has a number of recurrences, all of which readily respond to therapy. Complete assessment of the patient, including the psychiatric status, must enter into the process of deciding for or against possible surgery for ulcer.

The considerations of gastric ulcers are very similar to those for duodenal ulcers. In these, there is a greater incentive to be conservative, since the disease is more easily treated and the tendency to massive hemorrhage is not as high as with duodenal ulcer.

As possible prophylaxis against gastrointestinal tract irritation and bleeding, all transplant patients receive acid neutralizing preparations. Those patients with previous ulcer disease also receive cimetidine. Any gastrointestinal tract symptom is quickly investigated and treated.

Another site for gastrointestinal tract bleeding associated with immunosuppression and the stress of transplantation is the large bowel. Colonic ulcers due to fungi (often aspergillosis), bacteria, or protozoa (amebic dysentery) have been seen in the immunosuppressed patient. Parasitic diseases such as *Strongyloides* cause eosinophilia and occult blood loss in the host before transplant and may cause hemorrhage from the gastrointestinal tract and infest other systems to which they migrate after immunosuppressive therapy.

Aspergillosis may give multiple, superficial mucosal ulcerations that can bleed profusely. This bleeding is painless in a patient who may have no other systemic manifestations of the fungal infection. The bleeding mimics that of colonic polyps, diverticuli, or arteriovenous malformations. Mackel's diverticulum also may be considered.

Attention is to be directed to establishing the site of bleeding and the correct diagnosis. A simple expedient is to examine the stool for fungi by light microscopy and culture. Endoscopy and colonoscopy may be attempted. Arteriography may indicate the site if the rate of loss is great enough. Radionuclide scanning with tagged red blood cells is a very effective means of localizing colonic bleeding. This technique, however, suffers from inherent weaknesses when examining the flexures and the region of the colon adjacent to the transplanted kidney since these areas are not sensitive to this examination.

Treatment of continued colonic hemorrhage follows the same guidelines as in the nonimmunosuppressed patient. If the site of hemorrhage is established and the bleeding surpasses an agreed limit (such as 6 or 10 units in a 12 or 24 hour period), then the appropriate hemicolectomy is performed. If the cause of the hemorrhage is in fact due to unrecognized aspergillosis or other fungal diseases then surgical treatment may be a serious error. Invariably, the pathologist will establish the diagnosis upon microscopic examination of the ulcer base. By that time, it is likely that other regions of ulceration will have occurred and that renewed hemorrhage will be present. Medical therapy under these conditions may not salvage the patient.

Bacterial dysenteries in immunosuppressed patients are not common other than in the immediate post-transplant period. These patients have profound signs of systematic toxicity and colonic irritation, with bloody diarrhea, toxic dilated colon, and cardiopulmonary instability. Appropriate stains of stool specimens will usually guide the physician to the most appropriate antibiotic regimen, while cultures define the actual organism. *Staphyloccus*, clostridia, and shigella-salmonella are frequent causes of overwhelming bacterial forms of colitis that may cause profound bloody diarrhea. It is a safe approximation that any bacteria may produce these symptoms in an immunosuppressed patient.

REFERENCES

1. Castaldi PA, Rosenberg MC, Stewart JH. The bleeding disorder of uraemia: A qualitative platelet defect. *Lancet*. 1:66, 1966.
2. Stewart JH. Platelet numbers and life span in acute and chronic renal failure. *J Throm Diath Hemorrh*. 17:532, 1967.
3. Rabiner, SF. Uremic bleeding. In: *Progress in Hemostatis and Thrombosis*. Vol. 1. Spaet TH, Ed. New York, Grune and Stratton, 1972, pp. 233–250.
4. Ward CA, Forest TW. On the relation between platelet adhesion and the roughness of a synthetic biomaterial. *Ann Biomed Eng*. 4:184–207, 1976.
5. Madras PN, Morton WA, Petschek HE. Dynamics of thrombus formation. *Fed Proc*. 30:(5)1665–1676, 1971.
6. Craddock PR, Hammerschmidt D, White JG, Delmasso AP, Jacob HS. Complement (C5a)-induced granulocyte aggregation in vitro: A possible mechanism of complement-mediated leukostasis and leukopenia. *J Clin Invest*. 60:260-264, 1977.
7. Herzlinger GA, Cumming RD. Role of complement activation in cell adhesion to polymer blood contact surfaces. *Trans Am Soc Artific Intern Organs*. 26:165–171, 1980.
8. Herzlinger, GA, Bing, DH, Stein, R, Cumming, RD. Quantitative measurement of C_3 activation at polymer surfaces. *Blood*. 57:764–770, 1981.
9. Rabiner, SF, Drake, RF. Platelet function as an indicator of adequate dialysis. *Kidney Int*. 7(1) (Suppl. 2):s-144 to s-146, 1975.
10. Uldall, R. Subclavian cannulation for hemodialysis: the present state of the art. *Artif Organs*. 6:73–76, 1982.
11. Owens, ML, Wilson, SE, Maxwell, JG, Bordner, A, Smith, R, Ehrlich, R. Major arterial hemorrhage after renal transplantation. *Transplantation*. 27:285–287, 1979.

Chapter 16

Management of Hemodialysis in Patients at Risk for Hemorrhage

David C. Yoburn, M.D., and Murray M. Bern, M.D.

George Haas, a German investigator, first performed human dialysis from 1924 to 1928. Herodin, a preparation of crushed leech heads, was used as the anticoagulant. The bleeding that occurred from the surgical cannulation wound and from the gums of the patient clearly identified hemorrhage as a complication with which to contend during hemodialysis. In 1943, Willem Kolff used cellophane, a cellulose acetate material, on a rotating drum as the semipermeable membrane for dialysis. The heparin dosages ranged from 6,000 to 9,000 units and were usually administered prior to dialysis. Since then there have been improvements in the semipermeable membranes and anticoagulation techniques. However, the risk of excessive hemorrhage, especially in patients with anatomical defects or recent surgery, persists.

I. The Interface of Blood With Membranes

Modern hemodialysis requires a continuous 200 to 300 cc per minute blood flow. The blood is propelled by the arterial blood pressure and a roller pump through the artificial kidney and returned to the patient. Inside the artificial kidney, blood is separated from the dialysate fluid by semipermeable membranes constructed in one of three basic designs. A coil kidney is composed of two blood envelopes running parallel, spiralling from outside to inside, and supported on a plastic grid through which the dialysate is bubbled. The parallel plate dialyzer consists of multiple flat blood envelopes stacked one upon another and separated by a grid in which dialysate fluid is flowing. Hollow fiber kidneys consist of capillary-sized tubes that direct the blood through a bath of dialysate fluid, all sealed in a plastic container.

From Bern MM (ed.): *Urinary Tract Bleeding: Diagnosis and Control by Medical, Radiologic, and Surgical Techniques*. Mount Kisco, NY, Futura Publishing Co., Inc., 1985.

Regenerated cellulose is the most common material used for hemodialysis membranes. Different preparations of the regenerated cellulose can influence not only the dialysis characteristics but also their procoagulant properties. Different anticoagulant regimens are needed for these various preparations. Thus, indirectly, they influence the hemorrhagic risks. A short description of how it is prepared is thus appropriate. A solution of purified cellulose is prepared in sodium hydroxide and is made gelatinous by adding carbon disulfide. This is then dissolved in sodium hydroxide and formed into polymeric membranes in an acid bath, thus regenerating the cellulose. This final product is called cellophane. Cuprophane is made by using the regenerated cellulose, with an ammonium solution of cupric oxide to dissolve the cellulose. An acid bath again is used to regenerate the membrane. Cellulose acetate membranes are made from acetone-formamide mixtures. Polyacrylonitrile, a noncellulose dialysis membrane, is similar to Cuprophane but with the addition of increased permeability to certain molecular weight substances. Permeability factors of these membranes can be increased by partially regenerating the cellulose acetate by hydrolysis or by physically stretching the membranes to alter pore size.

The process of hemodialysis has many facets that can initiate coagulation. First is the exposure of blood to foreign surfaces included in the needles, tubing, and the artificial kidney itself. While these surfaces are relatively inert, they nevertheless do allow activation of coagulation and platelets (see Chapters 1 and 2). The possibility that the membranes activate coagulation causing consumption of factor XII, the Hageman factor, has been proposed and subsequently contested.[1,2] Second is the type of dialyzer. Artificial kidneys are designed to reduce turbulence in the blood as it flows from tubing to the dialysis membrane and back to the patient. Nevertheless, turbulence occurs, dependent somewhat upon the organization of the system. The organization of the blood path thus plays a role in the amount of anticoagulation needed for each artificial kidney. In the coil and parallel plate systems, the blood path is rather simply organized, and the risk for thrombosis is thought to be reduced. In the hollow fiber kidney, a high blood flow of 200 to 300 cc/min is subdivided from the large tubing into thousands of capillary-sized pathways, increasing the stress on the blood in such a fashion as to put the system at added risk for thrombosis. Third, the membrane type itself has certain characteristics that not only can initiate thrombosis but also hemolysis.

II. Therapeutic Index

Adequacy of anticoagulation can be determined by *in vitro* assays of coagulation, such as the ACT or PTT, as well as by watching the patient's clinical status and the machine's function. After all, the patient's clinical status is the parameter against which the efficacy of anticoagulation as measured by prolongation of *in vitro* clotting assay is measured. Blood flow throughout the artificial kidney is relatively well regulated, and clotting in the kidney system an be recognized as resistance to the flow through the system. Blood clots forming in the "clot trap" or beyond in the lines leading to the patient may significantly decrease the rate of blood flow despite pump pressure. Clotting of blood inside the artificial kidney can be evaluated by detecting change in the blood volume space in the artificial kidney at a certain fluid pressure after the artificial kidney has been rinsed with saline. More blood may be retained if anticoagulation is inadequate. This eventually leads to loss of dialysis efficiency.[3]

Hypoxia is a common complication in the initial stages of dialysis. How this relates to the coagulation scheme is very complex. It is unclear whether post-dialysis hypoxia is related more to leukostasis in the pulmonary arterioles following complement activation by the cellulose dialyzer membrane (but not polyacrylonitrile dialyzers), fluid shifts, small emboli composed of clots or platelets to the pulmonary circuit, or simply the removal of serum bicarbonate during dialysis.[2,4–7] However, if anticoagulation is inadequate, then it is very likely that dialysis-associated hypoxia is contributed to by clot embolizing to the lungs. These emboli may contain fibrin, platelet thrombi, or both.

Laboratory assays for the adequacy of anticoagulation may be as simple as looking at the peripheral blood smear for schistocyes or as refined as measuring the fibrinopeptide A, prothrombin fragments, or iron or red blood cell losses on the membranes.[8] However, due to the complex nature of coagulation, platelet function, and the vascular changes occurring in patients during hemodialysis, it is not adequate simply to measure a clotting assay as a monitor of safety. The balance between coagulation and hemorrhage, or therapeutic index, constantly changes depending on a patient's comorbid disease(s). Acute hemorrhage is an obvious indication of over-anticoagulation. However, slight or more subtle observations including bleeding at an access puncture site, occult GI bleeding, falling serum iron levels, or hematomas without trauma may be indications of over-anticoagulation.

There may be simple adjuvants to heparin in hemodialysis that may be overlooked. As an example, blood that drops forcibly onto the superior miniscus of blood in the chamber may denature and thus activate clotting by bubbling. Allowing the blood to flow along the side of chamber by tilting the chamber removes this problem. Minimizing vessel trauma at the access puncture site limits thrombin generation. By carefully securing the needles, trauma to the vascular access site is reduced, turbulence is reduced, and thrombin generation is reduced. Optimal control of the temperature of the blood in the lines as well as in the dialysis machinery may further help.[9,10]

III. Use of Heparin

Many laboratory assays exist to test the adequacy of heparin's anticoagulant activity with wide ranges for ease of performance, sensitivity, and reliability. Heparin, which acts by cofactoring with antithrombin III, is cleared by first order kinetics from the plasma and does not appear to be cleared by hemodialysis.[11,12] It is neutralized by platelet factor 4. The final anticoagulant effect depends upon the concentrations of these materials, plus its volume of distribution and rates of clearance. It is apparent, therefore, that the final anticoagulant effect must vary throughtout the dialysis run. As an example, AT3 may actually fall at the initiation of dialysis only to rise during the remainder of the treatment.[13] Platelet factor 4 may be released during dialysis as the platelets are induced to release their granules when interacting with the dialysis membranes. Thus, assays of activity should be studied for each patient throughout the dialysis run.

The original approach used to monitor heparin's activity revolved around whole blood coagulation as reflected by the Lee-White clotting time. Modern techniques can extend the assays of adequacy to measures of rates of fibrinogen consumption or of fibrinopeptide A generation,[8] or of heparin concentrations. Still, whole blood or plasma clotting times are reasonable assay systems. Whole blood thrombin time[15,16] or activated whole blood clotting times,[17–20] using either celite or bason as activators, are efficient assays and require only a few minutes to perform. They obviously do not need the time required for separation of plasma as called for in other clotting assays and can be performed at the patient's bedside. These assays have strong correlations with heparin levels. A whole blood activated clotting time (WBACT) of 150 to 200 seconds and a whole blood thrombin time (WBTT) of 6 to 10 seconds corresponds to a heparin level of .5 to 1.0 units per ml of blood.[15] No matter which assay is selected for the dialysis unit, it is important that the assay be systemically assayed in that dialysis unit to establish its reliability, its variability, and its limitations in a wide variety of clinical settings. All personnel in the dialysis unit must have the ability to make an accurate and reproducible appraisal of the patient based upon the clotting assay. This is essential when confronting problems of excessive bleeding or excessive thrombosis.

Heparin was first used as a single bolus of 6,000 to 9,000 units. This schedule was then modified to include a loading dose and a mid-dialysis bolus, and thereafter further modified to a loading dose followed by multiple hourly doses. Once established for any individual patient in routine hemodialysis, the dosages selected can be repeated with close attention to the patient's current clotting or bleeding. Studies measuring fibrinopeptide A as a measure of clotting in the kidney found little difference between heparin administration by loading dose, by continuous heparin introduced into the dialyzer, or by intravenous loading followed by continuous infusion of heparin dosed according to coagulation assays.[8] All three methods of administration appeared safe.

A distinction needs to be made between the acute effects of anticoagulation and the long-term effects of hypercoagulation and atherosclerotic diseases in patients with renal failure.[17,18] Chronic suppression of fibrinolysis, lowered AT3, and elevated factor VIII complex[19,20] are seemingly linked with atherosclerotic diseases. Although these events are not clearly alterable by changes in heparin dose, the day-to-day importance of anticoagulation, at present, exceeds the ability to manage the atherosclerotic risk. The addition of other agents, such as platelet-suppressing drugs including sulfinpyrazone, dipyridamole, or prostacyclin, may help prevent these long-term diseases.

IV. Management of High-Risk Patients

Although any patient is at risk for hemorrhage during hemodialysis,[25–28] certain patients are at higher risk. For some groups this is estimated to be as high as a 26% incidence of bleeding complications.[29] Beyond those with uremic pericarditis or other uremic-related disorders,[28,30] patients with renal lesions requiring surgery are particularly vulnerable in the first 24 to 48 hours.[27,28] In particular, patients with recent vascular procedures such as renal transplantation, renovascular repair, or cardiovascular surgery may require special attention. The history of recent trauma with or without hematomas also increases the risk associated with anticoagulation. Patients who are already bleeding, such as with urinary tract bleeding, gastrointestinal bleeding, hemoptysis, epistaxis, central nervous system bleeding, hemorrhagic effusions, or retroperitoneal bleeding require tailoring of their heparin therapy.[29–33] Nephrolithiasis and polycystic kidney disease may produce the scenario of urinary tract bleeding and uremia. Patients with hematologic or oncologic malignancies and those with thrombocytopenia, with DIC, thrombotic thrombocytopenia, or post-transfusion purpura also certainly constitute high-risk patients when hemodialysis is required. Diabetics are particularly vulnerable due to retinal vascular disease. To this group, one could add assorted patients with coagulopathies including those with true circulating anticoagulants as with systemic lupus, inherited coagulation defects, and those patients receiving third-generation cephalosporins and who acquire defects associated with vitamin K deficiency.

Most patients with uremia have coagulopathies associated with platelet and endothelial defects (see Chapters 1 and 2). The therapeutic index for anticoagulation for heparin must be established based upon these pre-existing lesions. Patients with thrombocytopathy, or possibly very high levels of endothelial PGI_2, may be bothered by excessive hemorrhage. In one report, the heparin used for dialysis was associated with elevation of PGI_2.[34] Likewise, those with congenital lesions such as Glanzman's disease will require special attention.

For these high-risk patients, a number of schemes for heparin administration have been proposed. Regional anticoagulation involves infusing heparin into the blood as the blood enters into the dialyzer and then infusing protamine sulfate, a heparin-neutralizing agent, into the blood as it exits the dialyzer. This allows the anticoagulation effect to be confined to the artificial kidney and avoidance of systemic anticoagulation.[35–43] Heparin has a longer biological *in vivo* survival than does protamine. This appears to be due to later redistribution of heparin from depot sites.[42] This method may, but not always, require the administration of protamine sulfate several hours after dialysis to prevent "rebound" anticoagulation.[38,41] Thus, this method is time consuming and technically more difficult. It requires careful laboratory monitoring as well as more technical assistance and equipment at the patient's bedside.

An alternative is to use low-dose continuous infusions of heparin, with or without an intravenous loading dose. This may be used to maintain thrombin clotting times at two to three times that of baseline. Heparin infusion can also be regulated by the Lee-White clotting time so as to keep it no higher than 25% over the predialysis levels. This approach is safe and apparently free of the heparin rebound phenomenon.[41] These are technically easier and they effectively lower the risks for patients at higher risk.[44–47]

Despite having good procedural control, Schwartz and Port[47] found that regional heparinization could still be associated with severe bleeding complications. Thus, they performed a perspective study of regional and low-dose heparin programs. For regional therapy, heparin was infused into the blood before it entered the dialyzer at 0.3 units heparin/ml of blood. Protamine sulfate was infused into the blood as it left the dialyzer at approximately 1 mg protamine sulfate per 100 units of heparin infused. The patient's thrombin times were monitored every 30 minutes and the doses of protamine were adjusted to keep the thrombin clotting times near baseline. Fifty milligrams of protamine sulfate was given also 3 hours after the dialysis was completed. Anticoagulation using the alternative approach of low-dose heparin was begun with 5 to 10 units of heparin per pound of body weight, followed by heparin infused at a rate of 10 units per pound body weight per hour into the blood as it entered into the dialyzer. This dose was adjusted to keep the thrombin time at two to three times baseline. In the patients with active bleeding at the time of dialysis, there was a 38% incidence of bleeding using low-dose heparin and a 47% incidence of bleeding using regional heparinization within 24 hours of dialysis. In patients with "high risk" defined as having had active bleeding within 3 days of dialysis, surgery or trauma within 3 days of dialysis, or dialysis-related perforation of a major vessel, there was a 23% incidence of bleeding with regional heparinization and an 11% incidence of bleeding with low-dose heparinization within 24 hours. Of all hemodialysis patients at all levels of risk for bleeding, regional heparinization resulted in a 19% incidence of further bleeding while low-dose heparinization resulted in only a 10% incidence. Both techniques led to a 3–5% incidence of dialyzer clotting. Thus, it appeared that the easier low-dose heparinization method was preferable in terms of hemorrhage.

In a second report, Schwartz[29] examined the "best" heparin dose by pretesting for the *in vitro* response of blood to the addition of heparin and then calculating the "ideal" dose for heparin base upon the previously acquired *in vitro* data. *In vitro*, 0.3 units of heparin was added to each ml of patient's blood. If the thrombin clotting time changed less than 150% of baseline, the loading dose of heparin given was 22 units/kg body weight given via the venous return needle. The same dose was then given by hourly infusions via the arterial needle. If the original *in vitro* response was more than 300% of baseline, the heparin dose was reduced by one-half and 11 units of heparin/kg body weight were given. Intermediate doses were given for intermediate *in vitro* clotting time responses found during the pretesting. Thereafter, heparin dosing was refined to keep the thrombin time near 200% of baseline.

A heparin pharmacokinetic model has been devised based on first order kinetics for elimination.[29,46,48–50] In this model, and individual patient's sensitivity (response according to clotting times versus heparin levels) and elimination of heparin are established before treating by giving one IV dose. Subsequently, the loading doses, infusion rates, and the duration of infusions can be determined so as to maintain minimal heparinization with a rapid termination phase of the anticoagulation near the end of dialysis.[45,49] Nomograms have been created, but still intermittent re-evaluation of individual patients is required.[48] The half-lives of heparin vary between 34 and 94 minutes.[49,51] The physiologic responses also vary but do not change simply due to repeated exposure to heparin.[50,51] This wide range of clearances has been found for nephrectomized and non-nephrectomized patients when measured either by bioassay or by 355-heparin clearance studies. Both groups cleared heparin in approximately the same fashion.[51,52] Of importance when using this system is to appreciate that the elimination of heparin from the plasma declines during the infusion period, thus causing an increase of the half-life with continued dose delivery.[53] Thus, when individualized, this system allows the dose of heparin to be reduced during dialysis and yet keep constant plasma levels. As the heparin level falls below .5 units/ml of blood, fibrin begins to form on the dialysis membrane, and fibrinopeptide A appears.[8] Nevertheless, patients can be managed with clinical safety at .3 units of heparin/ml of blood.[33,49,54] Shapiro et al. reduced heparin doses to as low as 2,000 units for a 5-hour dialysis with continuous infusion without the use of a loading dose.[44] Although individual modeling of heparin can considerably reduce the dose up to 38% in one series, it has been pointed out that some patients may actually require even less heparin when it is given as a single dose.[29,45,48,49]

For continuous infusions of heparin the body weight is equally used as the guide for dose selection. Unfortunately, there is overall a poor and inconsistent correlation between heparin dose based on body weight as evaluated by heparin clearance studies.[48,50] This may change even for the same patient on different days of dialysis.[50] This fluctuation and unreliability is due to changes of AT3 and the heparin-neutralizing substance platelet factor 4, both of which play major roles in the *in vivo* response to heparin. Also, the volumes of distribution and clearance for the heparin may change from day to day.[51–53] Thus, to base heparin doses simply on the patients' weights often will fail clinically. Also, response to heparin may also change with an acute illness or with changes in other medication. Thus, many variables affect the response and a patient must be surveyed periodically to insure constant efficacy as well as safety especially at low doses.

Many variations on these themes are available.[54] In our dialysis unit, we use the whole blood activated clotting time by tilt tube techniques as a rapid monitor of coagulation.[17] This allows dose adjustments of heparin. We normally employ a small loading dose of heparin followed by hourly boluses of intravenous heparin so as to maintain an activated clotting time at more than 2 minutes and 15 seconds. In patients at high risk for bleeding, we measure the initial whole blood activated clotting time (WBACT), and if normal, we give between 1,000 and 2,000 units of heparin intravenously. We then measure the WBACT at 15- to 30-minute intervals during dialysis and repeat the administration of heparin at doses of 250 to 1,000 units based on the results of the WBACT. For patients at particularly high risk for bleeding, we keep the WBACT at 90 to 120 seconds following repeated doses of heparin. Our philosophy may allow minor clotting of the artificial kidney in preference to significant anticoagulating in patients who are at particularly high risk.

V. Other Techniques for Patients at Risk During Hemodialysis

PGI_2 inhibits platelet activity without interfering with the soluble clotting system (see Chapter 2). Platelets have decreased sensitivity to prostacycline (PGI_2) during dialysis.[55] Recently PGI_2 has been used as a heparin-sparing or a heparin replacement agent in hemodialysis,[56,57] despite the increase of PGI_2 which seems to occur following heparinization and during hemodialysis.[34] It has a very short plasma half-life of 3–5 minutes and thus needs to be continuously infused. Doses studied in patients so far have been 4–5 mg/min. Hypotension due to the vasodilatory effects were encountered frequently and created the need for dose reduction to 0.25 mg/min, a dose that was still protective.

Heparin requirements go up as the level of the platelet factor 4 (PF4) goes up.[56] In dialysis, the PF4 and another platelet releasate, beta thromboglobulin (βTG), rises due to platelet damage on the membrane.[58] Buccianti et al.[58] showed that a reduction of βTG and platelet factor 4 occurred during dialysis, if Indobufen, a platelet inhibitor, was used along with heparin. If there is less PF4, there will be less need for heparin. Other platelet-suppressive drug programs such as sulfinpyrazone and aspirin[60–63] may also reduce the need for heparin. This may have the advantage of allowing reduced doses of heparin and thus less risk of hemorrhage and osteoporosis. Two reports are available in which no anticoagulant was used in a high-flow rate hemodialysis. When the flow rate was

300 ml/minute, dialyzer clearance was maintained. If the flow rate fell, clotting occurred in about 30% of dialyzer fibers.[64,65]

In the future, other antithrombogenic materials may be available for dialysis that need no systemic anticoagulation or platelet inhibition. These preparations will include polymers with attached heparin or heparinoids, prostaglandins, dipyridamole, or ditazole.[66,67,68] The physical properties of such synthetic materials will be altered so as to allow selective attachment *in vivo* of anticoagulating materials such as antithrombin 3 or macroglobulins. The configuration of these materials in the *ex vivo* system will be altered further so as to reduce thrombogenicity.[69] Another system for the future may be filters that allow the afferent blood to be heparinized while the efferent blood is cleared by bound heparinase.[70]

Recently a technique was described in which trisodium citrate at 2.5−7.5 mU final concentration was infused into the patient's blood in order to create regional anticoagulation. The dialysis was then conducted against a calcium-free dialysate, and calcium chloride was infused into the blood as it returned to the patient.[71] This technique required a somewhat more complicated dialysis since ultrafiltration was required in order to remove the additional 300−600 ml volume of citrate solution infused per hour. In the limited experience reported (i.e. 15 dialysis sessions for four patients), the clinical results were good with no thrombocytopenia or leukopenia. With greater experience other complications discussed by the authors may be encountered.[71]

Finally, there is the possibility of managing some patients without any anticoagulant during hemodialysis. In 29 patients at high risk of bleeding, 111 hemodialyses were performed by Casati et al.[72] The dialyzer was changed 11 times and the drip chamber 20 times. Fibrinopeptide A went up in these patients but other coagulation parameters did not change consistently.

VI. Platelet Counts During Hemodialysis

Functional platelet defects are commonly found in uremic patients (see Chapter 2). Thrombocytopenia also can occur during dialysis and may be another potential source of hemorrhage.[73] In a study by Lynch,[74] hollow fiber dialyzers reduced the platelet count 7% while the parallel flow dialyzers reduced the platelet count 31%. Platelet counts dropped markedly over the first half-hour of dialysis and slowly rose again during the third to sixth hour of dialysis. The fall in platelet count did not relate to patient's age, BUN, hematocrit, calcium, blood flow, or initial platelet count. Albumin priming or saline priming of the dialyzer made little difference. Jacobs et al.[75] found thrombocytopenia was more common with Cuprophane and cellulose acetate membranes than it was with polyacrilonitrile membranes. Adler and Berlyne found support for this observation when they reported that receiving hemodialysis with Cuprophane or regenerated cellulose acetate membranes differed from those using polyacrilonitrile. Dialysis with polyacrilonitrile membranes led to lower predialysis and intradialysis βTG levels, but the PF4 levels did not change.[76] Platelet-generated thromboxane B_2 (TxB_2) also goes up during dialysis, further indicating that platelets are damaged during hemodialysis. Ing et al.[77] demonstrated similar decreases in platelet counts in patients undergoing isolated ultrafiltration. This suggests that blood-membrane contact is the most likely factor in thrombocytopenia and not the process of dialysis itself. Thrombocytopenia does not necessarily mean that platelets are adhering to the dialyzer membrane. They may be sequestered in the lung after being released from the membrane. Thrombocytopenia could also result from temperature changes or from sheer-stress forces on the platelets.[9,78] These sheer forces could be ameliorated by the addition of agents that stabilize platelets, including agents such as theophylline or PGE_1. Combined aspirin and dipyridamole can reduce the thrombocytopenic effects of dialysis while reducing the deposition of platelets and fibrin on the membranes.[79] Sulfinpyrazone also can reduce the amount of thrombocytopenia encountered.[61] The heparin itself may be cause for thrombocytopenia.[80,81] The mechanisms involved may be immunologic, direct suppression of endothelial cell release of PGI_2, nonimmunoplatelet agglutination, or others yet to be described. This is a very dangerous situation and deserves prompt cessation of the source of heparin being used and institution of other forms of coagulation.

VI. Peritoneal Dialysis for Patients at Risk for Bleeding

In patients at particularly high risk for hemorrhage during dialysis, alternative means of dialysis may be employed. Peritoneal dialysis has a low risk of bleeding during chronic means of dialysis. Using automated peritoneal dialysis machinery and strict adherence to sterile technique, the incidence of infections can be kept to a minimum. The advantage of peritoneal dialysis in the context of this discussion is that it does not require systemic anticoagulation. While intraperitoneal heparin is used to prevent clotting of the peritoneal catheter, this heparin does not appear to affect systemic coagulation in any meaningful way. One hundred units of heparin are injected per 2 liters of peritoneal dialysate. Even after all 100 units were absorbed from the peritoneum, an event which is unlikely, there would be an approximate plasma concentration of 0.02 units heparin/ml of blood. This is over 10 times less heparin than is used for hemodialysis.

The risk of bleeding during peritoneal dialysis for these patients with systemic coagulopathies relates to peritoneal or extraperitoneal bleeding during and following catheter insertion. This is obviated generally by using careful surgical technique during the preparation of the insertion site. Small volumes of blood loss, as measured by hemoglobin determinations on the effluent dialysate, can be replaced if need be. In the setting of a minor coagulopathy, it is not necessarily recommended to use heparin in the dialysate since the patient is "auto-anticoagulated." The same is not necessarily true of those with thrombocytopenia.

VII. Opening Clotted Arterial Venous (AV) Shunts and Fistulas

Despite the coagulopathies of uremia and dialysis, it may become necessary to open thrombotic occlusions of AV shunts and fistulae. Fibrinolytic agents instilled locally into the shunt or fistula can re-open the conduit without worsening the systemic coagulopathy. This approach is an appealing alternative to the surgical management of these problems, especially when hemorrhage is a potential complication of the surgery (see Chapter 15).

Urokinase, a fibrinolytic activator, has been used successfully to dissolve clots in AV shunts.[83,84] Streptokinase, while useful in the same setting, had a higher incidence of side effects including hypersensitivity.[85]

Urokinase was also useful in opening clotted AV fistulae.[85] In the study by Mangiarotti et al.,[86] 50,000–100,000 units of urokinase, with 2,500 units of heparin, in 20 ml of 0.9% saline were injected intravenously into the thrombosed area over 15 minutes. If the clot was lysed, IV heparin was given for 24–48 hours. If the clot was only partially lysed, the procedure was repeated until lysis was complete up to 400,000 units over 2 hours. In this report there was no advantage to repeating the procedure when clots re-formed in less than 48 hours. In such cases, the primary cause for the clotting needed correction. If there is advanced fibrosis, surgery is then needed. Using this approach, changes in the systemic fibrinolysis or coagulation parameters must be monitored, though in the study reported no change or only minor changes occurred.[86]

REFERENCES

1. Wardle EN, Piercy DA. Studies of contact activation of blood in haemodialysis. *J Clin Pathol.* 25:1045–1049, 1972.
2. Vaziri ND, Toohey J, Paule P, Alikani S, Hung E. Effect of hemodialysis on contact group of coagulation factors, platelets and leukoyctes. *Am J Med.* 77:437–441, 1984.
3. Kramer P, Matthaci D, Go JG, Windsler K, Scheler F. Effect of blood factor depositor in reused dialyzers on the dialysance of middle-weight molecules. *Proc Eur of Dial Transplant Assoc.* 9:278–285, 1972.
4. Bischel MD, Orrell FL, Scoles BG, Mohler JG, Barbour BH. Effects of microemboli blood filtration during hemodialysis. *Trans Am Soc Artif Intern Organs.* 19:492–497, 1973.
5. Craddock PR, Fehr J, Brigham KL, Kronenberg RS, Jacob HS. Complement and leukocyte-mediated pulmonary dysfunction in hemodialysis. *N Engl J Med.* 296: 769–774, 1977.
6. Craddock PR, Fehr J, Dalmasso AP, Brigham KL, Jacob HS. Hemodialysis leukopenia—Pulmonary vascular leukostasis resulting from complement activation by dialyzer cellophane membranes. *J Clin Invest.* 59:879–888, 1977.
7. Shin J, Matsuo M, Shinko S, Fujita Y, Inoue S, Sakai R, Nishioka M. A study on hemodialysis luekopenia using various dialyzers. *J Dialysis.* 4:51–62, 1980.
8. Wilhelmsson S, Asaba H, Gunnarsson B, Kudryk B, Robinson D, Bergtrom J. Measurement of fibrinopeptide A in the evaluation of heparin activity and fibrin formation during hemodialysis. *Clin Nephrol.* 15:252–258, 1981.
9. Lederman DM, Cumming RD, Petschek HE, Levine PH, Krinsky NI. the effect of temperature on the intraction of platelets and leukocytes with materials exposed to flowing blood. *Trans Am Soc Artif Intern Organs.* 24:557–559, 1978.
10. Teilemans CL, Herbaut CR, Geurts JD, Dratwa M. Hemolysis and consumption coagulopathy due to overheated dialysate. *Nephron.* 30:190–191, 1982.
11. Olsson P, Lagergren H, Ek S. The elimination from plasma of intravenous heparin: An experimental study on dogs and humans. *Acta Med Scand.* 173:619–630, 1963.
12. Estes JW. The kinetics of heparin. *Ann NY Acad Sci.* 179:187–204, 1971.
13. Turney JH, Fewell M, Williams LC, Dodd N, Weston MJ. Paradoxical behavior of antithrombin III during hemodialysis and its prevention with prostacyclin. *Clin Nephrol.* 17:31–35, 1982.
14. Aronstam A, Dennis B, Friesen MJ, Clark WF, Linton Al, Lindsay RM. Heparin

neutralizing activity in patients with renal diseases on maintenance hemodialysis. *Thromb Haemostas.* 39:695–700, 1978.

15. Penner JA. Experience with a thrombin clotting time assay for measuring heparin activity. *Am J Clin Pathol.* 61:645–653, 1974.
16. Wilhelmsson S, Lins LE. Whole blood thrombin time: A bedside method for determination of heparin activity. *Clin Nephrol.* 6:523–525, 1976.
17. Shanklin N, Ploth DW. Evaluation of an activated clotting time technique for use in hemodialysis. *Dialysis and Transplantation.* 9:955–958, 1980.
18. Hattersley PG. Activated coagulation time of whole blood. *JAMA.* 196:436–440, 1966.
19. Baden JP, Sonnenfield M, Ferlic RM, Sellers RD. The Bason test: A rapid bedside test for control of heparin therapy. *Surg Forum.* 22:172–174, 1971.
20. Congdon JE, Kardinal CG, Wallin JD. Monitoring heparin therapy in hemodialysis: A report on activated whole blood coagulation time tests. *JAMA.* 226:1529–1533, 1973.
21. Warrell RP, Jr., Hultin MB, Coller BS. Increased factor VIII/von Willebrand factor antigen and von Willebrand factor activity in renal failure. *Am J Med.* 66:226–228, 1979.
22. Ruggeri ZM, Ponticelli C, Mannucci PM. Factor VIII and chronic renal failure (letter). *Br Med J.* 1:1085, 1977.
23. Larrson SO, Hedner U, Nilsson IM. On coagulation and fibrinolysis in conservatively treated chronic uremia. *Acta Med Scand.* 189:433–441, 1971.
24. Edward N. Fibrinolysis in patients on regular hemodialysis. *Clin Nephrol.* 1:97–100, 1972.
25. Talalla A, Halbrooks H, Barbour BH, Kurze T. Subdural hematoma associated with long-term hemodialysis for chronic renal disease. *JAMA.* 212:1847–1849, 1970.
26. Burn RA. Intraocular pressure during hemodialysis. *Br J Opthalmol.* 57:511–513, 1973.
27. Milutinovich J, Follette WC, Scribner BH. Spontaneous retroperitoneal bleeding in patients on chronic hemodialysis. *Ann Intern Med.* 86:189–192, 1977.
28. Alfrey AC, Goss JE, Ogden DA, Vogel JHK, Homes JH. Uremic hemopericardium. *Am J Med.* 45:391–400, 1966.
29. Swartz RD. Hemorrhage during high-risk hemodialysis using controlled heparinization. *Nephron.* 28:65–69, 1981.
30. Galen MA, Steinberg SM, Lowrie EG, Lazarus JM, Hampers CL, Merrill JP. Hemorrhagic pleural effusion in patients undergoing chronic hemodialysis. *Ann Intern Med.* 82:359–361, 1975.
31. Horner BA, Hunt JC, Kincaid OW, DeWeerd JH. Perirenal hematoma secondary to intrarenal microaneurysms of periarteritis nodosa, demonstrated radiographically. *Mayo Clin Proc.* 41:169–178, 1966.
32. Shaw RE. Spontaneous rupture of the kidney. *Br J Surg.* 45:68–72, 1957.
33. Kaden WS, Friedman EA. Obstructive uropathy complicating anticoagulant therapy. *N Engl J Med.* 265:283–284, 1961.
34. Ylikorkala O, Huttunen K, Jarvi J, Viinikka L. Prostacyclin and thromboxane in chronic uremia: Effect of hemodialysis. *Clin Nephrol.* 18:83–87, 1982.
35. Lindholm DD, Murray JS. A simplified method of regional heparinization during hemodialysis according to a predetermined dosage formula. *Trans Am Soc Artif Intern Organs.* 10:92–97, 1964.
36. Gordon LA, Simon ER, Rukes JM, Richards V, Perkins HA. Studies in regional heparinization. *N Engl J Med.* 255:1063–1066, 1956.
37. Maher JF, Lapierre L, Schreiner GE, Geiger M, Westervelt FB, Jr. Regional heparinization of hemodialysis: Technique and clinical experiences. *N Engl J Med.* 268:451–456, 1968.
38. Hampers CL, Blaufox MD, Merrill JP. Anticoagulation rebound after hemodialysis. *N Engl J Med.* 275:770–776, 1966.
39. Spencer P, Cozzi E, Easterling RE, Penner JA. Regional heparinization with the hollow fiber artificial kidney. *J Proc Am Assoc Nephrol Nurs Tech.* 4:69–74, 1977.

40. Shaldon S, Chiandussi L, Higgs B. Haemodialysis by percutaneous catheterisation of the femoral artery and vein with regional heparinization. *Lancet.* 2:857–859, 1961.
41. Kjellstrand CM, Buselmeier TJ. A simple method for anticoagulation during pre- and postoperative hemodialysis, avoiding rebound phenomenon. *Surgery.* 72:630–633, 1972.
42. Maher JF, Schreiner GE. Hazards and complications of dialysis. *N Engl J Med.* 273:370–377, 1965.
43. Nakamoto S, Holmes JH. Our experience in regional heparinization. *Trans Am Soc Artif Intern Organs.* 4:36–47, 1958.
44. Shapiro WB, Faubert PF, Porush JG, Chou S. Low-dose heparin in routine hemodialysis monitored by activated partial thromboplastin time. *Artif Organs.* 3:73–77, 1979.
45. Farrell PC, Ward RA, Schindhelm K, Gotch F. Precise anticoagulation for routine hemodialysis. *J Lab Clin Med.* 92:164–176, 1978.
46. Gotch FA, Keen ML. Precise control of minimal heparinization for high bleeding risk hemodialysis. *Trans Am Soc Artif Intern Organs.* 23:168–176, 1977.
47. Swartz RD, Port FK. Preventing hemorrhage in high-risk hemodialysis: Regional versus low-dose heparin. *Kidney Int.* 16:513–518, 1979.
48. Ward RA, Farrell PC. Precise anticoagulation for routine hemodialysis using normograms. *Trans Am Soc Artif Intern Organs.* 24:439–442, 1978.
49. Gunnarsson B, Asaba H, Dawidson S, Wilhelmsson S, Bergstrom J. The effects of three different heparin regimes on heparin concentrations in plasma and fibrin formation dialyzers. *Clin Nephrol.* 15:135–142, 1981.
50. Bern MM. Variable response of activated partial thromboplastin time to heparin therapy during hemodialysis. *Am J Clin Pathol.* 64:602–607, 1975.
51. Cameron JS, Fitzgerald D, Youssef AK, Ogg CS, Czorba T, Barkhan P. Heparin-^{35} S removal in anephric patients undergoing regular dialysis. *Proc Eur Dial Transplant Assoc.* 9:614–617, 1972.
52. Teien AN, Bjoonson J. Heparin elimination in uraemic patients on haemodialysis. *Scand J Haematol.* 17:29–35, 1976.
53. McAvoy TJ. Pharmacokinetics modeling of heparin and its clinical implications. *J Pharmacoenet Biopharm.* 7:331–354, 1979.
54. Buccianti G, Pogliani E, Valenti G, Cofrancesco E, Miradoli R, Vigo A. Clinical monitoring of heparin during hemodialysis a new method. *Dialysis and Transplantation.* 8:1118–1123, 1979.
55. Kristensen SD, Knudsen F, Nielsen AH, Ring T. Decreased platelet sensitivity to prostacyclin (epoprostenol) during hemodialysis. *Clin Nephrol.* 21:230–234, 1984.
56. Turney JH, Williams LC, Fewell MR, Parons V, Weston MJ. Platelet protection and heparin sparing with prostacyclin during regular dialysis therapy. *Lancet.* 2:224–226, 1980.
57. Zusman RM, Rubin RH, Cato AE, Concchetto DM, Crow JW, Tolkoff-Rubin N. Hemodialysis using prostacyclin instead of heparin as the sole antithrombotic agent. *N Engl J Med.* 304:904–939, 1981.
58. Buccianti G, Pogliani E, Miradoli R, Columbi MA, Valenti G, Lorenz M, Polli EE. Reduction of plasma levels of betathromboglobulin and platelet factor 4 during hemodialysis: A possible role for a short acting inhibitor of platelet aggregation. *Clin Nephrol.* 18:204–208, 1982.
59. Green D, Santhanam S, Krumlovsky FA, del Greco F. Elevated beta-thromboglobulin in patients with chronic renal failure: Effect of hemodialysis. *J Lab Clin Med.* 95:679–685, 1980.
60. Harter HR, Burch JW, Majerus PW, Stanford N, Delmez JA, Anderson CB, Weerts CA. Prevention of thrombosis in patients on hemodialysis by low-dose aspirin. *N Engl J Med.* 301:577–579, 1980.
61. Bern MM, Cavaliere BM, Lukas G. Plasma levels and effects of sulfinpyrazone in patients requiring chronic hemodialysis. *J Clin Pharmacol.* 20:107–116, 1980.
62. Bern MM, Green J. Effect of sulfinpyrazone upon antithrombin III and platelet factor 4 in chronic renal failure. *Thromb Res.* 27:457–466, 1982.

63. Woods HF, Ash G, Parsons V, Weston MJ. Reduction of dialyzer fibrin deposition with sulfinpyrazone. *Clin Nephrol.* 12:122–126, 1979.
64. Naito H, Miyazakai T, Shimizo M, Yoneada K, Yoshikawa K. Non-anticoagulant hemodialysis with synthetic EVAL HF artificial kidney. *Artif Organs.* 5 (Suppl) (A) 50(abs), July 1981.
65. Raja R, Kramer M, Rosenbaum JL, Bolisay C, Krug M. Thrombogenicity in hollow fiber (HF) kidney-use of Cordis Dow(CD)-3500 without heparin. *Artif Organs.* 5 (Suppl):58 (abstr), 1981.
66. Marconi W, Bartoli F, Mantovani E, Pittalis F, Sittembri L, Cordova C, Musca A, Alessandre C. Development of New Antithrombogenic surfaces by employing platelet aggregating agents: Preparation and characterization. *Trans Am Soc Artif Intern Organs.* 25:280–285, 1979.
67. Grode GA, Pitman J, Crowley JP, Leininger RD, Falb RD. Surface Immobilized prostaglandin as a platelet protective agent. *Trans Am Soc Artif Intern Organs.* 20A:38–41, 1974.
68. Schmer G, Teng LN, Vizzo JE, Graefe U, Miluintinovich J, Cole JJ, Scribner BH. Clinical use of a totally heparin grafted hemodialysis system in uremic patients. *Trans Am Soc Artif Intern Organs.* 23:177–184, 1977.
69. Cummings RD. Important factors affecting initial blood-material interactions. *Trans Am Soc Artif Internal Organs.* 26:304–308, 1980.
70. Langer R, Linhardt RJ, Hoffberg S, Larsen AK, Cooney CL, Tapper D, Klein M. An enzymatic system for removing heparin in extra corporeal therapy. *Science.* 217: 261–263, 1982.
71. Pinnick RV, Wiegmann TB, Diederich, DA. Regional citrate anticoagulation for hemodialysis in the patient at high risk for bleeding. *N Engl J Med.* 308:258–261, 1983.
72. Casati S, Moia M, Graziani G, Cantaluppi A, Citterio A, Mannucci PM, Ponticelli C. Hemodialysis without anticoagulants efficiency and hemostatic aspects. *Clin Nephrol.* 21:105, 1984.
73. Lindsay RM, Mason RG, Kim SW, Andrade JD, Hakim RM. Blood surface interactions. *Trans Am Soc Artif Intern Organs.* 26:603–610, 1980.
74. Lynch RE, Bosl RH, Streifel AJ, Ebben JP, Ehlers SM, Kjellstrand CM. Dialysis thrombocytopenia: Parallel plate vs hollow fiber dialyzers. *Trans Am Soc Artif Intern Organs.* 24:704–707, 1978.
75. Jacob AI, Gavellas G, Zarco R, Perez G, Bourgoignie JJ. Leukopenia, hypoxia, and complement function with different hemolysis membranes. *Kidney Int.* 18:505–509, 1980.
76. Adler AJ, Berlyne GM. B Thromboglobulin and platelet factor 4 levels during hemodialysis with polyacrilonitrile. *Am Soc Artif Intern Organs.* 3:100–102, 1981.
77. Ing TS, Chen WT, Weber DV, Daugirdas JT, Vilbar RM, Hano JE, Kwaan HC. Hematologic studies during isolated ultrafiltration. *Clin Nephrol.* 15:229–301, 1981.
78. Hardwick RA, Hellums JD, Maoke JL, Peterson DM. Alfrey CP. Effects of antiplatelet agents on platelets exposed to sheer stress. *Trans Am Soc Artif Intern Organs.* 26:179–183, 1980.
79. Salter MCP, Crow MJ, Donaldson DR, Roberts TG, Rajah SM, Davidson AM. Prevention of platelet deposition and thrombus formation on hemodialysis membranes: A double blind randomized trial of heperin and dipyridamole. *Artif Organs.* 8:57–61, 1984.
80. Rhodes GR, Dixon RH, Silver D. Heparin-induced thrombocytopenia with thrombotic and hemorrhagic manifestations. *Surg Gynecol Obstet.* 136:409–416, 1973.
81. Bell WR, Tomasulo PA, Alving BM, Duffy JP. Thrombocytopenia occurring during the administration of heparin: A prospective study of 52 patients. *Ann Int Med.* 85:155–160, 1976.
82. Watt DAL, Dunn BP, Livingstone WR, MacDougal AJ, MacKay RKS, Obineche EN, Rennie JB. The use of urokinase in declotting of arteriovenous shunts. *Proc EDTA.* 6:88–91, 1969.

83. Hartley LCY, Ellis FG, Rendall M, Cameron JS, Ogg CS. The use of urokinase in Scribner shunts. *Br J Urol.* 42:246–249, 1970.
84. Epstein I, Saker B, Marshall V, Kincaid-Smith A. Treatment of clotting in external arteriovenous shunts with a fibrinolytic enzyme. *Med J Aust.* 11:137–138, 1969.
85. Cocke TB, Burgos-Calderon RA, Gonzales FM. The use of streptokinase infusion for arteriovenous shunt declotting. *Trans Am Soc Artif Internal Organs.* 16:292–296, 1970.
86. Mangiarotti G, Canavese C, Theia A, Segoloni GP, Stratta P, Salomone M, Vercellone A. Urokinase treatment for arteriovenous fistulae declotting in dialyzed patients. *Nephron.* 36:60–64, 1984.

Index

(f) = figure; (t) = table